Bradykinin Antagonists

INFLAMMATORY DISEASE AND THERAPY

Series Editor

Daniel E. Furst
University of Medicine and Dentistry
of New Jersey
Robert Wood Johnson Medical School
New Brunswick, New Jersey
and Pharmaceuticals Division
CIBA-GEIGY Corporation
Summit, New Jersey

1. Methotrexate Therapy in Rheumatic Disease, *edited by William S. Wilke*
2. Therapy of Inflammatory Bowel Disease: New Medical and Surgical Approaches, *edited by Mark A. Peppercorn*
3. Platelet-Activating Factor in Endotoxin and Immune Disease, *edited by Dean A. Handley, Robert N. Saunders, William J. Houlihan, and John C. Tomesch*
4. Immunomodulators in the Rheumatic Diseases, *edited by Daniel E. Furst and Michael E. Weinblatt*
5. Bradykinin Antagonists: Basic and Clinical Research, *edited by Ronald M. Burch*
6. Drug Therapy for Headache, *edited by R. Michael Gallagher*

Additional Volumes in Preparation

Monoclonal Antibodies, Cytokines, and Arthritis: Mediators of Inflammation and Therapy, *edited by Thomas F. Kresina*

Behçet's Disease: Basic and Clinical Aspects, *edited by J. Desmond O'Duffy and Emre Kokmen*

Bradykinin Antagonists

Basic and Clinical Research

edited by

Ronald M. Burch
Nova Pharmaceutical Corporation
Baltimore, Maryland

MARCEL DEKKER, INC.   New York • Basel • Hong Kong

Library of Congress Cataloging-in-Publication Data

Bradykinin antagonists: basic and clinical research / edited by Ronald M. Burch.
p. cm. -- (Inflammatory disease and therapy; 5)
Includes index.
ISBN 0-8247-8310-7 (alk. paper)
1. Bradykinin--Antagonists. 2. Bradykinin--Antagonists--Therapeutic Use--Testing. I. Burch, Ronald M. II. Series.
[DNLM: 1. Adrenergic Beta Receptor Blockaders--pharmacology. 2. Bradykinin--antagonists & inhibitors. 3. Synaptic Receptors--physiology. W1 IN41LA v. 5 / QU 68 B8115]
RM666.B68B73 1991
615'.7--dc20
DNLM/DLC
for Library of Congress 90-13983
CIP

This book is printed on acid-free paper.

MARCEL DEKKER, INC.
270 Madison Avenue, New York, New York 10016

Current printing (last digit):
10 9 8 7 6 5 4 3 2 1

PRINTED IN THE UNITED STATES OF AMERICA

Series Introduction

As knowledge of inflammation has flourished over the last decade, understanding of the pathogenesis and therapy of inflammatory diseases has also improved. This has been particularly true in the rheumatic diseases, including infectious rheumatic diseases, those rheumatic diseases associated with gastrointestinal inflammation, immunologically mediated illnesses, various forms of vasculitis, and so forth.

Marcel Dekker, Inc., which specializes in high-quality monographs in a variety of focused medical disciplines, has supplied up-to-date, detailed, and practical information for the practicing physician and research scientist. The Inflammatory Disease and Therapy series will address a number of carefully chosen topics of interest to practicing physicians, rheumatologists, and research scientists.

Daniel E. Furst

Preface

This book is largely the result of the stimulus to bradykinin research of the pioneering work of John Stewart and Ray Vavrek, who in 1985 reported the first bradykinin analogs with antagonist activity at the B2 bradykinin receptor (see Chapter 3). In the short time since their report, several of these antagonists have been extensively used in studies of bradykinin receptor subtypes and of the role of bradykinin in blood pressure regulation, inflammatory diseases, pain, airway diseases, and endocrinological regulation.

Bradykinin has a long history as a putative mediator of blood pressure regulation and inflammation. A large body of literature has accumulated on the biochemistry and molecular biology of kinin metabolic enzymes. However, while attempts have been made to use inhibitors of kinin metabolic enzymes to elucidate the role of bradykinin in biological processes, poor specificity of many inhibitors, coupled with the large concentrations of substrate kininogens, and extraordinarily rapid degradation of products have dramatically hampered research on the final biological product, bradykinin.

A decade ago, it became apparent that at least two major classes of bradykinin receptors exist, B1 and B2 (Chapter 2). This was made possible by the development by Domenico Regoli and colleagues of specific agonists and antagonists of B1 receptors. While B1 receptors have been demonstrated in living animals, study of B1 receptors has remained largely an in vitro effort. On the other hand, B2 receptors have been implicated in most of the in vivo effects of bradykinin.

This book discusses the comparative pharmacology of bradykinin receptors, followed by discussions of structure-activity relationships among B1 receptor antagonists and B2 receptor antagonists. B2 antagonists have been identified in the literature using several systems. Structure is unambiguous but clumsy, so two alphanumeric systems have been used. The first, the "B" system, is that used by Stewart and Vavrek in their laboratory bookkeeping and refers to compound structure *and* batch; thus, a single compound may be—and has been in the literature—identified with more than a single number. Another alphanumeric system is "NPC," in which each compound is identified by a unique number; this is the system used in the present book. To facilitate comparisons with the existing literature, a listing of all structures, B numbers, and NPC numbers has been included (see Chapter 3).

Therapeutic utility of bradykinin antagonists will ultimately depend largely upon the availability of nonpeptide receptor antagonists that are metabolically stable and orally active. João Calixto and colleagues have discussed efforts to identify such compounds. Don Kyle and his associates have been involved in efforts to identify the common structural features of bradykinin, peptide bradykinin antagonists, and, recently, nonpeptide compounds. They describe their working hypothesis of the active conformation of bradykinin. A major stumbling block in the use of available peptide antagonists in vivo is their metabolic lability. Patrick Ward describes the metabolic pathways for bradykinin and analogs. Understanding of the susceptible bonds in the peptides may lead to metabolically stable compounds.

A group of chapters describes the activity of bradykinin antagonists in several systems for which many data have been collected. Haralambos and Irene Gavras discuss the cardiovascular system, Larry Steranka and Ronald Burch discuss pain and inflammation, and Stephen Farmer discusses the airway.

Clinical study of bradykinin receptor antagonists is ongoing in several areas. The first clinical trials using bradykinin antagonists studied the effects of the agents on the symptoms of rhinovirus infections. David Proud and colleagues describe the rationale for such studies and early clinical results. Bradykinin antagonists are being assessed for their ability to reduce the pain associated with burns. These studies are at a very early stage at this time, so results are not available. An exciting finding is that bradykinin antagonists are quite effective in inhibiting the late phase of allergic asthma in a sheep model. William Abraham and colleagues describe their results in the model. Because of the sheep results, in the first quarter of 1990, clinical studies were initiated to assess the utility of bradykinin antagonists in human patients with asthma. Also in 1990, clinical studies were planned to assess bradykinin antagonists in the cough associated with the use of angiotensin-converting enzyme inhibitors for hypertension and in inflammatory skin disorders.

A strong American bias may be inferred from the list of contributors. This was unintended, and the various chapters cite the many contributions of investigators in Europe. Some data are discussed in detail in more than one chapter. This has been encouraged since the study of bradykinin receptor antagonists is still in its early development, with available agents still in their "first generation"; thus, many interpretations must be considered preliminary and some, controversial.

Ronald M. Burch

Contents

Contributors

William M. Abraham, Ph.D. Associate Director, Department of Research, Mount Sinai Medical Center, Miami Beach, Florida

Paul R. Blake Graduate Student, Chemistry/Biochemistry, University of Maryland, Baltimore County, Baltimore, Maryland

Ronald M. Burch, M.D., Ph.D. Group Leader, Inflammation, Nova Pharmaceutical Corporation, Baltimore, Maryland

João B. Calixto, M.Sc., Ph.D. Senior Lecturer, Department of Pharmacology, Biological Sciences Center, Universidade Federal de Santa Catarina, Florianópolis, Santa Catarina, Brazil

Laurie Churchill, Ph.D. Postdoctoral Fellow, Department of Medicine, The Johns Hopkins University School of Medicine, Baltimore, Maryland

Stephen G. Farmer, Ph.D. Staff Scientist, Pain and Inflammation Group, Nova Pharmaceutical Corporation, Baltimore, Maryland

Haralambos Gavras, M.D. Professor, Department of Medicine, and Chief, Hypertension and Atherosclerosis Section, Boston University School of Medicine, Boston, Massachusetts

Irene Gavras, M.D. Clinical Professor, Department of Medicine, Boston University School of Medicine, Boston, Massachusetts

Rickey P. Hicks, Ph.D. Assistant Professor and Technical Director of MSU NMR Laboratory, Mississippi State University, Mississippi State, Mississippi

Valentine J. Klimkowski, Ph.D.* Senior Computational Chemist, Polygen Corporation, Waltham, Massachusetts

Donald J. Kyle, Ph.D. Senior Computational Chemist, Nova Pharmaceutical Corporation, Baltimore, Maryland

Francois Marceau, M.D., Ph.D.† Unité de Recherche Inflammation et Immunorhumatologie, Centre Hospitalier de l'Université Laval, Quebec City, Quebec, Canada

Yara S. Medeiros, M.D. Assistant Professor, Department of Pharmacology, Biological Sciences Center, Universidade Federal de Santa Catarina, Florianopolis, Santa Catarina, Brazil

Jacqueline A. Pongracic, M.D. Postdoctoral Fellow, Division of Clinical Immunology, Department of Medicine, The Johns Hopkins University School of Medicine, Baltimore, Maryland

David Proud, Ph.D. Associate Professor, Department of Medicine, Johns Hopkins Asthma and Allergy Center, The Johns Hopkins University School of Medicine, Baltimore, Maryland

Giles A. Rae, M.Sc., Ph.D. Senior Lecturer, Department of Pharmacology, Biological Sciences Center, Universidade Federal de Santa Catarina, Florianópolis, Santa Catarina, Brazil

Domenico C. Regoli, M.D., Ph.D. Professor, Department of Pharmacology, Medical School, University of Sherbrooke, Sherbrooke, Quebec, Canada

---

Present affiliations:
*Senior Computational Chemist, Supercomputer Applications and Molecular Design, Lilly Research Laboratories, Eli Lilly and Company, Indianapolis, Indiana.
†Assistant Professor, Department of Pharmacology, Centre de Recherche de l'Hôtel-Dieu de Québec, Quebec City, Quebec, Canada.

Larry R. Steranka, Ph.D. Executive Director of Research, Pain and Inflammation Program, Nova Pharmaceutical Corporation, Baltimore, Maryland

John M. Stewart, Ph.D. Professor, Department of Biochemistry, University of Colorado School of Medicine, Denver, Colorado

Raymond J. Vavrek, Ph.D. Assistant Professor, Department of Biochemistry, University of Colorado School of Medicine, Denver, Colorado

Patrick E. Ward. Ph.D. Professor, Department of Physiology, College of Medicine, The Ohio State University, Columbus, Ohio

Rosendo A. Yunes, Ph.D. Professor, Department of Chemistry, Centro de Ciências Físicas e Matemáticas, Universidade Federal de Santa Catarina, Florianópolis, Santa Catarina, Brazil

Bradykinin Antagonists

1

The Pharmacology of Bradykinin Receptors

Stephen G. Farmer and Ronald M. Burch
Nova Pharmaceutical Corporation
Baltimore, Maryland

I. INTRODUCTION

A. Bradykinin

Bradykinin (BK) is a nonapeptide (Arg-Pro-Pro-Gly-Phe-Ser-Pro-Phe-Arg), generated as a result of the activity of kallikreins, a group of proteolytic enzymes present in most tissues and body fluids, on kininogens. Once released, kinins produce many physiological responses, including pain and hyperalgesia by stimulating C- and A-fibers in the periphery (1-7). There is also considerable evidence that kinins contribute to the inflammatory response (8,9) (see Chapter 8). After local injection into skin, BK produces all of the cardinal signs of inflammation. Additional evidence supporting the participation of BK in inflammatory reactions comes from studies indicating activation of the kallikrein-kinin system in various pathological conditions characterized by inflammation, and including thermal and chemical injury, allergic reactions, rheumatoid, psoriatic and gouty arthritis, asthma, pancreatitis, viral rhinitis, and inflammatory disease of the colon (9-11).

In addition to its algesic and pro-inflammatory effects, BK is a vasodilator. Because of its ability to lower blood pressure, BK has been implicated in the pathogenesis of several shock syndromes, particularly septic or endotoxic shock (10,12-16). BK is also a potent bronchoconstrictor in animals and asthmatic subjects, and it has been implicated as a contributor to the pathogenesis of airway inflammatory conditions such as allergic asthma and rhinitis (see Chapters 9, 10, and 11)

Detailed discussions of the molecular genetics, structure, synthesis, release, and degradation of kallikreins and kinins, in addition to their physiological effects in health and disease, can be found in several books (17-19) and literature reviews (6,8,9,11,20-28), as well as in the present volume. The present chapter will review the pharmacology of BK receptors and their mediation of the many effects of kinins.

1. Other Endogenous Kinins

Lys-BK, or kallidin, is a physiological kinin released by tissue kallikreins in humans but not in other species examined (25). Kallidin and BK have very similar or identical effects in all tissues studies. Ile-Ser-BK (T-kinin) was recently isolated from rat plasma and is an endogenous kinin unique to this species (25,29). T-kinin is a B2 receptor agonist, as it displaces $[^3H]$-BK binding in guinea pig ileum (R. M. Burch, unpublished observation).

Another endogenous kinin is hydroxy-Pro^3-BK (Hyp^3-BK) (30-31), which has been reported to account for about one-third and three-quarters of the kinin contained, respectively, in human and monkey high molecular weight kininogens (30). Similarly, incubation of human plasma with trypsin yields both BK and Hyp^3-BK, whereas incubation of plasma with human urinary kallikrein results in production of kallidin and Hyp^3-KD (kallidin) (25,32). Hyp^3-BK binds to B2 receptors with affinity similar to BK itself (33) (R. M. Burch, unpublished observation). Curiously, this kinin cannot be detected in any of the other species, including several rodents and cattle, examined (30).

Ala^3-BK and desPro^3-BK have also been reported as endogenous kinins in man, although they probably represent artifacts of analysis (31). Similarly, Met-kallidin has been reported as an endogenous kinin. It can be isolated only from urine samples and is now thought to be an artifactual product resulting from the action of pepsin on urinary kininogen (25).

II. BRADYKININ RECEPTORS

A. B1 and B2 Receptors

As in most other biological systems, kinin receptors have been classified according to the relative potencies of series of agonists or antagonists. In their now classical review, Regoli and Barabé (20) described their many studies, wherein kinin receptors were classified in isolated vascular smooth muscle preparations and subdivided into two classes, B1 and B2. B2 receptors exhibit the following rank order of agonist potency in rabbit jugular vein:

Kallidin > [Tyr(Me)^8]-BK > BK > desArg^{10}-KD > desArg^9-BK

Dog carotid artery exhibits a similar rank order, except that BK and [Tyr(Me)^8]-BK (a synthetic analog) are equipotent as spasmogens, and both are slightly more potent than kallidin (21). It is perhaps noteworthy that in a recent review, Regoli (21) lists a slightly different rank order than that given above. However, reference to Table 1 in that report (p. 275), as well as to the Regoli and Barabe reviews (20, p. 22), indicates that kallidin is indeed marginally more potent in causing contraction of rabbit jugular vein than either BK or [Tyr(Me^8)]-BK. Most effects of BK in vivo and in isolated tissue preparations are mediated by B2 receptors.

By comparison, B1 receptors (see also Chapter 2) in rabbit aorta or mesenteric vein exhibit almost the opposite rank order of sensitivity:

desArg^{10}-KD > desArg^9-BK > kallidin > BK > [Tyr(Me)^8)]-BK

More generally, B2 receptors exhibit much higher affinity for kallidin or BK than for the kininase I metabolites, desArg^{10}-KD or desArg^9-BK, whereas B1 receptors are more sensitive to the desArg metabolites. Indeed, investigators often utilize the relative potencies of BK or kallidin and desArg^9-BK to classify a particular response as B1 or B2.

B. B2 Receptor Heterogeneity

Recently, a great deal of evidence for heterogeneity among B2 receptors has been produced, in addition to indications that there are BK receptor subtypes other than the well-characterized B1 and B2 receptors. For example, in rat duodenum, desensitization to the contractile but not relaxant effects of BK can be demonstrated (34). However, this phenomenon may, at least partly, be explained by the fact that much lower concentrations of the kinin are required to elicit relaxation than contraction. In addition, different signal transduction systems certainly mediate the two different effects, and it may be a transducer, rather than a receptor, that was desensitized. DesArg^9-BK was inactive in rat duodenum, unless experiments were carried out following an incubation period of at least 4 hours. After this time high concentrations of the B1 agonist elicited contractions but not relaxations. The requirement for a relatively long incubation may indicate induction of B1 receptors similar to that described later in this review. The differential ability of the tissue to develop tachyphylaxis to BK's contractile effect, along with the relative potency in BK's ability to cause relaxation as opposed to contraction, led Boschcov and coworkers (34) to the conclusion that contraction and relaxation are mediated by different receptors. That desArg^9-BK was largely inactive confirms that rat duodenum normally lacks B1 receptors.

In the rat vas deferens BK elicits contraction by a direct effect on the smooth muscle cells and potentiates neurogenic contractions via a prejunctional influence on intrinsic sympathetic nerve endings (35). DesArg^9-BK is inactive, and neither the smooth muscle nor the neuronal effects of BK are inhibited by desArg^9[Leu^8]-BK, a B1 receptor antagonist. Thus, rat vas deferens does not contain B1 receptors. Nevertheless, Llona and coinvestigators (35) provided evidence that the smooth muscle effects of BK are mediated by a different receptor than the neuronal effects. The ability of several BK analogs to cause contraction presents the following rank order of potency:

BK = kallidin > Met-Lys-BK = [Tyr(Me)^8]-BK

By contrast, the ability of these analogs to potentiate prejunctional norepinephrine release is different:

Met,Lys-BK > BK > kallidin > [Tyr(Me)^8]-BK > NPC 431

In addition, NPC 431, a B2 antagonist, while inhibiting neuronal effects of BK (with a pA_2 value of 5.60), behaved as an agonist, causing smooth muscle contraction (35). It was proposed that in rat vas deferens there are B2 receptors but not B1 receptors. Moreover, the different structure-activity relationships for smooth muscle stimulation as compared with increasing transmitter release led to the further suggestion that the B2 receptors in this tissue could be subdivided. This was substantiated by the observation that NPC 431 behaved as an agonist prejunctionally (35). Interpretation of the latter observation should perhaps be a little cautious, since there is no evidence that the "agonist" effect of NPC 431 is mediated by an action on kinin receptors.

Additional studies have corroborated the existence of different types of B2 receptors on nerves and smooth muscle cells. NPC 394 was fivefold more potent as an antagonist of the postjunctional effects of BK than of the prejunctional effects (36). In contrast, NPC 349 was approximately fourfold more potent as an antagonist of BK's prejunctional effects. Unlike NPC 431, neither NPC 349 nor NPC 394 exhibited agonist activity in the vas deferens (36). These studies, therefore, provide evidence in favor of the hypothesis that rat vas deferens contains pre- and postjunctional B2 receptors of different subtypes.

Recent studies indicate that there may be multiple B2 receptors in other tissues. Whereas NPC 361 is a weak agonist in rat uterus, it antagonizes BK-induced contraction in guinea pig ileum (pA_2, 5.00) (37,38). This contrasts with other BK analogs NPC 420 and NPC 431, which are B2 antagonists in both preparations. Furthermore, while NPC 361 and NPC 431 actually stimulate phosphoinositide turnover in N1E-115 neuroblastoma cells, NPC 348, NPC 349, NPC 394, and NPC 420 inhibit BK-induced phosphoinositide turnover (39). The effect of NPC 349 in the study by Braas and colleagues (39) is contradicted in a more recent report that this analog is a full agonist in N1E-115 cells (40). We have consistently found, however, that NPC 349 is a relatively potent BK antagonist (4,6,41). The differential effects of the BK analogs in separate bioassay procedures, along with the observation that desArg^9-BK was largely inactive, led to the suggestion that there are multiple B2 receptors (39).

However, while these BK analogs bind with varying nanomolar affinities to ileal or N1E-115 cell membranes, again there is no direct evidence that the "agonist" effects of NPC 361 in N1E-115 cells or rat uterus and of NPC 431 in N1E-115 cells is mediated via BK receptors. Interestingly, we have found that NPC 567 elicits spasmogenic activity in rat uterus and guinea pig trachea in addition to its well-known B2 receptor antagonist effect (41,42). Again, however, whether the stimulation of smooth muscle reflects a receptor mechanism remains to be determined.

In another cultured line of hybrid, dorsal root ganglion neural cells (F-11) (43), several BK antagonists were tested. NPC 349 was the most potent antagonist of BK-induced inositol trisphosphate formation, elevated intracellular Ca^{2+} concentration, and cyclic GMP formation, with a pA_2 value of 10.40 (44,45). Several other BK analogs inhibited all three second messengers over a broad potency range (44). In one report, NPC 362 was listed as an agonist (45), while in another (44) NPC 362 was a pure, albeit weak, antagonist.

1. *[D-Arg^1, D-Phe^7]-Substituted Bradykinin Analogs*

In contrast to the apparent "ileum selectivity" of NPC 361 as a B2 antagonist, NPC 573, a [D-Arg^1]-substituted analog, inhibits BK-induced contractions of rat uterus (pA_2, 5.60) but is inactive against BK-induced contraction of guinea pig ileum (4). Moreover, this analog does not significantly displace [^{3}H]-BK binding from ileal or N1E-115 membranes. Therefore, NPC 573 is not a B2 receptor antagonist in guinea pig ileum. Unlike several other BK antagonists (NPC 349, NPC 414, NPC 566, NPC 567, and NPC 722), NPC 573 has no effect on BK-induced vascular pain in vivo. The apparent "uterus selectivity" of NPC 573 resulted in the proposal that B2 receptors in ileum are different from those in uterus (4).

We examined further the ability of several [D-Arg^1,D-Phe^7]-substituted analogs, including NPC 573, to antagonize BK-induced effects. It was confirmed that unlike the B1 and B2 receptor antagonist NPC 567, NPC 573 inhibited BK-induced contraction in uterus but not ileum (41). Binding studies revealed that 11 [D-Arg^1]-substituted analogs, including NPC 573, were either inactive or displaced very weakly [^{3}H]-BK binding in ileum or uterus. These data imply that the inhibitory action of NPC 573 on BK effects in uterus is not mediated by BK receptors. NPC 573, unlike NPC 567, also inhibited vasopressin-induced uterine contractions although neither analog bound to vasopressin receptors. [Arg^1]-substituted analogs, therefore, are not BK or vasopressin receptor antagonists (41).

2. *A Bradykinin B3 Receptor?*

Recently, we have examined the abilities of several B1 and B2 receptor antagonists to inhibit BK-induced contraction and to displace [^{3}H]-BK binding in airway smooth muscle in vitro. B1 or B2 receptor antagonists have little, if any, effect on BK-induced tracheal contraction, or on [^{3}H]-BK binding, and the evidence for a third, novel BK binding site in airway smooth muscle, the B3 receptor, is discussed in Chapter 9 of this volume (42).

III. BRADYKININ RECEPTOR SIGNAL TRANSDUCTION

It has been proposed that receptor subclassification should include consideration of the signal transduction pathways activated by particular agonists (46). Such classification is inappropriate for kinin receptors, at least for the present time, since B1 and B2 receptor responses can be mediated by the same transduction mechanisms. Activation of B2 receptors in virtually all tissues so far described leads to stimulation of the activity of phosphatidylinositol-specific phospholipase C, resulting in the formation of inositol phosphates and diacylglycerol (28,40,47-52). In most tissues, eicosanoid synthesis is also enhanced, potentially by release of arachidonic acid from the diacylglycerol produced by inositol lipid hydrolysis. In several tissues, however, inositol lipid hydrolysis is pharmacologically independent of arachidonate release and has been proposed to result from activation of phospholipase A_2 (53,54). Both B2 receptor-mediated inositol lipid hydrolysis and eicosanoid release are dependent on coupling of the receptors to guanine nucleotide binding proteins (G proteins) (45,53, 55,56), suggesting that B2 BK receptors belong to the class of receptors composed of seven hydrophobic transmembrane domains which, at present, is known to include adrenoceptors, muscarinic receptors, and receptors for serotonin, neurokinins, and dopamine (57).

In addition, B2 receptor activation often leads to enhanced cellular accumulation of cyclic AMP (58,59). This is often due to stimulation of the biosynthesis of eicosanoids, which subsequently bind to their respective receptors and activate adenylate cyclase (59), but in certain tissues the BK receptor may be directly coupled to adenylate cyclase by G_S (59a).

The transduction pathways activated by B1 receptor stimulation are less clear. In rabbit vascular smooth muscle, eicosanoid synthesis is apparently not stimulated as inhibitors of fatty acid cyclooxygenase are without effect on desArg^9-BK-induced contraction (20). Similarly, in murine macrophages (60) and human fibroblasts (61), desArg^9-BK does not stimulate eicosanoid synthesis. Conversely, eicosanoid production by B1 agonists has been reported in endothelial cells and other tissues (62-65).

IV. INDUCTION OF B1 RECEPTORS IN INFLAMMATION

A. Vascular Smooth Muscle

A particularly interesting characteristic of B1 receptors is their apparent induction following various pathological insults in vitro or in vivo. This subject was reviewed extensively a few years ago (8) and will be alluded to with particular reference to recent studies in the present article (see also Chapter 8).

In some isolated tissues, especially rabbit vascular smooth muscle, B1 receptors are generated de novo in a time-dependent manner. This phenomenon was first reported by Regoli and colleagues (66) using rabbit anterior mesenteric vein, in which responsiveness to the contractile effect of desArg^9-BK, initially nonexistent, increases with time of incubation in the organ bath, being maximal at around 6 hours. The increase in responsiveness to desArg^9-BK is not mediated by endogenous prostanoids, but is abolished by treating the tissues with cycloheximide or actinomycin, to inhibit protein synthesis or RNA synthesis, respectively (66). Ligand binding studies in the same tissue provided further evidence that the time-dependent increase in responsiveness to desArg^9-BK was due to de novo synthesis of B1 receptors (67). Incubation of chopped mesenteric artery for 24 hours caused an almost 13-fold increase in specific binding of desArg^9-BK, an effect which was also completely inhibited by cycloheximide. DesArg^9-BK binding was competed for by desArg^9-[Leu^8]-BK with a pA_2 value of 6.86. In veins removed from animals pretreated with *Escherichia coli* endotoxin, a procedure previously shown to enhance the effects of desArg^9-BK both in vitro and in vivo (68), there was a greater number of desArg^9-BK binding sites than in tissues from untreated rabbits (67). Interestingly, a significant correlation was also established between the time-dependent increase in contractile activity of desArg^9-BK and the increase in binding.

More recently, Deblois and Marceau (65) found that if strips of rabbit mesenteric artery are precontracted with the α-adrenoceptor agonist phenylephrine, the ability of desArg^9-BK to elicit *relaxation* also increases in a time-dependent fashion. Relaxation responses were not detectable for at least 60 minutes, but became evident after 2.5 hours and were maximal at 6 hours. Unlike contractile responses to desArg^9-BK (in the absence of phenylephrine), relaxations were abolished by the cyclooxygenase inhibitor indomethacin and, in fact, inhibition of prostanoid synthesis unmasked a time-dependent contraction superimposed on the phenylephrine-induced tone. It is now well established that BK-induced relaxation of vascular smooth muscle is endothelium-dependent (69). That relaxation to desArg^9-BK was markedly reduced by indomethacin, or by removing the endothelial layer, indicates that it is mediated largely by prostanoids originating from the endothelium (65). As with the development of contractions over time, however, cycloheximide prevented entirely the onset of relaxations without affecting phenylephrine-induced tone.

In contrast to mesenteric artery, rabbit celiac artery appears to contain B1 receptors which mediate relaxations independently of the endothelium (70). In celiac arterial smooth muscle, precontracted with phenylephrine, desArg^{10}-KD, a B1 receptor agonist, and BK both cause endothelium-independent relaxations which are inhibited by a B1 antagonist (desArg^{10}-[Leu^9]-KD) (70). A B1 and B2 antagonist, [β-Thi^{6,9},D-Phe^8]-KD, also inhibited the relaxations, but was less potent than the selective B1 antagonist. As in mesenteric artery (65), responses to kinins in celiac artery were also inhibited by a cyclooxygenase inhibitor (70).

It should be emphasized, however, that certain vascular beds express B1 receptors under apparently normal circumstances and without pathological insult. In conscious dogs, for example, infusion of BK into the saphenous vein causes venoconstriction secondary to thromboxane synthesis (71). This response is mediated by a B1 receptor, since desArg^9-[Leu^8]-BK is a potent antagonist. Additionally, the mixed B1 and B2 receptor antagonist, NPC 431, blocked BK-induced venoconstriction (71).

B. Nonvascular Smooth Muscle

Rat bladder smooth muscle has B1 and B2 receptors, desArg^9-BK and [Tyr-(Me^8)]-BK both mediating contraction, although only responses to the former are inhibited by desArg^{10}[Leu^9]-KD (72). As in rabbit vascular smooth muscle, responsiveness of rat bladder to desArg^9-BK, but not [Tyr(Me^8)]-BK, increases with time of incubation from an initial null level to a maximal contraction after 4 hours (72). The same study reported that the induction of responsiveness to desArg^9-BK was inhibited by cycloheximide. indicating the de novo synthesis of B1 receptors. Furthermore, inflammation of the bladder in vivo, caused by intravesicular injection of Triton X-100 several hours prior to sacrifice, while having no effect on responses to [Tyr(Me^8)]-BK or substance P, resulted in a dramatic increase in responsiveness to desArg^9-BK. This phenomenon was evident at the beginning of the experiment, where no response to desArg^9-BK is seen in controls, and after 2.5 hours incubation. The effect of Triton X-100 appeared to be localized to the inflamed bladder as responses of mesenteric veins from the same animals were unchanged (72).

Marceau and colleagues (8) suggested that de novo synthesis of B1 receptors is a result of tissue trauma, such as that produced either during tissue isolation and incubation, or by inflammation. It was further proposed that the induction of these responses may represent a regulatory mechanism during the inflammatory response whereby formation of B1 receptors could unmask local responses to normally inactive C-terminal desArg^9 metabolites of kinins.

Circular smooth muscle of human colon also develops responses to desArg^9-BK during incubation at 37 °C for at least 5 hours (73). Contractions were inhibited by desArg^{10}[Leu^9]-KD, confirming their mediation by B1 receptors. By contrast, storage of these tissues at 4 °C for periods of up to 44 hours did not result in an initial response to desArg^9-BK in the tissue (at 37 °C), perhaps indicating that the processes involved in B1 receptor induction are temperature-dependent. Similar to the bladder effects described above, inflammation of rat colon in vivo, induced by instillation of acetic acid 8 days previously, induces an approximately 100% increase in the maximal response to desArg^9-BK-induced C1-ion secretion by the mucosa in vitro (74). Responses to BK and substance P were unaffected by this procedure.

C. Mechanisms of B1 Receptor Induction

Recently, Marceau and coworkers have attempted to elucidate the mechanisms underlying induction of B1 receptors in rabbit aorta (75,76). A variety of substances cause an increase in the rate of specific sensitization of the smooth muscle to the contractile effect desArg^9-BK or a relatively higher concentration of BK in vitro. Application of *E. coli* endotoxin caused an approximately 100% increase in contraction magnitude at 3 and 6 hours as compared with untreated controls (75). Aortic strips prepared from rabbits treated 5-20 hours previously with endotoxin also exhibit enhanced B1 responsiveness (68,77). In addition, intravenous des-

Arg^9-BK has a hypotensive effect in endotoxin-treated rabbits, but not in controls (12,68,75,77).

Since endotoxin exerts many of its pathophysiological effects via stimulation of tissue macrophage protein synthesis (78-80), the effects of other macrophage stimulants on induction of B1 receptors was examined. Muramyldipeptide (MDP) and, to a lesser degree, phorbol-12-myristate-13-acetate each enhanced B1 receptor mediated contraction at 3 (MDP only) and 6 hours incubation (75). Moreover, the effects of these substances were selective for the kinins, as responses to neither norepinephrine nor histamine were affected.

Subsequent studies by Deblois et al. (76) provided further evidence that interleukin 1 (IL-1) and possibly IL-2 are involved in induction of B1 receptors in vitro. IL-1 was potent in its stimulation of responses to desArg^9-BK, and it is notable that endotoxin and MDP both promote IL-1 synthesis and release from macrophages (79,80) and fibroblasts (81). That IL-1 may be important in induction of aortic responses to desArg^9-BK was evidenced by the observation that glucocorticoid treatment of these tissues inhibited the development of B1 responsiveness (76). Glucocorticoids, among their myriad pharmacological actions, inhibit IL-1 synthesis (82).

Recent studies in our own laboratory provide further, albeit indirect, evidence for a role for IL-1 in induction of B1 receptors. Antigen arthritis in rabbits (induced by human fibrin) was associated with induction of bradykinin B1 receptors in isolated aorta smooth muscle 24 h following injection of antigen into the knee joint of sensitized animals (S. G. Farmer and R. M. Burch, unpublished observations). The arthritis was characterized by acute phase protein synthesis and joint swelling. Even at the beginning of experiments, vascular smooth muscle from these animals, unlike that from controls, exhibited responsiveness to desArg^9-BK and BK in vitro. In addition, the time-dependent increase in B1 responsiveness was greater in tissues from arthritic rabbits than from controls. In contrast, responses to another spasmogen, phenylephrine, were unaffected by antigen challenge. This is the first demonstration of induction of smooth muscle B1 receptors associated with an immune complex disease. The observation that fibrin challenge, administered locally, induced responsiveness to desArg^9-BK at a distant site implies that circulating cytokines are involved in inducing B1 receptors during inflammation.

V. BRADYKININ RECEPTOR ANTAGONISTS

A. B1 Antagonists

Several peptide antagonists of BK exhibit selectivity for the B1 receptor. Thus, various analogs of desArg^9-BK or desArg^{10}-KD have pA$_2$ values in the range of 6.00 to 8.40 as antagonists of desArg^{9}-BK-induced contraction in rabbit aorta (20). Probably the two most extensively utilized (and most potent) B1 antagonists are those in which Phe^{8} is substituted with Leu in the desArg^{9} analogs, desArg^{9}[Leu^{8}]-BK and desArg^{10}[Leu^{9}]-KD. These antagonists are B1-selective and do not antagonize the effects of BK mediated via B2 receptors, e.g., in rabbit jugular vein, dog carotid artery, guinea pig ileum (33,41,42), and rat (74) and human colon (73).

Substitution of Phe^{5} or Phe^{6} with L-carboranyl-Ala (Car^{5} or Car^{6}) in the above structures results in B1 antagonists with more prolonged durations of action, possibly due to increased resistance to kininase II (angiotensin converting enzyme, ACE) (83,84). Carboranyl-Ala is an amino acid containing a rigid ring of 10 boron atoms, which occupies a volume similar to that occupied by a phenyl nucleus (as in Phe^{5}) (20).

Although B1 receptors have so far been described primarily in vascular smooth muscle tissues, particularly those isolated from rabbits (20), desArg^{9}-BK elicits effects in nonvascular tissue also. For example, under certain conditions (see above), intestinal tissues from rats and humans, as well as rat bladder, express B1 receptors (34,72-74). B1 receptors have also been demonstrated in human fetal lung fibroblasts, wherein desArg^{9}-BK induces collagen formation, protein synthesis, and proliferation which are inhibited by desArg^{9}[Leu^{8}]-BK, whereas BK also stimulates prostaglandin formation, an effect which is not blocked by the B1 antagonist (61). It would seem, therefore, that these cells contain both BK receptor subtypes.

In bovine pulmonary artery endothelial cells in culture, BK and desArg^{9}-BK both stimulate synthesis of prostacyclin (62-64), platelet activating factor (62), and endothelium-derived relaxant factor (64). Nevertheless, higher concentrations of desArg^{9}-BK are necessary to induce these responses (62-64). These effects of BK and desArg^{9}-BK are inhibited by NPC 431 (62) or NPC 567 (63). In contrast, the B1 antagonist, desArg^{9}[Leu^{8}]-BK, inhibits only the effects of desArg^{9}-BK (63,64). Thus, like rat renal vasculature (85) and duodenum (34) and human fetal lung fibroblasts (61), various cell types in bovine pulmonary artery appear to contain B1 and B2 BK receptors (62-64). Other tissues containing both BK receptor subtypes include rabbit vena cava, renal vein and trachea, rat mesenteric vein, stomach and urinary bladder, and canine jugular and mesenteric veins, vena cava and subclavian artery (20).

B. B2 Antagonists

B2 receptors mediate BK-induced responses in most isolated smooth muscles and other tissues, and the effects of antagonists at these receptors are discussed later in the present review. It is interesting that, even though B2 receptors are perhaps the most ubiquitous subtype, until fairly recently the B1 receptor was more pharmacologically characterized. However, the discovery by Stewart and Vavrek (37) (see Chapter 3) that substitution with D-Phe for L-Pro in position 7 of the BK sequence conferred the ability to inhibit B2 receptor-mediated effects led to the first description of B2 receptor antagonists. Since 1985, hundreds of antagonist sequences, based on D-Phe^7-BK (NPC 361), have been synthesized (6,28,37,38,86,87). The peptide B2 receptor antagonists have contributed greatly to our appreciation of the role of this receptor subtype in the physiology and pathophysiology of BK. The pharmacology of B2 receptor antagonists is discussed in the following paragraphs. For detailed analyses of the structure-activity considerations of these agents, the reader is referred to other reviews (6, 28,37,38,88) and to Chapter 3.

C. Nonpeptide Bradykinin Antagonists

Drapeau et al. recently described a synthetic BK analog ([Phe^8-*psi*(CH$_2$-NH)-Arg^9]-BK) which is not metabolized either by kininase I or II (89, 90). This agent was claimed to be a B2 receptor agonist both in vivo and in vitro, although no antagonists were assessed. Nevertheless, no effect on B1 receptors (in rabbit aorta) was evident (89). This BK analog may provide clues to the synthesis of B2 receptor antagonists of similar metabolic stability.

Over the years, many reports of nonpeptide BK "antagonists" have been published. Rather disappointingly, however, the majority of these substances actually inhibit transduction pathways, such as cyclooxygenase, subsequent to BK receptor activation, or exhibit nonspecific cell membrane perturbing activity. Thus, since the agents described to date are merely functional antagonists of BK, and quite nonspecific in their actions, they will not be considered further here. A description of the rather varied assortment of such drugs is included in Chapter 4 and in a recent review (28).

VI. PHARMACOLOGY OF BRADYKININ ANTAGONISTS

As discussed earlier, much of the classification of BK receptors into B1 and B2 subtypes was carried out in isolated vascular smooth muscle (20, 21). Although there are many reports on the effects of kinins on a diversity of isolated tissue preparations, and their modification by various pharmacological interventions, relatively less is known about effects of specific BK antagonists in these types of study. The purpose of the present section is to provide a summary of the pharmacology of kinin antagonists.

A. Antagonist Specificity

In isolated vascular preparations, the B1 antagonist desArg^9[Leu^8]-BK is quite specific for B1 receptors (20). Although the D-Phe^7-substituted BK analogs are usually referred to as "B2-antagonists," in most tissues they are nonselective for B1 and B2 receptors (60,63,71,91,92). Under certain conditions, this can be due to tissue conversion of the antagonists to their desArg metabolites by carboxypeptidases (91,93). In other preparations, however, B1 receptor antagonism occurs in the absence of metabolism of the D-Phe^7 analogs (60,63).

In addition to their effects on kinin receptors, some of the D-Phe^7-substituted analogs (NPC 349, NPC 392, and NPC 414) have the ability to inhibit human kallikrein (94). The authors stated that the ability of these analogs to inhibit kallikrein is consistent with the inhibitory activity of other BK analogs, with Lys instead of Arg at position 1, and bulky substituents at position 3, on human urinary kallikrein (95,96).

B. Cardiovascular Effects

1. *Effects on Vascular Smooth Muscle*

BK increases microvascular permeability, contributing to the acute inflammatory response (see Chapters 8 and 9). Similarly, studies on the induction of B1 receptors, carried out mainly in vascular smooth muscle, are reviewed in Section IV and Chapter 4.

D'Orléans-Juste and colleagues (92) reported that endothelium-dependent relaxation of canine carotid artery induced by BK is mediated by B2 receptors, since it was not inhibited by desArg^{10}[Leu^9]-KD. Regoli et al. (91) demonstrated that BK-induced relaxations of the same tissue, as well as contractions of rabbit jugular vein, are inhibited by NPC 431 or [Thi^{6,9}, D-Phe^8]-KD, confirming the presence of B2 receptors. Moreover, desArg^9-BK was inactive in these smooth muscle preparations.

BK, injected close-arterially in the submandibular gland of the cat, causes vasodilation (97). The B2 antagonist NPC 349 inhibits this response, without affecting vasodilation elicited with acetylcholine or nerve stimulation.

In rat perfused kidneys, kallidin causes vasodilation followed, 4-7 minutes later, by a vasoconstrictor effect, whereas BK elicits only vasodilation (85). Indomethacin abolishes the vasodilation, but not the vasoconstriction, suggesting a role for endogenous prostanoids. The B1 antagonist desArg^9[Leu^8]-BK inhibited kallidin-induced renal vasoconstriction, but had no effect on vasodilation. In addition, desArg^9-BK also increased renal vascular resistance, and this too was abolished by the B1 antagonist. Thus, rat renal vasculature appears to contain B1 and B2 receptors (85).

There are very few reports on the effects of kinins on human isolated vascular preparations (98-100) and, to our knowledge, only one study which utilized BK antagonists (101). Whalley and associates recently analyzed the rank order of potency of various BK analogs in causing endothelium-dependent relaxation of human basilar artery. Since BK was considerably more potent than desArg^9-BK (which was essentially inactive), and since BK-induced relaxation was inhibited by NPC 431, it was concluded that BK-induced relaxation of human basilar artery is mediated by B2 receptors (101).

2. *Effects on Blood Pressure*

Many laboratories have examined BK as a potent hypotensive agent and whether kinins exert a physiological role in blood pressure control. A recent review by Margolius provides a comprehensive description of possible roles for kinins and kallikreins in hypertension and diabetes (25). Similarly, there is a brief review on the role for BK in blood pressure regulation (22). Finally, Gavras discusses the potential role of BK in hypertensive diseases in Chapter 7.

Regulation of Blood Pressure in Normal Animals. Many studies have examined the possibility that BK plays a physiological role in blood pressure regulation in animals and man. There have been several demonstrations that urinary kallikrein excretion is low in hypertensive patients, suggesting that kinins may play a role in maintaining normal blood pressure. It is now clear, however, that kallikrein dysregulation in hypertension is quite complex (22,25,28).

Several studies have failed to find any effect of the peptide BK antagonists NPC 349 and NPC 394 on blood pressure in normal rats, following administration of doses that block the blood pressure-lowering effect of BK (102,103). However, a very high dose of NPC 349 (4 mg/kg) injected into the ascending aorta of conscious, restrained rats caused a transient, biphasic effect on blood pressure, consisting of a pressor effect (7 mmHg) followed by a depressor effect (-20 mmHg), returning to baseline by 2 minutes (104). The pressor effect of NPC 349 was not affected by nephrectomy, adrenalectomy, vasodepressin V1-receptor antagonists, ganglionic and α- and β-adrenoceptor antagonists, histamine H1- and H2-receptor antagonists, or indomethacin. However, nephrectomy or indomethacin blocked the secondary depressor activity, suggesting that the BK antagonist elicited prostaglandin release from the kidney. NPC 394, when injected as a large dose (1 mg) also caused a transient rise in blood pressure of 12-15 mmHg (105).

In another study, NPC 349 at a dose of 400 μg i.v. (a dose that was shown to block the reduction in blood pressure elicited by BK) was administered to conscious, normotensive rats with no effect on blood pressure. However, if the rats were given nonpressor doses of angiotensin II or methoxamine, or pressor doses of vasopressin or methoxamine, NPC 349 significantly *increased* blood pressure by 9-16 mmHg (103).

Since it has been suggested that a component of the hypotensive effect of ACE inhibitors might be mediated by elevated BK concentration, NPC 349 was administered to rats that had also received captopril (106). NPC 349 had no effect on blood pressure in these animals. A similar study was conducted in spontaneously hypertensive rats (SHR) that had also been fed a salt-deficient diet for 10 days prior to the experiment (14). In these animals, BK seemed to play a role in blood pressure regulation, since NPC 567 caused an increase in blood pressure. However, as in the normal rats, captopril did not increase further the effect of the antagonist, nor did saralasin, a competitive angiotensin II antagonist.

Since NPC 349 had a hypertensive effect in salt-deprived SHRs, further studies were conducted to assess the interactions between the renin-angiotensin system and the kallikrein-kinin system. In order to cause acute salt-depletion and stimulate renin secretion, animals were pretreated with furosemide. In these animals, the hypertensive effects of NPC 349 were augmented (14). In rats receiving furosemide, the effect of NPC 349 was accompanied by bradycardia and decreased splanchnic nerve activity, suggesting that the effects of the kinin antagonist were peripheral and not mediated by increased sympathetic discharge (14).

In another study of the role of BK in the hypotensive effects of kininase II inhibitors, NPC 394 was used (15). In normotensive rats, the antagonist alone had no effect on blood pressure, although it was able to antagonize the hypotensive effects of a bolus of BK. NPC 394 was then tested in renovascular hypertensive rats. When these animals received enalapril, blood pressure fell by about 36 mmHg. NPC 394 increased blood pressure 12 mmHg in the enalapril-treated animals. When the renovascular hypertensive animals received saralasin, blood pressure fell by 25 mmHg, and NPC 394 had no effect in the presence of saralasin. Interestingly, the effect of NPC 394 in the enalapril-treated animals was about the same as the difference in effect of saralasin and enalapril, suggesting to the authors that increased BK concentration may account for one-third of the antihypertensive effect of ACE inhibitors (15).

NPC 392 (500 $\mu g^{-1} \cdot kg^{-1} \cdot min^{-1}$, i.a.) elicited a rise in blood pressure of 15 mmHg within 1 minute, an effect which increased gradually by another

10 mmHg over the next 4 minutes (15). Blood pressure was also increased by NPC 392 in nephrectomized animals, but the rise was only about one-half that observed in the intact animals. When plasma catecholamines were measured after administration of the kinin analog, norepinephrine and epinephrine were both elevated. The blood pressure response to NPC 392 was mediated by epinephrine acting on vascular α_1 adrenoceptors, since it was changed to a blood pressure-lowering effect by the α_1 adrenoceptor antagonist prazosin. Blockade of both α and β_1 adrenoceptors antagonized the ability of NPC 392 to alter blood pressure, as did adrenal enucleation (107). Adrenalectomy blocked the rise in circulating epinephrine in response to NPC 392, confirming the site of its release, but did not block norepinephrine release (107). Thus, relation of the effect of NPC 392 to BK antagonism is questionable.

In a related study on the role for BK in the hypotensive activity of ACE inhibitors, it was found that enalapril stimulated production of aortic PGI_2, and that this was blocked by prior infusion of NPC 349 (108). It was proposed, therefore, that the hemodynamic effects of ACE inhibitors may result, at least in part, form decreased degradation of kinins by ACE (kininase II). The increase in kinin levels subsequently stimulate vascular endothelial phospholipase A_2, which in turn results in increased production of the vasodilator PGI_2 (108).

Renal Hemodynamics. A recent study provided evidence that both the renin-angiotensin and kallikrein-kinin systems participate in regulating renal blood flow in rats (109). Animals were injected with enalapril (an ACE inhibitor) and phosphoramidon (a neutral endopeptidase 24.11 inhibitor), along with sodium bicarbonate solution, to inhibit degradation of endogenous kinins and increase urinary kallikrein activity, respectively. This procedure resulted in an increase in papillary blood flow, urine production, and sodium excretion. Administration of intravenous NPC 349 completely reversed the increase in blood flow, while having no effect on urine flow or sodium excretion. Administration of NPC 349 itself also produced a 20% decrease in renal papillary blood flow without altering cortical blood flow or glomerular filtration rate (GFR). These data suggest that endogenous kinins exert a vasodilator effect in the medullary circulation of the kidneys, and may play a role in regulating renal papillary blood flow (109).

In salt-restricted dogs, infusion of NPC 349 (50 μg/min) into the renal artery abolished renal vasodilation elicited by BK (110). During normal renal perfusion, intrarenal infusion of NPC 349, was also found to decrease renal blood flow without affecting systemic blood pressure, GFR, or sodium excretion. The decreased blood flow was due to a renal vasoconstrictor effect of the kinin antagonist, possibly due to increased renin secretion. This effect of NPC 349 on renin secretion may have resulted from a partial agonist effect, although this was thought unlikely (110). The effect of NPC 349 on renal blood flow was eliminated by the ACE inhibitor captopril.

Under conditions of decreased renal perfusion, autoregulation ensured that renal blood flow and GFR were well maintained, in the absence and presence of NPC 349 (110). In contrast, as perfusion pressure was decreased even further, the kinin antagonist blocked autoregulation, as evidenced by a marked decrease in GFR and filtration fraction. Under these circumstances, NPC 349 had no effect on renal blood flow. It was thus suggested that inhibition of endogenous kinins, as renal perfusion decreases to within the range of autoregulation, results in a reduction in renal coefficient of filtration. This in turn diminishes GFR autoregulation, even when blood flow is maintained, and it was proposed that kinins have a homeostatic effect in the balance of factors regulating glomerular filtration. Furthermore, this regulatory action of kinins seems to become increasingly apparent as the kidneys adapt to maintain normal function (110).

Angina Pectoris. Studies have also suggested that BK may have a role in stimulating cardiac sympathetic afferent neurons, thus contributing to the pain associated with myocardial ischemia and reflex cardiovascular responses during angina (111-113). Application of capsaicin, potassium chloride or BK to the myocardium of anesthetized dogs, results in reflex tachycardia and hypertension, whereas desArg^9-BK is without effect. Similarly, perfusion of the myocardium with desArg^9[Leu^8]-BK has no effect on reflex responses to epicardial BK, although the response is inhibited by NPC 349 (114). Another B2 receptor antagonist, [Thi^{6,9},D-Phe^8]-KD, also blocked responses to BK. Thus, the ability of BK to stimulate cardiac sympathetic reflexes appears to be mediated via activation of B2 receptors. Interestingly, BK also stimulates capsaicin-sensitive sensory nerves in guinea pig myocardium, via prostanoid release, although the nature of the BK receptor was not examined (115). A B2 antagonist, therefore, may find utility in some aspect of symptomatic relief from the pain associated with angina pectoris. It is important to note though, that this pain serves a purpose in stopping a patient's exertions, thereby reducing cardiac load.

Central Pressor Effects of Bradykinin. In addition to peripheral, hypotensive effects, BK causes marked and sustained hypertension following i.c.v. administration (116-119). The site of the hypertensive effect of BK in the brain has been proposed to lie in the lateral septal area (117), the ventral portion of the third ventricle (120), or in sites on the dorsal surface of the medulla (118,119). A recent study examined the nature of receptors mediating the central pressor effect of kinins in rats, and reported that desArg^9-BK was without effect (119). However, the pressor effects of i.c.v. BK or T-kinin were abolished by the B2 antagonist NPC 349, but unaffected by the B1 antagonist, desArg^9[Leu^8]-BK (119).

Overall, use of BK receptor antagonists has suggested that BK does not play an active role in the regulation of systemic blood pressure in normal rats. However, the kinin may act to blunt the hypertensive effects of a variety of pressor hormones, both administered acutely, and in disease states in which these hormones act to increase blood pressure. It will be important for future studies to address the role of BK in blood pressure regulation in other species. Finally, since some of the antagonists may have actions other than at BK receptors (28), including stimulation of renal prostaglandin synthesis and release of adrenal epinephrine, results obtained with the antagonists, especially when they are administered at high doses, should be interpreted with caution.

Endotoxic Shock. Endotoxic shock is caused by interaction of lipopolysaccharides (endotoxins) of certain bacterial walls with reticuloendothelial cells. An acute effect of endotoxin administration is a profound fall in mean arterial pressure within a few minutes, which recovers, and then falls again as the animals approach death. A rather large body of literature concerning the putative role of kinins in septic shock has accumulated (10). In many studies, it was determined that the kallikrein-kinin system is activated in human sepsis and experimental endotoxic shock. However, without the availability of kinin receptor antagonists, the studies could only correlate metabolic and physiologic changes with changes in components of the kallikrein-kinin system.

There are two recent reports using bradykinin antagonists in animals during endotoxin shock. In the first, rats were given an intravenous bolus of endotoxin 5 minutes after the beginning of a continuous infusion of NPC 413 ($100 \mu g \cdot kg^{-1} \cdot min^{-1}$, i.v.) (13). NPC 413 infusion continued for a further 20 minutes. Endotoxin caused a rapid, nearly 50% fall in blood pressure at 6 minutes. In the presence of NPC 413, however, blood pressure fell only slightly. In this study, no other concentrations of the antagonist were assessed, and its effect on survival was not determined. In the other study, NPC 567 infusion into the jugular vein of rats was initiated 30 minutes prior to endotoxin (16). Endotoxin was then administered as an infusion for 10 minutes, along with NPC 567. NPC 567 infusion was continued for an additional 90 minutes. Under these circumstances, endotoxin caused a biphasic fall in blood pressure, the first phase reaching its nadir at 1 hour, recovering gradually by 2.5 hours, and falling again, until the animals died. Endotoxin caused a 38% fall in mean arterial pressure at 1 hour, an effect which was inhibited approximately 60% by infusion of NPC 567. During the second phase of hypotension, the effects of NPC 567 were monitored to 4 hours after endotoxin, at which time NPC 567 completely blocked the hypotensive effect of endotoxin, even though infusion of the antagonist was discontinued 2.5 hours previously. Even more striking than the effects of NPC 567 on blood pressure was its effect on mortality. At 24 hours, 100% of animals receiving endotoxin had died, compared to only 50% of the animals that received NPC 567 (16).

C. Pain and Inflammation

The potent analgesic and inflammatory effects of kinins are discussed in detail in Chapter 8. Similarly, the involvement of kinins in inflammatory conditions of the upper and lower airways are the topics of Chapters 9, 10, and 11.

D. Gastrointestinal Effects

As discussed earlier, Boschcov et al. (34) suggested that BK-induced contraction and relaxation of rat duodenum are mediated by different receptor subtypes. Neither type of response involved B1 receptors, however, as desArg^9-BK had little effect. Similarly, in guinea pig ileal smooth muscle, there is evidence that, although the predominant receptor for BK is the B2 subtype, the possibility of a multiplicity of B2 receptors exists in this tissue (4,33,91). For example, Manning and colleagues (33) reported that there are two distinct binding sites for BK in guinea pig ileal, heart, and kidney membranes. This study examined a large number of BK analogs for their ability to displace radiolabeled BK from its receptors. DesArg^9-BK had no effect, indicating an absence of B1 receptors, but these workers showed that there were two specific BK binding sites with different affinities (33). Regoli and associates (91) reported the effects of NPC 361, NPC 431, and [Thi^{6,9}, D-Phe^8]-KD (B2 antagonists) in several smooth muscle tissues including guinea pig ileum. BK-induced contractions were antagonized by NPC 361 (pA_2, 5.85), NPC 431 (pA_2, 5.90), and [Thi^{6,9}, D-Phe^8]-KD (pA_2, 5.93), although the latter analog exhibited weak stimulatory effects in this tissue. In addition, the three peptides were specific for BK, having no effect on contractile activity produced by substance P and angiotensin II. Higher concentrations of each of the three antagonists also inhibited B1 receptor-mediated contractions of rabbit aorta to desArg^9-BK (91). These data confirm those of Vavrek and Stewart (37), who also demonstrated that NPC 361 and NPC 431 were competitive B2 antagonists (with respective pA_2 values of 5.00 and 6.30) in guinea pig ileum. NPC 431 also exhibited similar antagonist activity against BK-induced contractions in rat uterus, whereas NPC 361 displayed weak stimulatory effects (37).

Vavrek and Stewart have synthesized several analogs of NPC 361 which are B2 antagonists in guinea pig ileum (38). These studies are discussed elsewhere in this volume. In addition, studies in our laboratory have confirmed that NPC 349, NPC 414, and NPC 567 are B2 receptor antagonists both in guinea pig ileum and rat uterus (41). Another report also confirms that several B2 receptor antagonists, NPC 348, NPC 349, NPC 394, NPC 420, and NPC 431, inhibit BK-induced ileal contractions (121).

Recent studies confirm that the receptors mediating kinin-induced mucosal electrolyte secretion in rat colon and guinea pig ileum are of the B2 subtype. The pharmacology of BK-induced intestinal secretion is discussed in a recent review (26). NPC 361, but not desArg^9[Leu^8]-BK, inhibited the effect of BK in these preparations in a competitive fashion (122). In ileal smooth muscle, the same group also demonstrated the presence of B2 receptors, as NPC 361 but not desArg^9[Leu^8]-BK inhibited BK-induced contraction (pA_2, 5.40) (123). Similarly, another B2 receptor antagonist, NPC 349, inhibits BK-induced Cl^- ion secretion by rat colonic mucosa in vitro (124). In addition, B2 receptors also appear to mediate BK-induced contraction of guinea pig taenia caeci, since this response is unaffected by desArg^9[Leu^8]-BK (125). The recent description of nonpeptide, competitive BK antagonists, isolated from plant extracts, in intestinal smooth muscle from several species (126-128) is discussed in Chapter 4.

E. Pulmonary Effects

The reader is referred to Chapters 9, 10, and 11 in the present volume for reviews of the pulmonary pharmacology of kinins and their antagonists.

F. Other Effects

Studies with BK antagonists in neurogenic contractions of isolated vasa deferentia are discussed in the section on BK receptor heterogeneity (35, 36), as are effects in isolated uterus smooth muscle (4,39,41). Regoli and colleagues (91) confirmed that, as in the rat, canine bladder smooth muscle responses to BK are mediated by B2 receptors. In this tissue, NPC 431 and [Thi^{6,9},D-Phe^8]-KD were potent BK antagonists, whereas desArg^9-BK was inactive.

In isolated iris smooth muscle, BK-induced contraction is mediated by substance P released from intrinsic nerve endings (129). It was demonstrated recently that NPC 415 exhibits BK-induced stimulation of substance P release from trigeminal nerve endings in rabbit isolated iris (pA_2, 7.59), suggesting the involvement of B2 receptors (2).

B1, and perhaps also B2, receptors mediate resorption of bone in the mouse calvarium, as both BK and desArg^9-BK, in a dose-dependent fashion, cause calcium and matrix degradation (130). DesArg^9[Leu^8]-BK inhibits desArg^9-BK-induced resorption, whereas cyclooxygenase inhibitors abolished BK-induced resorption, although their effects on the B1 agonist were not reported.

In porcine-cultured articular chondrocytes, BK causes increased inositol phosphate generation, intracellular free calcium ions, and prostaglandin biosynthesis (131). Since these effects are not mimicked by desArg^9-BK, but are blocked by NPC 431, they are mediated by B2 receptors.

Both BK and desArg^9-BK stimulate IL-1 and tumor necrosis factor release from the mouse macrophage-like cell line, RAW264.7 (60). These effects of the kinins are not eicosanoid-dependent. Although the effects are blocked both by NPC 567 and desArg^9[Leu^8]-BK, suggesting that the receptor involved is a B1 receptor, it is interesting that BK and desArg^9-BK are almost equipotent (60).

Recent studies compared the effects of BK and kallikrein, both of which cause contractions, in rat isolated uterus (132,133). Whereas one study found that kallikrein-induced uterine contraction was not blocked by an antibody to BK (132), the other reported that NPC 349 did inhibit the effect of kallikrein (133). It was thus concluded that the oxytocic effect of kallikrein was, at least in part, due to release of endogenous kinins the effects of which, presumably on B2 receptors, were antagonized by NPC 349 (133). Alternatively, if kallikrein has a specific receptor, it is possible that activation of that receptor involves kallikrein's enzymatic activity, and this enzymatic activity may be blocked by NPC 349.

In rabbit ovary, perfused in situ, infusion of BK caused a dose-dependent increase in ovulation, as well as elevating 6-keto-$PGF_{1\alpha}$ and $PGF_{2\alpha}$ within 1 hour of administration (134). By 4 hours and 24 hours, respectively, PGE_2 and TxB_2 production were also increased. Whereas neither indomethacin nor NPC 349 inhibited BK-induced ovulation, NPC 431 did block the effects of BK. In addition, ovulation induced by human chronic gonadotropin (hCG) was inhibited by NPC 431, and it was suggested that kinins may be involved in follicle rupture during ovulation (134). Indeed, it was demonstrated earlier that kinin-generating activity is increased in pregnant mare serum gonadotropin/hCG-primed rats (135).

VII. CONCLUDING REMARKS

Most effects of kinins, in vivo and in vitro, are mediated by specific receptors. Nevertheless, while our knowledge concerning receptor heterogeneity, tissue and organ receptor distribution, and pharmacological effects of receptor activation has burgeoned in the past decade or so, we still have a great deal to learn. The development of peptide antagonists have been, and will continue to be, significant in this regard, although these agents have restricted practical utility, due to low potency and metabolic instability. It is often overlooked that the current peptide bradykinin antagonists represent "first-generation" compounds.

We look forward to future development of specific, potent, and stable nonpeptide drugs, which are antagonists (and, perhaps, agonists) at the various subtypes of kinin receptors. These agents will not only contribute tremendously to understanding of the pharmacology, physiology and pathophysiology of kinins, but may also represent powerful instruments in our struggles to relieve pain and inflammation associated with many diseases in animals and man.

REFERENCES

1. Clark, W. G. Kinins and peripheral and central nervous system, in: *Bradykinin, Kallidin and Kallikrein. Handbook of Experimental Pharmacology, Volume XXV, Supplement* (E. G. Erdös, ed.). Springer-Verlag, New York, pp. 311-356 (1979).
2. Griesbacher, T., and F. Lembeck. Effect of bradykinin antagonists on bradykinin-induced plasma extravasation, venoconstriction, prostaglandin E_2 release, and nociceptor stimulation and contraction of the iris sphincter muscle in the rabbit. *Br. J. Pharmacol.* **92**:333-340 (1987).
3. Taiwo, Y. O., and J. D. Levine. Characterization of the arachidonic acid metabolites mediating bradykinin and noradrenaline hyperalgesia. *Brain Res.* **458**: 402-406 (1988).
4. Steranka, L. R., D. C. Manning, C. J. Dehaas, J. W. Ferkany, S. A. Borosky, J. R. Connor, R. J. Vavrek, J. M. Stewart, and S. H. Snyder. Bradykinin as a pain mediator: Receptors are localized to sensory neurons, and antagonists have analgesic actions. *Proc. Natl. Acad. Sci. USA* **85**:3245-3249 (1988).
5. Dray, A., J. Bettaney, P. Forster, and M. N. Perkins. Bradykinin-induced stimulation of afferent fibres is mediated through protein kinase C. *Neurosci. Lett.* **91**:301-307 (1988).
6. Steranka, L. R., S. G. Farmer, and R. M. Burch. Antagonists of B2 bradykinin receptors. *FASEB J.* **3**:2019-2025 (1989).

7. Haley, J. E., A. H. Dickenson, and M. Schachter. Electrophysiological evidence for a role of bradykinin in chemical nociception in the rat. *Neurosci. Lett.* **97**:198-202 (1989).
8. Marceau, F., A. Lussier, D. Regoli, and J. P. Giroud. Pharmacology of kinins: Their relevance to tissue injury and inflammation. *Gen. Pharmacol.* **14**:209-229 (1983).
9. Proud, D., and A. P. Kaplan. Kinin formation: Mechanisms and role in inflammatory disorders. *Annu. Rev. Immunol.* **6**:49-84 (1988).
10. Colman, R. W. and P. Y. Wong. Kallikrein-kinin system in pathologic conditions, in: *Bradykinin, Kallidin and Kallikrein, Handbook of Experimental Pharmacology, Volume XXV, Supplement* (E. G. Erdös, ed.). Springer-Verlag, New York, pp. 569-607 (1979).
11. Greaves, M. W. Inflammation and mediators. *Br. J. Dermatol.* **119**:419-426 (1988).
12. Marceau, F., A. Lussier, and S. St-Pierre. Selective induction of cardiovascular responses to des-Arg^9-bradykinin by bacterial endotoxin. *Pharmacol.* **29**: 70-74 (1984).
13. Weipert, J., H. Hoffman, M. Siebeck, and E. T. Whalley. Attenuation of arterial blood pressure fall in endotoxin shock in the rat using the competitive bradykinin antagonist Lys-Lys-[Hyp^2, $Thi^{5,8}$, D-Phe^7]-BK (B4148). *Br. J. Pharmacol.* **94**:282-284 (1988).
14. Waeber, B., J.-F. Aubert, J.-P. Flükiger, J. Nussberger, R. J. Vavrek, J. M. Stewart, and H. R. Brunner. Role of endogenous bradykinin in blood pressure control of conscious rats. *Kidney International* **34(Suppl.26)**:S63-S68 (1988).
15. Gavras, I., and H. Gavras. Anti-hormones and blood pressure: Bradykinin antagonists in blood pressure regulation. *Kidney International* **34(Suppl.26)**: S60-S62 (1988).
16. Wilson, D. D., L. de Garavilla, W. Kuhn, J. Togo, R. M. Burch, and L. R. Steranka. D-Arg-[Hyp^3-D-Phe^7]-bradykinin, a bradykinin antagonist, reduces mortality in a rat model of endotoxic shock. *Circ. Shock* **27**:93-101 (1989).
17. *Bradykinin, Kallidin and Kallikrein, Handbook of Experimental Pharmacology, Volume XXV, Supplement* (E. G. Erdös, ed.). Springer-Verlag, New York, pp. 1-817 (1979).
18. *Kinins IV. Advances in Experimental Medicine and Biology, Volume 198A* (L. M. Greenbaum and H. S. Margolius, eds.). Plenum Press, New York, pp. 1-590 (1986).
19. *Kinins IV. Advances in Experimental Medicine and Biology, Volume 198B* (L. M. Greenbaum and H. S. Margolius, eds.). Plenum Press, New York, pp. 1-572 (1986).
20. Regoli, D., and J. Barabé. Pharmacology of bradykinin and related kinins. *Pharmacol. Rev.* **32**:1-46 (1980).

21. Regoli, D. Kinins. *Br. Med. Bull.* **43**:270-284 (1987).
22. Sharma, J. N. Interrelationship between the kallikrein-kinin system and hypertension: a review. *Gen. Pharmacol.* **19**:177-187 (1988).
23. Kozin, K., and C. G. Cochrane. The contact activation system of plasma: biochemistry and pathophysiology, in: *Inflammation: Basic Principles and Clinical Correlates* (J. I. Gallin, I. M. Goldstein, and R. Snyderman, eds.). Raven Press, Ltd., New York, pp. 101-120 (1988).
24. Fuller, R. W., and P. J. Barnes. Kinins, in: *Asthma: Basic Mechanisms and Clinical Management* (P. J. Barnes, I. W. Rodger, and N. C. Thomson, eds.). Academic Press Ltd., London, pp. 259-272 (1988).
25. Margolius, H. S. Tissue kallikreins and kinins: Regulation and roles in hypertensive and diabetic diseases. *Annu. Rev. Pharmacol. Toxicol.* **29**:343-364 (1989).
26. Gaginella, T. S., and J. F. Kachur. Kinins as mediators of intestinal secretion. *Am. J. Physiol.* **256**:G1-G15 (1989).
27. Erdos, E. G. and R. A. Skidgel. Neutral endopeptidase 24.11 (enkephalinase) and related regulators of peptide hormones. *FASEB J.* **3**:145-151 (1989).
28. Burch, R. M., S. G. Farmer, and L. R. Steranka. Bradykinin receptor antagonists. *Med. Res. Rev.* **10**:237-269 (1990).
29. Okamoto, H., and L. M. Greenbaum. Isolation and structure of T-kinin. *Biochem. Biophys. Res. Commun.* **112**:701-708 (1983).
30. Emjyoji, K.-I., and H. Kato. Hydroxyprolyl^3-bradykinin in high molecular mass kininogen: Presence in human and monkey kininogens, but not in kininogens from bovine, rat, rabbit, guinea pig and mouse plasmas. *FEBS Lett.* **238**:1-4 (1988).
31. Maeda, H., Y. Matsumura, and H. Kato. Purification and identification of [hydroxyprolyl^8]bradykinin in ascitic fluid from a patient with gastric cancer. *J. Biol. Chem.* **263**:16051-16054 (1988).
32. Mindroiu, T., O. A. Carretero, D. Proud, D. Walz, and A. G. Scicli. A new kinin moiety in human plasma kininogens. *Biochem. Biophys. Res. Commun.,* **152**:519-526 (1988).
33. Manning, D. C., R. Vavrek, J. M. Stewart and S. H. Snyder. Two bradykinin binding sites with picomolar affinities. *J. Pharmacol. Exp. Ther.* **237**:504-512 (1986).
34. Boschcov, P., A. C. M. Paiva, T. B. Paiva, and S. I. Shimuta. Further evidence for the existence of two receptor sites for bradykinin responsible for the diphasic effect in the rat isolated duodenum. *Br. J. Pharmacol.* **83**:591-600 (1984).
35. Llona, I., R. Vavrek, J. Stewart, and J. P. Huidobro-Toro. Identification of pre- and postsynaptic bradykinin receptor sites in the vas deferens: Evidence for different structural prerequisites. *J. Pharmacol. Exp. Ther.* **241**:608-614 (1987).

36. Rifo, J., M. Pourrat, R. J. Vavrek, J. M. Stewart, and J. P. Huidobro-Toro. Bradykinin receptor antagonists used to characterize the heterogeneity of bradykinin-induced responses in rat vas deferens. *Eur. J. Pharmacol.* **142**:305-312 (1987).
37. Vavrek, R. J., and J. M. Stewart. Competitive antagonists of bradykinin. *Peptides* **6**:161-164 (1985).
38. Stewart, J. M., and R. J. Vavrek. Bradykinin competitive antagonists for classical kinin receptors, in: *Kinins IV. Advances in Experimental Medicine and Biology, Volume 198A* (L. M. Greenbaum and H. S. Margolius, eds.). Plenum Press, New York, pp. 537-542 (1986).
39. Braas, K. M., D. C. Manning, D. C. Perry, and S. H. Snyder. Bradykinin analogues: Differential agonist and antagonist activities suggesting multiple receptors. *Br. J. Pharmacol.* **94**:3-5 (1988).
40. Fergus, J. H., R. F. Bruns, and D. T. Dudley. Differential effect of bradykinin analogues on phosphatidylinositol turnover in JH4 and N1E-115 cells. *Soc. Neurosci. Abst.* **14**:979 (1988).
41. Farmer, S. G., R. M. Burch, D. J. Dehaas, J. Togo, and L. R. Steranka. [Arg^1 $DPhe^7$]-substituted analogs of bradykinin inhibit vasopressin- and bradykinin-induced contractions of uterine smooth muscle. *J. Pharmacol. Exp. Ther.* **248**:667-681 (1989).
42. Farmer, S. G., R. M. Burch, S. N. Meeker, and D. E. Wilkins. Evidence for a pulmonary bradykinin B3 receptor. *Mol. Pharmacol.* **36**:1-8 (1989).
43. Francel, P. C., K. Harris, M. Smith, M. C. Fishman, G. Dawson, and R. J. Miller. Neurochemical characterization of a novel dorsal root ganglion X neuroblastoma hybrid cell line, F-11. *J. Neurochem.* **48**:1621-1631 (1987).
44. Francel, P. C., R. J. Miller, and G. Dawson. Modulation of bradykinin-induced inositol triphosphate release in a novel neuroblastoma X dorsal root ganglion sensory neuron cell line (F-11). *J. Neurochem.* **48**:1632-1639 (1987).
45. Francel, P. C., J. F. Keefer, and G. Dawson. Bradykinin analogs antagonize bradykinin-induced second messenger production in a sensory neuron cell line. *Mol. Pharmacol.* **35**:34-38 (1989).
46. Kenakin, T. P. Challenges for receptor theory as a tool for a drug receptor classification. *Trends Pharmacol. Sci.* **10**:18-22 (1989).
47. Higashida, H., and D. A. Brown. Ca^{2+}-dependent K^+ channels in neuroblastoma hybrid cells activated by intracellular inositol trisphosphate and extracellular bradykinin. *FEBS Lett.* **238**:395-400 (1988).
48. Portilla, D., J. Morrissey, and A. R. Morrison. Bradykinin-activated membrane-associated phospholipase C in Madin-Darby canine kidney cells. *J. Clin. Invest.* **81**:1896-1902 (1988).
49. Volonté, C., G. S. Parries, and E. Racker. Stimulation of inositol incorporation into lipids of PC12 cells by nerve growth factor and bradykinin. *J. Neurochem.* **51**:1156-1162 (1988).

50. Chuang, D.-M. Neurotransmitter receptors and phosphoinositide turnover. *Annu. Rev. Pharmacol. Toxicol.* **29**:71-110 (1989).
51. Kaya, H., G. M. Patton, and S. L. Hong. Bradykinin-induced activation of phospholipase A_2 is independent of the activation of polyphosphoinositide-hydrolyzing phospholipase C. *J. Biol. Chem.* **264**:4972-4977 (1989).
52. Perney, T. M., and R. J. Miller. Two different G-proteins mediate neuropeptide Y and bradykinin-stimulated phospholipid breakdown in cultured rat sensory neurons. *J. Biol. Chem.* **264**:7317-7327 (1989).
53. Burch, R. M., and J. Axelrod. Dissociation of bradykinin-stimulated arachidonic acid release from inositol phosphate formation in Swiss 3T3 fibroblasts. Evidence for a G protein-dependent coupled phospholipase A_2. *Proc. Natl. Acad. Sci. USA* **84**:6374-6378 (1987).
54. Slivka, S. R., and P. A. Insel. Phorbol ester and neomycin dissociate bradykinin receptor-mediated arachidonic acid release and polyphosphoinositide hydrolysis in Madin-Darby canine kidney cells. Evidence that bradykinin mediates noninterdependent activation of phospholipases A_2 and C. *J. Biol. Chem.* **263**:14640-14647 (1988).
55. Higashida, H., R. A. Streaty, W. Klee, and M. Nirenberg. Bradykinin-activated transmembrane signals are coupled via N_0 or N_i to production of inositol 1,4,5-triphosphate, a second messenger in NG108-15 neuroblastoma-glioma hybrid cells. *Proc. Natl. Acad. Sci. USA* **83**:942-946 (1986).
56. Murayama, T., and M. Ui. Phosphatidic acid may stimulate membrane receptors mediating adenylate cyclase inhibition and phospholipid breakdown in 3T3 fibroblasts. *J. Biol. Chem.* **262**:5522-5529 (1987).
57. Frielle, T., M. G. Kobilka, R. S. Lefkowitz, and M. G. Caron. Human β_1- and β_2-adrenergic receptors: Structurally and functionally related receptors derived from distinct genes. *Trends Neurosci.* **11**:321-324 (1988).
58. Stoner, J., V. C. Maganiello, and M. Vaughan. Effects of bradykinin and indomethacin on cyclic GMP and cyclic AMP in lung slices. *Proc. Natl. Acad. Sci. USA* **70**:3830-3833 (1973).
59. Brunton, L. L., R. A. Wiklund, P. M. Van Arsdale, and A. G. Gilman. Binding of [^{3}H]prostaglandin E_1 to putative receptors linked to adenylate cyclase of cultured cell clones. *J. Biol. Chem.* **251**:3037-3044 (1976).

59a. Liebmann, C., S. Riessmann, P. Robberecht, and H. Arold. Bradykinin action in the rat duodenum: Receptor binding and influence on the cyclic AMP system. *Biomed. Biochim. Acta* **46**:469-478 (1987).

60. Tiffany, C. W., and R. M. Burch. Bradykinin stimulates tumor necrosis factor and interleukin 1 release from macrophages. *FEBS Lett.* **247**:189-192 (1989).
61. Goldstein, R. H., and M. Wall. Activation of protein formation and cell division by bradykinin and Des-Arg^9-bradykinin. *J. Biol. Chem. 259*:9263-9268 (1984).
62. Cahill, M., J. B. Fishman, and P. Polgar. Effect of des arginine^9-bradykinin and other bradykinin fragments on the synthesis of prostacyclin and the binding of bradykinin by vascular cells in culture. *Agents Actions* **24**:224-231 (1988).

63. Conklin, B. R., R. M. Burch, L. R. Steranka, and J. Axelrod. Distinct bradykinin receptors mediate stimulation of prostaglandin synthesis by endothelial cells and fibroblasts. *J. Pharmacol. Exp. Ther.* **244**:646-649 (1988).
64. Sung, C.-P., A. J. Arleth, K. Shikano, and B. A. Berkowitz. Characterization and function of bradykinin receptors in vascular endothelial cells. *J. Pharmacol. Exp. Ther.* **247**:8-13 (1988).
65. Deblois, D., and F. Marceau. The ability of des-Arg^9-bradykinin to relax rabbit isolated mesenteric arteries is acquired during in vitro incubation. *Eur. J. Pharmacol.* **142**:141-144 (1987).
66. Regoli, D., F. Marceau, and J. Barabé. *De novo* formation of vascular receptor for bradykinin. *Can. J. Physiol. Pharmacol.* **56**:674-677 (1978).
67. Barabé, J., C. Babiuk, and D. Regoli. Binding of [^{3}H]des-Arg^9-BK to rabbit anterior mesenteric vein. *Can. J. Physiol. Pharmacol.* **60**:1551-1555 (1982).
68. Regoli, D., F. Marceau, and J. Lavigne. Induction of B1 receptors for kinins in the rabbit by a bacterial lipopolysaccharide. *Eur. J. Pharmacol.* **71**:105-115 (1981).
69. Furchgott, R. F., and P. M. Vanhoutte. Endothelium derived relaxing and contracting factors. *FASEB J.* **3**:2007-2018 (1989).
70. Ritter, J. M., H. S. Doktor, and E. J. Cragoe. Actions of bradykinin and related peptides on rabbit coeliac artery rings. *Br. J. Pharmacol.* **96**:23-28 (1989).
71. Müller-Schweinitzer, E. Changes in the venous compliance by bradykinin and angiotensin II and its significance for the vascular effects of cyclosporine A. *Naunyn-Schmiedeberg's Arch. Pharmacol.* **338**:699-703 (1988).
72. Marceau, F., J. Barabé, S. St-Pierre, and D. Regoli. Kinin receptors in experimental inflammation. *Can. J. Physiol. Pharmacol.* **58**:536-542 (1980).
73. Couture, R., J. Mizrahi, D. Regoli, and G. Devroede. Peptides and the human colon: An *in vitro* pharmacological study. *Can. J. Physiol. Pharmacol.* **59**:957-970 (1982).
74. Kachur, J. F., W. Allbee, and T. S. Gaginella. Effect of bradykinin and des-Arg^9-bradykinin on ion transport across normal and inflamed rat colonic mucosa. *Gastroenterol.* **90**:1481 (1986).
75. Bouthillier, J., D. Deblois, and F. Marceau. Studies on the induction of pharmacological responses to des-Arg^9- bradykinin *in vitro* and *in vivo*. *Br. J. Pharmacol.* **92**:257-264 (1987).
76. Deblois, D., J. Bouthillier, and F. Marceau. Effect of glucocorticoids, monokines and growth factors on the spontaneously developing responses of the rabbit isolated aorta to des Arg^9 bradykinin. *Br. J. Pharmacol.* **93**:969-977 (1988).
77. Nwator, I. A. A., and E. T. Whalley. Angiotensin converting enzyme inhibitors and expression of des-Arg^9-BK (kinin B_1) receptors in vivo. *Eur. J. Pharmacol.* **160**:125-132 (1989).
78. Kawakami, M., P. H. Pekala, M. D. Lane, and A. Cerami. Lipoprotein lipase suppression in 3T3-L1 cells by an endotoxin-induced mediator from exudate cells. *Proc. Natl. Acad. Sci. USA* **79**:912-916 (1982).

79. Dinarello, C. A., and J. M. Krueger. Induction of interleukin 1 by synthetic and naturally occurring muramyl peptides. *Fed. Proc.* **45**:2545-2548 (1986).
80. Warren, S. H., R. F. Vogel, and L. A. Chedid. Current status of immunological adjuvants. *Annu. Rev. Immunol.* **4**:369-388 (1986).
81. Iribe, H., T. Koga, S. Kotani, S. Kusumoto, and T. Shiba. Stimulating effect of MDP and its adjuvant-active analogues on guinea-pig fibroblasts for the production of thymocyte-activating factor. *J. Exp. Med.* **157**:2190-2195 (1983).
82. Altiere, R. J., and L. Diamond. Comparison of vasoactive intestinal peptide and isoproterenol relaxant effect in isolated cat airways. *J. Appl. Physiol.* **56**:986-992 (1984).
83. Couture, R., J.-N. Drouin, O. Leukart, and D. Regoli. Biological activities of kinins and substance P-octapeptides (4-11) in which phenylalanine residues have been replaced with L- carbonylalanine. *Can. J. Physiol. Pharmacol.* **57**:1437-1442 (1979).
84. Drouin, J.-N., P. Gaudreau, S. St-Pierre, and D. Regoli. Biological activities of kinins modified at the N- or at the C- terminal end. *Can. J. Physiol. Pharmacol.* **57**:1018-1023 (1979).
85. Guimaraes, J. A., M. A. R. Vieira, E. Eich, and T. Maack. Effects of kinins on the isolated perfused rat kidney and evidence for the presence of renal B1 receptors, in: *Kinins IV. Advances in Experimental Medicine and Biology,* Volume 198A (L. M. Greenbaum and H. S. Margolius, eds.). Plenum Press, New York, pp. 559-562 (1986).
86. Vavrek, R. J., and J. M. Stewart. Smooth muscle selectivity in bradykinin analogs with multiple D-amino acid substitutions, in: *Kinins IV. Advances in Experimental Medicine and Biology,* Volume 198A (L. M. Greenbaum and H. S. Margolius, eds.). Plenum Press, New York, pp. 543-548 (1986).
87. Steranka, L. R., R. M. Burch, R. J. Vavrek, J. M. Stewart, and S. J. Enna. Multiple bradykinin receptors: results of studies using a novel class of receptor antagonists, in: *Receptor Mechanisms of Neurotransmitters and Neuropeptides* (S. Kito, ed.). Plenum Press, New York, pp. 111-127 (1988).
88. Regoli, D. Kinins, receptors, antagonists, in: *Kinins IV. Advances in Experimental Medicine and Biology,* Volume 198A (L. M. Greenbaum and H. S. Margolius, eds.). Plenum Press, New York, pp. 549-558 (1986).
89. Drapeau, G., N.-E. Rhaleb, S. Dion, D. Jukic, and D. Regoli. [Phe^8psi(CH_2-NH)Arg^9]bradykinin, a B2 receptor selective agonist which is not broken down by either kininase I or kininase II. *Eur. J. Pharmacol.* **155**:193-195 (1988).
90. Drapeau, G., and D. Regoli. Synthesis of bradykinin analogs. In *Chemotaxis and Inflammation: Methods in Enzymology,* Vol. 163 (G. Di Sabato, ed.). Academic Press, New York, pp. 263-272 (1988).
91. Regoli, D., G. Drapeau, P. Rovero, P. D'Orléans-Juste, and J. Barabé. The actions of kinin antagonists on B_1 and B_2 receptor systems. *Eur. J. Pharmacol.* **123**:61-65 (1986).
92. D'Orléans-Juste, P., S. Dion, J. Mizrahi, and D. Regoli. Effects of peptides and non-peptides on isolated arterial smooth muscles: Role of endothelium. *Eur. J. Pharmacol.* **114**:9-21 (1985).

93. Regoli, D., G. Drapeau, P. Rovero, S. Dion, N.-E. Rhaleb, J. Barabé, P. D'Orléans-Juste, and P. Ward. Conversion of kinins and their antagonists into B1 receptor activators and blockers in isolated vessels. *Eur. J. Pharmacol.* **127**:219-224 (1986).
94. Spragg, J., R. J. Vavrek, and J. M. Stewart. The inhibition of glandular kallikrein by peptide analog antagonists of bradykinin. *Peptides* **9**:203-206 (1988).
95. Okunishi, H., J. Burton, and J. Spragg. Specificity of substrate analogue inhibitors of human urinary kallikrein. *Hypertension* **7**:I-72-I-75 (1985).
96. Okunishi, H., J. Spragg, and J. Burton. The design of substrate analogue tissue kallikrein inhibitors. *Hypertension* **8**:I-114-I-118 (1986).
97. Barton, S., E. Karpinski, and M. Schachter. The effect of a bradykinin antagonist on vasodilator responses with particular reference to the submandibular gland of the cat. *Experientia* **44**:897-898 (1988).
98. Toda, N. Actions of bradykinin on isolated cerebral and peripheral arteries. *Am. J. Physiol.* **232**:H267-H274 (1977).
99. Wahl, M., A. R. Young, L. Edvinsson, and F. F. W. Wagner. Effects of kininase II inhibitors on the vasomotor response to bradykinin of feline intracranial and extracranial arteries in vitro and *in vivo*. *J. Cereb. Blood Flow Metabol.* **3**:339-345 (1983).
100. Hardebo, J. E., J. Hanko, J. Kahrstrom, and C. Owman. Endothelium dependent relaxation in cerebral arteries. *J. Cereb. Blood Flow Metabol.* **5(Suppl.1)**:5533-5534 (1985).
101. Whalley, E. T., Y. O. Amure, and R. H. Lye. Analysis of the mechanism of action of bradykinin on human basilar artery *in vitro*. *Naunyn-Schmiedeberg's Arch. Pharmacol.* **335**:433-437 (1987).
102. Benetos, A., H. Gavras, J. M. Stewart, R. J. Vavrek, S. Hatinoglou, and I. Gavras. Vasodepressor role of endogenous bradykinin assessed by a bradykinin antagonist. *Hypertension* **8**:971-974 (1986).
103. Aubert, J.-F., B. Waeber, J. Nussberger, R. J. Vavrek, J. M. Stewart, and H. R. Brunner. Influence of endogenous bradykinin on blood pressure response to vasopressors in normotensive rats assessed with a bradykinin antagonist. *J. Cardiovasc. Pharmacol.* **11**:51-55 (1988).
104. Carbonell, L. F., O. A. Carretero, P. Madeddu, and A. G. Scicli. Effects of a kinin antagonist on mean blood pressure. *Hypertension* **11(Suppl. I)**: 84-88 (1988).
105. Benetos, A., I. Gavras, and H. Gavras. Hypertensive effect of a bradykinin antagonist in normotensive rats. *Hypertension* **8**:1089-1092 (1986).
106. Aubert, J.-F., B. Waeber, J. Nussberger, R. J. Vavrek, J. M. Stewart, and H. R. Brunner. Lack of role of circulating bradykinin in blood pressure response to acute angiotensin converting enzyme inhibition in rats. *Agents Actions* **Suppl. 22**:349-351 (1987).
107. Mulinari, R., A. Benetos, I. Gavras, and H. Gavras. Vascular and sympathoadrenal responses to bradykinin and a bradykinin analogue. *Hypertension* **11**:754-757 (1988).

108. Beierwaltes, W. H., and O. A. Carretero. Kinin antagonist reverses converting enzyme inhibitor-stimulated vascular prostaglandin I_2 synthesis. *Hypertension* **13**:754-758 (1989).
109. Roman, R. J., M. L. Kaldunski, A. G. Scicli, and O. A. Carretero. Influence of kinins and angiotensin II on the regulation of papillary blood flow. *Am. J. Physiol.* **255**:F690-F698 (1988).
110. Beierwaltes, W. H., O. A. Carretero, and A. G. Scicli. Renal hemodynamics in response to a kinin analogue antagonist. *Am. J. Physiol.* **255**:F408-F414 (1988).
111. Staszewska-Barczak, J., S. H. Ferreira, and J. R. Vane. An excitatory nociceptive cardiac reflex elicited by bradykinin and potentiated by prostaglandins and myocardial ischemia. *Cardiovasc. Res.* **10**:314-327 (1976).
112. Staszewska-Barczak, J., and G. J. Dusting. Sympathetic cardiovascular reflex initiated by bradykinin-induced stimulation of cardiac pain receptors. *Clin. Exp. Pharmacol. Physiol.* **4**:443-452 (1977).
113. Johnson, A. R. Effects of kinins on organ systems, in: *Bradykinin, Kallidin and Kallikrein, Handbook of Experimental Pharmacology,* Volume XXV Supplement (E. G. Erdös, ed.). Springer-Verlag, New York, pp. 357-399 (1979).
114. Staszewska-Woolley, J., G. Woolley, and D. Regoli. Specific receptors for bradykinin-induced cardiac sympathetic chemoreflex in the dog. *Eur. J. Pharmacol.* **156**:309-314 (1988).
115. Manzini, S., F. Perretti, L. De Benedetti, P. Pradelles, C. A. Maggi, and P. Geppetti. A comparison of bradykinin- and capsaicin-induced myocardial and coronary effects in isolated perfused heart of guinea-pig: Involvement of substance P and calcitonin gene-related peptide release. *Br. J. Pharmacol.* **97**:303-312 (1989).
116. Correa, F. M. A., and F. G. Graeff. Central mechanism of the hypertensive action of intracerebroventricular bradykinin in the unanesthetized rat. *Neuropharmacology* **13**:65-75 (1974).
117. Correa, F. M. A., and F. G. Graeff. Central site of the hypertensive action of bradykinin. *J. Pharmacol. Exp. Ther.* **192**:670-676 (1975).
118. Lindsey, C. J., K. Fujita, and D. T. O. Martins. The central pressor effect of bradykinin in normotensive and hypertensive rats. *Hypertension* **2**:126-129 (1988).
119. Lindsey, C. J., C. R. Nakaie, and D. T. O. Martins. Central nervous system kinin receptors and the hypertensive response mediated by bradykinin. *Br. J. Pharmacol.* **97**:763-768 (1989).
120. Lewis, R. E., and M. I. Phillips. Localization of the central pressor action of bradykinin to the cerebral third ventricle. *Am. J. Pathol.* **247**:63-68 (1984).
121. Schachter, M., D. J. Uchida, D. J. Longridge, T. Labedz, E. T. Whalley, R. J. Vavrek, and J. M. Stewart. New synthetic antagonists of bradykinin. *Br. J. Pharmacol.* **92**:851-855 (1987).
122. Gaginella, T. S., and J. F. Kachur. Bradykinin as a mediator of mucosal secretion in IBD, in: *Inflammatory Bowel Disease: Current Status and Fu-*

ture Approach (R. P. MacDermott, ed.). Elsevier Science Publishers B. V., Cambridge, pp. 383-390 (1988).

123. Kachur, J. F., W. Allbee, W. Danho, and T. S. Gaginella. Bradykinin receptors: Functional similarities in guinea-pig gut muscle and mucosa. *Regul. Pept.* **17**:63-70 (1987).
124. Baron, D. A., H. S. Margolius, D. H. Miller, J. M. Stewart, and R. J. Vavrek. Antagonists of bradykinin-induced chloride secretion and concomitant morphological change. *Br. J. Pharmacol.* **91**:485P (1987).
125. Den Hertog, A., A. Nelemans, and J. Van den Akker. The multiple action of bradykinin on smooth muscle of guinea-pig taenia caeci. *Eur. J. Pharmacol.* **151**:357-363 (1988).
126. Calixto, J. B., M. Nicolau, and R. A. Yunes. Antagonistic effect of *Mandevilla velutina* extract on kinin- induced contractions of guinea-pig and cat ileum longitudinal smooth muscle. *Gen. Pharmacol.* **19**:595-599 (1988).
127. Calixto, J. B., G. H. Strobel, A. B. Cruz, and R. A. Yunes. Blockade of bradykinin-evoked diphasic responses of isolated rat duodenum by the crude extract of and compounds obtained from *Mandevilla velutina. Braz. J. Med. Biol. Res.* **21**:1015-1018 (1988).
128. Calixto, J. B., M. G. Pizzolatti, and R. A. Yunes. The competitive antagonistic effect of compounds from *Mandevilla velutina* on kinin-induced contractions of rat uterus and guinea pig ileum *in vitro. Br. J. Pharmacol.* **94**:1133-1142 (1988).
129. Ueda, N., I. Muramatsu, and M. Fujiwara. Capsaicin- and bradykinin-induced substance P-ergic responses in the iris sphincter muscle of the rabbit. *J. Pharmacol. Exp. Ther.* **230**:469-473 (1984).
130. Lerner, U. H., I. L. Jones, and G. I. Gustafson. Bradykinin, a new potential mediator of inflammation-induced bone resorption. *Arthritis Rheum.* **30**:530-540 (1987).
131. Benton, H. P., T. R. Jackson, and M. R. Hanley. Identification of a novel inflammatory stimulant of chondrocytes. *Biochem. J.* **269**:861-867 (1989).
132. Chao, J., J. Buse, K. Shimamoto, and H. S. Margolius. Kallikrein-induced uterine contraction independent of kinin formation. *Proc. Natl. Acad. Sci. USA* **78**:6154-6157 (1981).
133. Orce, G. G., O. A. Carretero, G. Scicli, and A. G. Scicli. Kinins contribute to the contractile effects of rat glandular kallikrein on the isolated rat uterus. *J. Pharmacol. Exp. Ther.* **249**:470-475 (1989).
134. Yoshimura, Y., L. Espey, Y. Hosoi, T. Adachi, S. J. Atlas, R. B. Ghodgaonker, N. H. Dubin, and E. E. Wallach. The effects of bradykinin on ovulation and prostaglandin production by the perfused rabbit ovary. *Endocrinology* **122**:2540-2546 (1988).
135. Epsey, L. L., D. H. Miller, and H. S. Margolius. Ovarian increase in kinin-generating capacity in the PMSG/hCG-primed rat. *Am. J. Physiol.* **251**: E362-E369 (1986).

2
Kinin Receptors of the B1 Type and Their Antagonists

Francois Marceau*
Centre Hospitalier de l'Université Laval
Quebec City, Quebec, Canada
Domenico C. Regoli
University of Sherbrooke
Sherbrooke, Quebec, Canada

I. THE B1 RECEPTOR TYPE

Kinins are blood-derived peptides that are suspected to be inflammatory mediators. Their pharmacologic profiles strongly suggest such a role in the inflammatory process. Vasodilation, increased vascular permeability, and pain perception are produced when synthetic bradykinin is injected in normal tissues (1), showing that this single peptide mimics several distinct inflammatory events. However, human leukocytes appear to be generally refractory to kinins, which are not chemotactic for phagocytes (2) and fail to modulate several types of function in lymphocytes (R. Roy and F. Marceau, unpublished observations), despite the fact that some effects have been described in leukocytes from rodent species (3). The prominent

**Present affiliation*: Centre de Recherche de l'Hôtel-Dieu de Québec, Quebec City, Quebec, Canada.

effect of kinins on the circulation, notably in the kidney, also suggest possible roles in the cardiovascular system as endogenous vasodilator and hypotensor factors (4).

The structure-activity relationship of kinins, namely bradykinin and kallidin (Lys-bradykinin), has been extensively studied. Much of the available information is derived from isolated smooth muscle preparations. Bioassay tissues, while of questionable selectivity to quantify kinins in biological fluids, provide valuable quantitative evaluation of potency and intrinsic activity when dealing with synthetic analogs produced by the solid phase peptide synthesis. Contractions of the rabbit jugular vein (5) and relaxation of canine arteries, e.g., the carotid artery (6), are obtained at very low concentrations, as is the case for other classical preparations contracted by kinins (rat uterus, guinea pig ileum (7)). It was realized early that kinin fragments without the C-terminal Arg residue, e.g., desArg^9-bradykinin (desArg^9-BK), were several orders of magnitude less potent than the native sequences in such bioassays (7), as well as in other tests such as pain production in the human skin (blister base) (8).

The identification in 1962 of a blood carboxypeptidase that cleaves bradykinin into desArg^9-BK was then interpreted as the discovery of an inactivation pathway ("kininase I") (9). This enzyme, also termed carboxypeptidase N, is now recognized as a key regulator of the complement anaphylatoxins (10) and is also able to hydrolyze a basic C-terminal amino acid residue from a number of potential substrates generated in blood (11). A carboxypeptidase (kininase II or angiotensin converting enzyme) present on the luminal surface of endothelial cells is regarded as more important to inactivate circulating kinins, but this type of enzyme activity is not prominent in plasma, and therefore in inflammatory exudates. It can be predicted that the soluble kininase I will predominate over the membrane-bound kininase II activity in inflammatory exudates, and, in fact, this has been verified in the nasal lavage fluid of patients with allergic rhinitis (12) or in the synovial fluid of patients with inflammatory arthritis (13). Thus, the formation of desArg^9-BK and of desArg^{10}-KD (desArg^{10}-kallidin), from BK and KD, respectively, is possible in an inflammatory environment.

The biological importance of such fragments was not clear until it was shown that they are the selective agonists for a distinct type of kinin receptor found initially in the isolated rabbit aorta (14). The vascular preparation is contracted by bradykinin and, unexpectedly, the study of the effects of kinin fragments showed that desArg^9-BK was more potent that the complete sequence in this preparation (Table 1). The same holds true for the pair kallidin and desArg^{10}-KD, as the latter is more potent than the

Table 1 Pharmacologic Parameters of Kinins, Some of Their Metabolites, and Some Antagonists

Preparation, receptor type parameters[a]	Rabbit aorta, B1			Rabbit jugular vein, B2		
	pD_2	R.A.	pA_2	pD_2	R.A.	pA_2
Analogs						
Bradykinin	6.22	8	—	8.46	100	—
Kallidin	7.27	95	—	8.63	150	—
desArg^9-BK	7.29	100	—	4.39	0.01	—
desArg^{10}-KD	8.61	2100	—	5.33	1.0	—
desArg^9,desPhe^8-BK	4.29	0.1	—		<0.01	—
desArg^{10},desPhe^9-KD	4.30	0.1	—	4.78	0.01	—
[Tyr(Me)^8]-BK	4.70	0.24	—	8.59	140	—
desArg^9[Leu^8]-BK	—	—	7.27	—		I[b]
desArg^{10}[Leu^9]-KD	—	—	8.37	—		I
[Thi^{5,8},D-Phe^7]-BK	—	—	6.20		+[c]	6.7
[Thi^{5,9},D-Phe^8]-KD	—	—	6.30		+	6.9

[a]Parameters: pD_2 = −log of concentration of agonist producing 50% of the maximum contraction; R.A. = relative affinity in percent of that of the reference compound (data underlined); pA_2 = −log of the concentration of antagonist that reduces the effect of a double dose of agonist to that of a single dose (49).
[b]I = compound inactive as an antagonist.
[c]+ indicates that the compound has some residual agonistic activity.
Source: From Refs. 43, 45, 50.

the former. More recent investigations have shown that the effect of bradykinin and kallidin in this preparation is largely due to conversion into desArg forms in situ by a tissue enzyme similar to kininase I (15,16). Therefore, the real affinity of bradykinin and kallidin for kinin receptors in the rabbit aorta is probably lower than initially thought, and these receptors would exhibit a high selectivity toward kinin fragments generated by carboxypeptidase N.

A first line of evidence for the existence of a distinct receptor type in the rabbit aortic preparation was a typical order of agonist potency, different from the one observed with classical preparations and with more recently characterized bioassay tissues, such as the rabbit jugular vein (Table 1). The second and decisive type of evidence was the development of selective and competitive antagonists based on the structure of desArg^9-BK. Replacing the C-terminal Phe residue in this octapeptide with a residue possessing an aliphatic side chain was sufficient to obtain these antagonists (14). The prototype of this new class of compounds was desArg^9[Leu^8]-BK. These compounds were the first bradykinin-related sequences to show selective antagonist properties against kinins, although it was clear that they did not antagonize kinins in commonly used bioassays, e.g., the contraction of the rat isolated uterus and the acute hypotensive effect in the blood pressure assay. This class of antagonists was, however, very important in defining for the first time a type of kinin receptor using the pharmacologic criteria proposed by Schild (17): the order of agonist potency and the affinity of the antagonists. The type of receptor mediating the contraction of the rabbit aortic strip was then termed the B1 type, in reference to the fact that it was more completely defined. Receptors in the other preparations, e.g., the rabbit jugular vein (Table 1), were said to belong to the B2 type, which was not fully defined pharmacologically, even if it was physiologically prominent. The development of antagonists for the B2 receptor type based on the structure of [D-Phe^{7}]-BK in recent years (18) has consolidated the classification of kinin receptors into B1 and B2 types. Recently, it has been proposed that the B2 type of receptors should be further subdivided, on the basis of discrepancies in potency and in the agonist/antagonist behavior of newer bradykinin analogs (19). This controversy does not affect the definition of the B1 type, which is the subject matter of the present chapter.

II. OCCURRENCE, REGULATION, AND ROLE OF B1 RECEPTORS

Receptors of the B1 type are found in a small subset of smooth muscle preparations sensitive to kinins, including several rabbit isolated blood vessels, but also tissues from rat, dog, and in strips of human colon (Table 2). In many instances the B1 type coexists with the B2 type and is better demonstrated by a stimulant effect of desArg^{9}-BK that is antagonized selectively by desArg^{9}[Leu^{8}]-BK or a similar antagonist. The function mediated by this type of receptor is usually smooth muscle contraction, although interesting vasorelaxant effects mediated by B1 receptors on the rabbit isolated mesenteric artery and dog renal artery have been reported (20,21).

DesArg^{9}-BK also elicits effects in a variety of cultured cells (Table 3). An intriguing mitogenic effect has been reported on a line of human fibroblasts (IMR-90) (22,23) and on a minority of fibroblast lines derived from rabbit dermis and cultured for a long time (24). The mediation of this trophic effect on cultured cells by the B1 type of receptors is further documented by the antagonist effect of desArg^{9}[Leu^{8}]-BK (22,24). Three cell types present in the bovine pulmonary artery (endothelium, smooth muscle, fibroblasts) were cultured, passaged, and shown to releaser prostaglandins in response to desArg^{9}-BK (25). In fact, some lines of bovine

Table 2 Smooth Muscle Preparations Responsive to desArg^9-BK, a Selective B1 Agonist

	Response to desArg^9-BK			
Preparation	Type[a]	Sensitization	Use of B1 antagonists	Ref.
Rabbit anterior mesenteric vein	Contr.	Yes	Yes	32
Rabbit basilar artery	Contr.	Yes	Yes	36
Rabbit aorta	Contr.	Yes	Yes	14
	Contr.	Yes	—	34, 41
Rabbit mesenteric artery	Relax.	—	Yes	20
	Contr.[b]	—	Yes	48
	Relax. or Contr.[b]	Yes	—	38
Rat mesenteric /portal veins	Contr.	Yes	—	33
Rat urinary bladder	Contr.	Yes	Yes	33
Rat duodenum	Contr.	Yes	—	37
Cat arteries (several)	Contr.	—	Yes	J. Barabé and D. Regoli, unpublished
Human colon	Contr.	Yes	Yes	35
Human urinary bladder	Contr.	Yes	—	D. Regoli, unpublished
Dog renal artery	Relax.	No	Yes	21

[a]Abbreviations used: Contr. = contraction; Relax. = relaxation.
[b]Contraction in indomethacin-treated tissues.

endothelial cells are reported to release vasoactive mediators (PGI_2 or endothelium-derived relaxing factor) when exposed to desArg^9-BK (26, 27), but not all of them (28); however, all these cell lines respond to bradykinin via B2 receptors. Calvarium bones from embryonic mice maintained in vitro were responsive to desArg^9-BK (Table 3).

DesArg^9-BK has very little effect in vivo on the blood pressure assay in rats (30) or rabbits (5); the antagonists of the desArg^9[Leu^8]-BK type exert no or only marginal effects in these assays against bradykinin (5). Bradykinin elicits an increase in vascular permeability to blood proteins when injected in the rabbit skin (31), and this effect is not antagonized by desArg^{10}[Leu^9]-BK, one of the most potent B1 antagonists. Therefore, the

Table 3 Effects of desArg⁹-BK on Cultured Cells

Type of cell	Observed effects[a]	Use of B1 antagonists	Ref.
IMR-90 (human embryonic fibroblasts)	DNA and collagen synthesis (NOT prostanoid synthesis)	yes	22
	DNA synthesis	no	23
R51, transformed rabbit fibroblasts	DNA synthesis, PGE_2 synthesis	yes	24
Freshly isolated lines of human dermis fibroblasts	DNA synthesis	no	47
Bovine vascular cells (endothelial, smooth muscle, fibroblasts)	PG synthesis	yes	25
Bovine endothelial cells	PGI_2 and EDRF release	yes	26,27
Organotypic culture of mouse embryo bones	PG-dependent bone resorption	no	29

[a]Abbreviations used: PG = prostaglandin; EDRF = endothelium-derived relaxing factor.

B1 type of kinin receptor is best demonstrated in vitro and its physiological significance remained very elusive until its regulation in isolated tissues was studied.

One distinctive feature of B1 kinin receptors is their apparent upregulation following some types of tissue injury. Most isolated smooth muscle preparations responsive to desArg⁹-BK cannot respond to the octapeptide in the first hour of incubation in vitro; the preparations become gradually responsive during the following hours. This was originally reported in the rabbit isolated mesenteric vein (32), the rat urinary bladder (33), the rabbit aorta (14,34) and confirmed using the human colon (35), the rabbit basilar artery (36), and the rat isolated duodenum (37). Moreover, this sensitization behavior is selective for kinins and totally preventable by pretreatment in vitro with cycloheximide, an inhibitor of protein synthesis (32-34,36). A possible explanation of this is a de novo synthesis of receptors triggered by injury to tissues. The original report on the prostaglandin-dependent relaxant effect of desArg⁹-BK on the rabbit mesenteric artery did not mention this sensitization behavior (20); complementary experiments performed recently using this preparation in another laboratory showed that the response to desArg⁹-BK was in fact acquired in vitro as in the contractile systems (38).

The view that no pharmacological preparation is responsive to desArg⁹-BK outside a tissue injury context has been generally verified but may have important exceptions. The response to desArg^9-BK in cell lines (Table 3) may well fall into the category of injury-induced responses because the cultured cells are not in a normal environment and, in fact, may exhibit changes in their responsiveness to desArg^9-BK as a function of time (24). Documented exceptions are the dog isolated renal artery (21), which appears to show a constitutive population of B1 receptors from the beginning of the in vitro incubation, and the perfused kidney from normal rats and dogs. A subtle vasoconstrictor effect is elicited in fresh kidneys from normal rats when selective agonists of the B1 receptors are perfused (39); the segmental and systemic circulations are also affected when desArg^9-BK is infused in the renal artery of anesthetized dogs (G. Plante and D. Regoli, unpublished observations). The role of desArg^9-BK in normal cardiovascular physiology clearly needs to be addressed.

The hypothetical upregulation of B1 receptors in vivo by tissue injury has been supported mainly by cardiovascular model in the rabbit: Animals injected intravenously with a sublethal dose (10 μg) of bacterial lipopolysacchardie (LPS) exhibit 5 hours later dose-related hypotensive responses to exogenous intraarterial desArg^9-BK or desArg^{10}-KD (Fig. 1). By contrast, control animals do not respond to desArg^9-BK and only minimally to desArg^{10}-KD, owing to some residual activity of the latter peptide as an agonist on B2 receptors (Table 1). In the extensively studied model (34,40) it was shown that (a) LPS pretreatment does not modify the basal blood pressure or the hypotensive response to bradykinin (mediated by B2 receptors) or to another, unrelated hypotensive peptide, substance P; (b) LPS given immediately before anesthesia does not induce the responsiveness to desArg^9-BK, indicating a minimal lag time possibly necessary for protein synthesis; (c) tissues removed from LPS-treated animals, e.g., rabbit aortic strips, exhibit contractile responses to desArg^9-BK within the first hour of incubation in vitro, suggesting that the response was acquired in vivo before sacrifice; (d) desArg^9-BK is a vasodilator of the coronary arteries only in hearts removed from LPS-treated animals and perfused in vitro using the Langendorf technique. This model suggests that the cardiovascular system of the rabbit can be sensitized to the bradykinin fragment without modifying the preexisting population of B2 receptors or receptors for other agents. In addition, experimental neutropenia did not prevent the inducer effect of LPS on the in vivo responsiveness to desArg^9-BK, suggesting that this type of leukocyte is not involved in the upregulation process (34).

The mechanism of tissue sensitization to desArg^9-BK has been explored in the rabbit isolated aorta preparation, as this blood-free system appears to possess all components necessary to spontaneously exhibit the upregu-

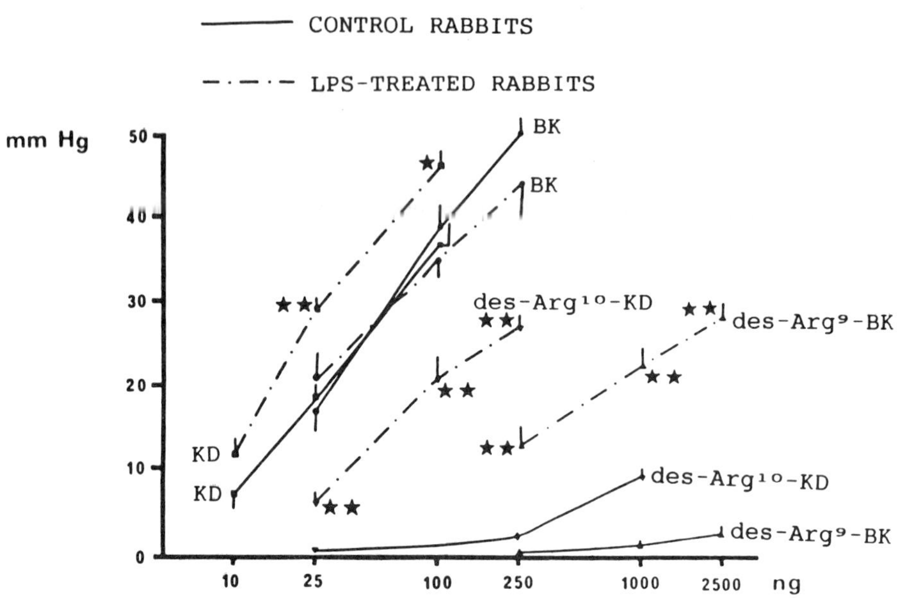

Figure 1 Dose-response curves for the hypotensive effect of four kinins in anesthetized control or endotoxin-treated rabbits. The endotoxin-pretreated animals were injected with 10 μg of *E. coli* LPS 5 hours before anesthesia. Peptides were injected intraarterially as boluses. Abcissa: dose of peptide (ng per animal); ordinate: fall of the mean arterial blood pressure, mmHg. Points are mean ± SEM of 5-18 determinations. The values for each dose and each peptide were compared between the control and the LPS-treated groups using Student's *t*-test. $^{\star}p < 0.05$; $^{\star\star}p < 0.001$.

lation phenomenon (34,41). It was found that the LPS action most likely to be linked with the upregulation of tissue responses to kinins was the release of cytokines from immunocompetent cells (macrophages and lymphocytes). Interleukins 1 and 2 were potent stimulants of the upregulation in vitro, whereas glucocorticoids were selective inhibitors of that process, consistent with the hypothesis. Thus, the major field of application of the B1 receptor upregulation theory could be immunopathology.

The de novo synthesis of B1 receptors has been postulated to explain the cycloheximide-sensitive upregulation of response to kinins (32). However, information on the number of receptors present in the preparations cannot be derived from biologic responses, and there are alternate explanations for that phenomenon. There is an evident need to address this problem with a binding assay for B1 receptors. A limited study of [^{3}H]-desArg^9-BK binding to fragments of rabbit mesenteric veins preincubated in Krebs media has been reported by Barabé et al. (42). A certain number of methodological problems can be identified in the design of the experiments: The low affinity ligand was extensively rinsed, dense fragments of tissue were used with potential diffusion problems, the binding was established at 37°C on living pieces of tissues, no protease inhibitors were used. Even under these conditions, a saturable binding (cellular uptake?) of [^{3}H]-desArg^9-BK was shown and was increased by either preincubating the tissues in vitro or by pretreating rabbits with LPS 5 hours before sacrifice; the uptake was reduced by preincubation with cycloheximide, consistent with the biologic data. There may be a valid basis in these experiments if binding to the B1 receptors is followed by receptor-ligand complex internalization, as it is the case with many peptide hormones. The "specific" binding would represent cellular uptake of the ligand, which would be saturable, but not reversible on washing.

III. STRUCTURE-ACTIVITY RELATIONSHIPS OF B1 ANTAGONISTS

The basic manipulation for obtaining a selective and competitive antagonist for kinins on the B1 receptor systems is to replace the aromatic residue Phe^8 in desArg^9-BK (or Phe^9 in desArg^{10}-KD) by an amino acid possessing an aliphatic side chain, Leu being optimal (14,43). However, Ala, Ile, cyclohexylAla, norLeu, and D-Leu substitutions also yield B1 antagonists of lower affinity but with no measurable residual agonist activity on the rabbit aortic preparation (Table 4). This suggests that the aromatic nature of the Phe^8 residue is primarily involved in the agonist action on the B1 receptor, but not the bulky and hydrophobic properties of its side chain, because substitution with the saturated analog cyclohexylAla, which is bulky and hydrophobic, produces a pure antagonist. Esterification of the C-terminal carboxylic acid, as in desArg^9[Leu(OMe)^8]-BK, or addition of an additional C-terminal residue, as in [Leu^8]-BK, which possess a C-terminal Arg residue, is tolerated but results in a variable loss of affinity (43).

Partial agonists or antagonists of B1 receptors can also be developed by substituting other positions, besides Phe^8. DesArg^9-[Ala^7]-BK is an example, with an intrinsic activity of 0.61 (43). The importance of this will be further discussed below and is related to the nonselectivity of B2 type antagonists whose structure is based on [D-Phe^7]-BK.

Table 4 Structure-Activity Relationship of B1 Antagonists on the Rabbit Isolated Aorta

Parameter[a] agonist used	pA_2 desArg⁹-BK	pA_2 BK	$pA_2 - pA_{10}$ desArg⁹-BK
desArg⁹[Ala⁸]-BK	4.40	3.95	—
desArg⁹[Nle⁸]-BK[b]	6.35	6.31	0.83
desArg⁹[Ile⁸]-BK	6.40	6.25	1.02
desArg⁹[Leu⁸]-BK	7.27	6.75	1.00
desArg⁹[Leu.NH_2]-BK	6.70	6.66	0.92
desArg⁹[D-Leu⁸]-BK	6.44	6.22	1.06
desArg⁹[Cha⁸]-BK	6.42	5.67	1.05
desArg¹⁰[Leu⁹]-KD	8.37	—	1.10
desArg¹¹[Leu¹⁰]-MLBK	8.22	—	1.05

[a]Parameters: pA_2 as in Table 1; $pA_2 - pA_{10}$ calculated to obtain a rough evaluation of antagonist competitiveness (47).
[b]Abbreviations: Nle = norLeu; Cha = cyclohexylAla; MLBK = Met, Lys-bradykinin.
Source: From Ref. 43.

The effect of prolonging the N-terminal sequence of desArg⁹[Leu⁸]-BK by a Lys residue, resulting in desArg¹⁰[Leu⁹]-KD, increases the pA_2 by 1.1 (Table 4); this is reasonably well correlated to the increased apparent affinity seen with agonists, desArg¹⁰-KD being more potent than desArg⁹-BK.

B1 antagonists are effective in the rabbit isolated aorta against the contractions induced by either BK or desArg⁹-BK with a similar apparent affinity, as assessed by the calculation of the pA_2 (Table 4). The nature of the antagonism exerted by these compounds is competitive, as shown by the application of numerical models developed by Schild and coworkers (14,43). Notably, the difference $pA_2 - pA_{10}$ is close to unity (Table 4), which is consistent with competitiveness (47). Importantly, these sequence-related antagonists are selective for kinins and do not affect aortic contractions induced by norepinephrine, serotonin, histamine, and angiotensin II (14). The latter finding is significant because desArg⁹-BK is an octapeptide which possesses some similarity of primary structure with the octapeptide angiotensin II (Asp-Arg-Val-Tyr-Ile-His-Pro-Phe) and because angiotensin antagonists are obtained in a very similar manner: by substituting the Phe⁸ residue with an aliphatic amino acid (44). It is clear that B1 receptors are not angiotensin receptors in the aortic preparation or in any other system. The antagonists of the type desArg⁹-BK are ineffective in the classical uterine and intestinal bioassays for bradykinin (7,43), this finding supporting the strong evidence for the existence of the distinct B2 receptor type.

IV. CONVERSION OF B2 ANTAGONISTS INTO THE B1 TYPE

Soon after the introduction of B2 antagonists based on [D-Phe^7]-BK (18) it was realized that these new compounds also antagonized the effect of bradykinin and desArg^9-BK on the rabbit aortic strip (45). [$Thi^{5,8}$,D-Phe^7]-BK and [$Thi^{6,9}$,D-Phe^8]-KD were almost as potent on B1 preparations as on B2 ones: The pA_2 values were between 6 and 7 for both peptides on both types of preparations (Table 1). Indirect evidence was later produced to show that desArg metabolites of these antagonists were largely responsible for the activity on the B1 type aortic preparation, but not on a tissue representing the B2 type receptors, the rabbit isolated jugular vein (16). Incubation of rabbit aorta with a selective blocker of kininase I, DL-mercaptomethyl-3-guanidinoethylthiopropanoic acid (MERGETPA) reduced the pA_2 values of [$Thi^{5,8}$,D-Phe^7]-BK and [$Thi^{6,9}$,D-Phe^8]-KD by more than one unit; by contrast the potency of desArg^9[Leu^8]-BK was not significantly affected by MERGETPA (Table 5). Moreover, the latter peptidase inhibitor did not change the apparent affinity of B2 antagonists on the jugular vein. The reduction in activity observed with B2 antagonists on the aortic preparation in the presence of MERGETPA is similar to the one observed with the agonists bradykinin and kallidin, which are metabolized in situ into more potent B1 agonists by a peptidase activity

Table 5 Apparent Affinities of Kinins and Some Antagonists as Measured in the Absence and Presence of the Carboxypeptidase Inhibitor MERGETPA

	Rabbit aorta				Rabbit jugular vein			
	Control		MERGETPA		Control		MERGETPA	
Compound	pD_2	pA_2	pD_2	pA_2	pD_2	pA_2	pD_2	pA_2
desArg^9-BK	7.27	—	7.30	—	4.40	—	4.35	—
Bradykinin	6.22	—	4.70	—	8.46	—	8.50	—
desArg^9[Leu^8]-BK	—	7.82	—	8.09	—	I[a]	—	I
[$Thi^{5,8}$,D-Phe^7]-BK	—	6.23	—	4.92	+[b]	6.53	+	6.53
[$Thi^{6,9}$,D-Phe^8]-KD	—	6.36	—	5.27	+	6.85	+	6.91

[a]I = inactive as an antagonist.
[b]+ indicates that the compound has some residual agonistic activity.
Source: From Ref. 16.

similar to kininase I (15,16). This suggests that [Thi^{5,8},D-Phe^7]-BK and its analogs have some selectivity for the B2 systems at the receptor level, but that their respective desArg metabolites have significant B1 receptor antagonist activity. The consequence of this lack of selectivity remains to be established if this type of kinin antagonists ever reach clinical use.

V. APPLICATIONS OF B1 ANTAGONISTS IN VITRO AND IN VIVO

Several groups have used selective B1 antagonists in vitro, chiefly desArg^9-[Leu^8]-BK, to identify the receptor type involved in kinin effects on isolated tissues (Table 2) and cultured cells (Table 3). These compounds are obviously useful to describe functions mediated by B1 receptors because this type of receptor is defined operationally, in part, by their effectiveness. It is not possible to predict accurately from these reports the effects of B1 antagonists against endogenously produced kinins, especially during the course of pathologies. Whether B1 antagonists possess any therapeutic potential is unknown but could be suspected, as the B1 agonist, desArg^9-BK, promotes either vasodilation or vasoconstriction, hypotension, prostanoid release from tissue, and activation of various cell functions (Table 3) under defined experimental conditions. It seems that the activation of B1 receptors by desArg^9-BK usually duplicates the effects of bradykinin through the activation of preexisting B2 receptors in many systems, with some exceptions. Notably, desArg^9-BK is consistently ineffective to produce pain, as opposed to the easily demonstrated algogenic effect of bradykinin in man and animals (8,46). The analgesic potential of B2 antagonists (46) is probably not shared by B1 antagonists.

The cardiovascular model of desArg^9-BK-induced hypotension in endotoxin-treated rabbits can be used to illustrate the effects of B1 antagonists in vivo (Fig. 2). The antagonists, when infused intraarterially at a constant rate of 10 μg/minute, were without effect on the basal blood pressure and antagonized only the acute hypotensive responses to desArg^9-BK. B1 antagonists did not antagonize a selective B2 agonist, [Tyr(Me)^8]-BK (Table 1), or an unrelated hypotensive neuropeptide, substance P. The effects of three antagonists are illustrated in Figure 2: desArg^9[D-Leu^8]-BK is not clearly effective at the dose tested, whereas desArg^9[D-Leu^8]-BK is partially effective and desArg^{10}[Leu^9]-KD totally prevents the effects of exogenously administered desArg^9-BK. This order of potency is clearly related to the respective pA_2 values of the compounds as measured on the isolated rabbit aorta (6.4, 7.3, and 8.4, respectively (43)). The effect of the most potent antagonist is rapidly reversible after the end of the infusion, prob-

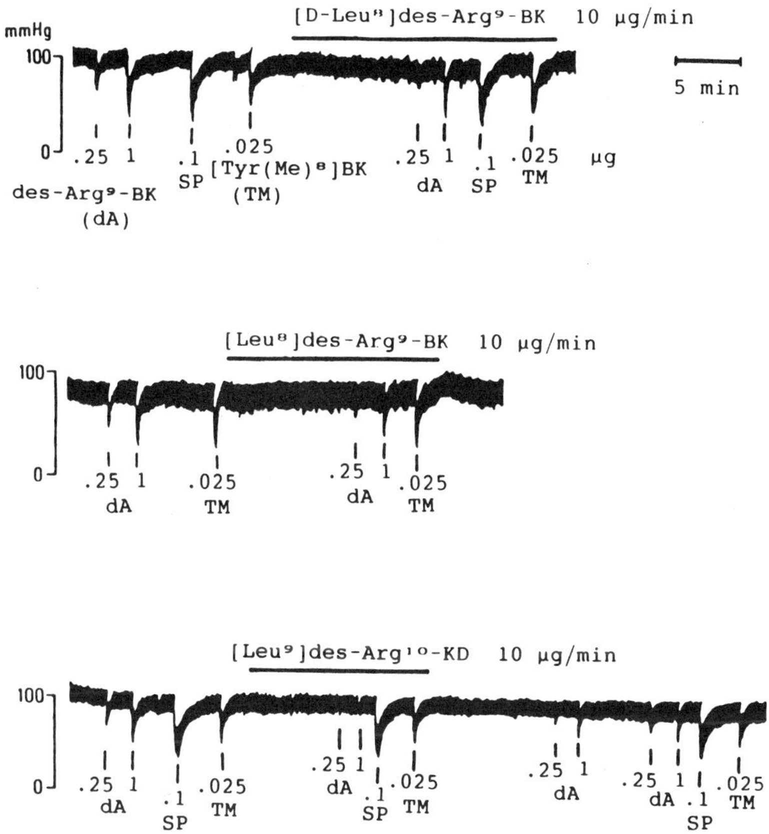

Figure 2 Effect of the infusion of three antagonists of the B1 receptors on the acute hypotension induced by peptides in LPS-pretreated rabbits. Three animals were injected i.v. with 10 μg of LPS 5 hours before anesthesia. DesArg⁹-BK (dA), [Tyr(Me)⁸]-BK (TM), and substance P (SP) were injected as boluses i.a. and antagonists were infused i.a. at a constant rate (10 μg/min) during the periods indicated by horizontal bars. Abcissa: time; ordinate: arterial blood pressure, mmHg. Lower tracing from (40).

ably due to proteolytic inactivation of the compound in blood or tissues (Fig. 2, lower tracing). In this model, only a sublethal dose of endotoxin is used and the animals do not develop cardiovascular shock; the effect of B1 receptor antagonism on the development of endotoxic shock has not been studied but could be an interesting application.

In conclusion, the B1 type of receptor for kinins is becoming a well-accepted pharmacological entity, as numerous reports of biologic activities for its selective agonist desArg^{9}-BK are contributed from around the world. Their pharmacologic definition is unambiguous, resting firstly on the selective agonist action of the kinin fragments without the C-terminal Arg residue, and secondly on the development of selective antagonists (prototype desArg^{9}[Leu^{8}]-BK). The function of B1 receptors is not prominent in vivo although some incompletely characterized cardiovascular effects can be recorded following stimulation of B1 receptors in some systems. However, they are apparently upregulated following some types of tissue injury and immunocompetent cells may be involved in this process. The B1 antagonists are a distinctive group of synthetic peptides that may possess a therapeutic potential, notably in the field of immunopathology; the proper evaluation of this potential will be dependent on the development of more stable, perhaps nonpeptide analogs.

ACKNOWLEDGMENTS

Supported by the Medical Research Council of Canada (MRCC). FM and DR are respectively Scholar and Career Investigator of the MRCC.

REFERENCES

1. Elliot, D. F., E. W. Horton, and C. P. Lewis. Actions of pure bradykinin. *J. Physiol.* **153**:473-480 (1960).
2. Kaplan, A., A. N. Kay, and K. F. Austen. A pre-albumin activator of prekallikrein. III. Appearance of chemotactic activity for human neutrophils by the conversion of human prekallikrein to kallikrein. *J. Exp. Med.* **135**:81-97 (1972).
3. Marceau, F., A. Lussier, D. Regoli, and J. P. Giroud. Pharmacology of kinins: Their relevance to tissue injury and inflammation. *Gen. Pharmacol.* **14**: 209-229 (1983).
4. Benetos, A., H. Gavras, J. M. Stewart, R. J. Vavrek, S. Hatinoglou, and I. Gavras. The vasodepressor contribution of endogenous bradykinin as assessed by a specific bradykinin antagonist. *Hypertension* **8**:971-974 (1986).
5. Barabé, J., F. Marceau, B. Thériault, J. N. Drouin, and D. Regoli. Cardiovascular actions of kinins in the rabbit. *Can. J. Physiol. Pharmacol.* **58**:536-542 (1980).
6. Couture, R., P. Gaudreau, S. St-Pierre, and D. Regoli. The common carotid artery: A sensitive bioassay for studying vasodilator effects of substance P and of kinins. *Can. J. Physiol. Pharmacol.* **58**:1234-1244 (1980).
7. Barabé, J., J. N. Drouin, D. Regoli, and W. K. Park. Receptors for bradykinin in intestinal and uterine smooth muscle. *Can. J. Physiol. Pharmacol.* **55**: 1270-1285 (1977).

8. Armstrong, D. Pain. *Handb. Exp. Pharmacol.* **25**:434-481 (1970).
9. Erdös, E. G., and E. M. Sloane. An enzyme in human blood plasma that inactivates bradykinin and kallidins. *Biochem. Pharmacol.* **11**:585-592 (1962).
10. Bokish, V. A., and H. J. Müller-Eberhard. Anaphylatoxin inactivator of human plasma: its isolation and characterization as a carboxypeptidase. *J. Clin. Invest.* **49**:2427-2436 (1970).
11. Skidgel, R. A. Basic carboxypeptidases: Regulators of peptide hormone activity. *Trends Pharmacol. Sci.* **9**:299-304 (1988).
12. Proud, D., C. R. Baumgarten, R. M. Nacleiro, and P. E. Ward. Kinin metabolism in human nasal secretions during experimentally induced allergic rhinitis. *J. Immunol.* **138**:428-434 (1987).
13. Chercuitte, F., A. D. Beaulieu, P. Poubelle, and F. Marceau. Carboxypeptidase N (kininase I) activity in blood and synovial fluid from patients with arthritis. *Life Sci.* **41**:1225-1232 (1987).
14. Regoli, D., J. Barabé, and W. K. Park. Receptors for bradykinin in rabbit aortae. *Can. J. Physiol. Pharmacol.* **55**:855-867 (1977).
15. Babiuk, C., F. Marceau, S. St-Pierre, and D. Regoli. Kininases and vascular responses to kinins. *Eur. J. Pharmacol.* **78**:167-174 (1982).
16. Regoli, D., G. Drapeau, P. Rovero, S. Dion, R. Nour-Eddine, and J. Barabé. Conversion of kinins and their antagonists into B1 receptor activators and blockers in isolated vessels. *Eur. J. Pharmacol.* **127**:219-224 (1986).
17. Schild, H. O. Receptor classification with special reference to beta-adrenergic receptors, in: *Drug Receptors* (H. P. Rang, ed.). University Park Press, Baltimore, pp. 29-36 (1973).
18. Vavrek, R. J., and J. M. Stewart. Competitive antagonists of bradykinin. *Peptides* **6**:161-164 (1985).
19. Braas, K. M., D. C. Manning, D. C. Perry, and S. H. Snyder. Bradykinin analogues: Differential agonist and antagonist activities suggesting multiple receptors. *Br. J. Pharmacol.* **94**:3-5 (1988).
20. Churchill, L., and P. E. Ward. Relaxation of isolated mesenteric arteries by des-Arg^9-bradykinin stimulation of B1 receptors. *Eur. J. Pharmacol.* **130**: 11-18 (1986).
21. Rhaleb, N. E., S. Dion, J. Barabé, N. Rouissi, D. Jukic, G. Drapeau, and D. Regoli. Receptors for kinins in dog isolated arterial vessels. *Eur. J. Pharmacol.,* In press.
22. Goldstein, R. H., and M. Wall. Activation of protein formation and cell division by bradykinin and des-Arg^9-bradykinin. *J. Biol. Chem.* **259**:9263-9268 (1984).
23. Straus, D. S., and K. J. Pang. Effects of bradykinin on DNA synthesis in resting NIL8 hamster cells and human fibroblasts. *Exp. Cell. Res.* **151**:87-95 (1984).
24. Marceau, F., and B. Tremblay. Mitogenic effect of bradykinin and of des-Arg^9-bradykinin on cultured fibroblasts. *Life Sci.* **39**:2351-2358 (1986).
25. Cahill, M., J. B. Fishman, and P. Polgar. Effect of des-arginine^9-bradykinin and other bradykinin fragments on the synthesis of prostacyclin and the bind-

ing of bradykinin by vascular cells in culture. *Agents Actions* **24**:224-231 (1988).

26. D'Orleans-Juste, P., G. De Nucci, D. Regoli, and J. R. Vane. Characterization of kinin receptors on bovine aortic endothelial cells. *Br. J. Pharmacol.* **95**:546P (1988).
27. Sung, C. P., A. J. Arleth, K. Shikano, and B. A. Berkowitz. Characterization and function of bradykinin receptors in vascular endothelial cells. *J. Pharmacol. Exp. Ther.* **247**:8-13 (1988).
28. Crutchley, D. J., J. W. Ryan, U. S. Ryan, and G. H. Fisher. Bradykinin-induced release of prostacyclin and thromboxanes from bovine pulmonary endothelial cells. *Biochim. Biophys. Acta* **751**:99-107 (1983).
29. Lerner, U. H., I. L. Jones, and G. T. Gustafson. Bradykinin, a new potential mediator of inflammation-induced bone resorption. *Arthritis Rheum.* **30**:530-540 (1987).
30. Park, W. K., S. A. St-Pierre, J. Barabé, and D. Regoli. Synthesis of peptides by the solid-phase method. III. Bradykinin: Fragments and analogs. *Can. J. Biochem.* **56**:92-100 (1978).
31. Marceau, F., M. Knap, and D. Regoli. Pharmacological characterization of the vascular permeability-enhancing effects of kinins in the rabbit skin. *Can. J. Physiol. Pharmacol.* **59**:921-926 (1981).
32. Regoli, D., F. Marceau, and J. Barabé. *De novo* formation of vascular receptors for kinins. *Can. J. Physiol. Pharmacol.* **56**:674-677 (1978).
33. Marceau, F., J. Barabé, S. St-Pierre, and D. Regoli. Kinin receptors in experimental inflammation. *Can. J. Physiol. Pharmacol.* **58**:536-542 (1980).
34. Bouthillier, J., D. Deblois, and F. Marceau. Studies on the induction of pharmacological responses to des-Arg^9-bradykinin *in vitro* and *in vivo*. *Br. J. Pharmacol.* **92**:257-264 (1987).
35. Couture, R., J. Mizrahi, D. Regoli, and G. Devroede. Peptides and the human colon: An *in vitro* pharmacological study. *Can. J. Physiol. Pharmacol.* **59**:957-964 (1981).
36. Whalley, E. T., H. Fritz, and R. Geiger. Kinin receptors and angiotensin converting enzyme in rabbit basilar arteries. *N. S. Arch. Pharmacol.* **324**:296-301 (1983).
37. Boschcov, P., A. C. M. Paiva, T. B. Paiva, S. I. Shimuta. Further evidence for the existence of two receptor sites for bradykinin responsible for the diphasic effect in the rat isolated duodenum. *Br. J. Pharmacol.* **83**:591-600 (1984).
38. Deblois, D., and F. Marceau. The ability of des-Arg^9-bradykinin to relax rabbit isolated mesenteric arteries is acquired during in vitro incubation. *Eur. J. Pharmacol.* **142**:141-144 (1987).
39. Guimaraes, J. A., M. A. R. Vieira, M. J. F. Camargo, and T. Maack. Renal vasoconstrictive effect of kinins mediated by B1-kinin receptors. *Eur. J. Pharmacol.* **130**:177-185 (1986).
40. Regoli, D. C., F. Marceau, and J. Lavigne. Induction of B1-receptors for kinins in the rabbit by a bacterial lipopolysaccharide. *Eur. J. Pharmacol.* **71**:105-115 (1981).

41. Deblois, D., J. Bouthillier, and F. Marceau. Effect of glucocorticoids, monokines and growth factors on the spontaneously developing responses of the rabbit isolated aorta to des-Arg[9]-bradykinin. *Br. J. Pharmacol.* **93**:969-977 (1988).
42. Barabé, J., C. Babiuk, and D. Regoli. Binding of [^{3}H]des-Arg[9]-BK to rabbit anterior mesenteric vein. *Can. J. Physiol. Pharmacol.* **60**:1551-1555 (1982).
43. Regoli, D., and J. Barabé. Pharmacology of bradykinin and related kinins. *Pharmacol. Rev.* **32**:1-46 (1980).
44. Regoli, D., W. K. Park, and F. Rioux. Pharmacology of angiotensin. *Pharmacol. Rev.* **26**:69-123 (1974).
45. Regoli, D., G. Drapeau, P. Rovero, S. Dion, P. d'Orléans-Juste, and J. Barabé. The actions of kinin antagonists on B1 and B2 receptor systems. *Eur. J. Pharmacol.* **123**:63-65 (1986).
46. Steranka, L. R., D. C. Manning, C. J. DeHaas, J. W. Ferkany, S. A. Borosky, J. R. Connor, R. J. Vavrek, J. M. Stewart, and S. H. Snyder. Bradykinin as a pain mediator: Receptors are located to sensory neurons, and antagonists have analgesic actions. *Proc. Natl. Acad. Sci. USA* **85**:3245-3249 (1988).
47. Baud, L., J. Perez, M. Denis, and R. Ardaillou. Modulation of fibroblast proliferation by sulfidopeptide leukotrienes: Effect of indomethacin. *J. Immunol.* **138**:1190-1195 (1987).
48. Churchill, L., and P. E. Ward. Conversion of B1 kinin receptor-mediated vascular relaxation to contraction. *Hypertension* **9**:1-5 (1987).
49. Schild, H. O. pAx, a new scale for measuring drug antagonism. *Br. J. Pharmacol.* **2**:189-206 (1947).
50. Regoli, D. Kinins. *Br. Med. Bull.* **43**:270-284 (1987).
51. Plummer, T. H., and T. J. Ryan. A potent mercapto biproduct analog inhibitor of carboxypeptidase N. *Biochem. Biophys. Res. Comm.* **98**:448-453 (1981).

3

Chemistry of Peptide B2 Bradykinin Antagonists

John M. Stewart and Raymond J. Vavrek
University of Colorado School of Medicine
Denver, Colorado

I. INTRODUCTION

Effective competitive antagonists are essential for the study of actions of molecules involved in biological communication. Hormones, neurotransmitters, and neuromodulators can produce effects on their receptors which make accurate evaluation difficult, if not impossible. In addition, rapid destruction of agonists causes serious problems in estimation of their presence in biological systems and of their potencies in assays. These problems are exacerbated in the cases of those agents that are produced and act locally, for these molecules are rapidly inactivated, frequently by a variety of processes. Properly designed antagonists can overcome these problems. For example, antagonists should not cause downregulation of receptors, nor should antagonist-receptor complexes be internalized. Moreover, antagonists can be designed with features to inhibit enzymatic degradation. Frequently it is only with antagonists that the existence of receptor classes or subclasses is recognized. The naturally occurring kinins, bradykinin, kallidin, and related peptides, exemplify to the highest degree all the problems of working with agonists. Kinins are involved in regulation of all the major physiological systems. They interact with essentially the entire known range of second messenger systems in target tissues. Several of these functions and interactions have become apparent only since the advent of antagonists able to block kinin actions.

Synthesis of analogs of bradykinin for structure-activity studies began shortly after announcement of the structure of bradykinin in 1960. Structures and biological activities of several hundred analogs were summarized in the reviews of Schroder (1) and of Stewart (2). Among these analogs, none having antagonist activity against the action of bradykinin on the classical bradykinin-responsive tissues, such as rat uterus, guinea pig ileum, and rat blood pressure, was reported. The surprisingly potent action of desArg^9-bradykinin on isolated rabbit aorta had already been reported, and antagonists of this system, designated by Regoli as "B1," had been described (3). DesArg^9[Leu^8]bradykinin was described as an antagonist of desArg^9-bradykinin in this system. As has been amply demonstrated since that time, this B1 system shows no crossover with the standard bradykinin responsive tissues, and the discovery of desArg^9[Leu^8] bradykinin was not helpful in the search for antagonists of bradykinin responses in other tissues (4). The bradykinin B1 system and antagonists for that system are described in Chapter 2 of this volume and will not be further discussed here.

Although no antagonists were found during the first two decades of bradykinin research, several analogs were found to behave as superagonists in certain tissues. For example, the analog containing thienylalanine (Thi) in place of Phe at positions 5 and 8 had remarkable agonist potency (5), and analogs having N-terminal extensions with basic amino acids, such as D-Arg or Lys-Lys, were found to be especially potent in systems where kinin action was severely limited by action of kininases (2) (see Table 1, Section A). These N-terminal extended analogs were shown to be resistant to the action of kininases, especially angiotensin converting enzyme in lung (6,7). Replacement of Pro residues in positions 2 and 3 by 4-hydroxyproline (Hyp) led to potent agonists with tissue selectivity favoring rat uterus (8). These kinds of structure modifications were shown to increase affinity for bradykinin receptors and were especially useful later for improving the potency of bradykinin antagonists (9).

The first report of bradykinin analogs able to antagonize the action of bradykinin on standard kinin assay systems came in 1985, with the description of [DPhe^7]bradykinin and [Thi^{5,8},DPhe^7]bradykinin (4). The critical change conferring bradykinin antagonist activity upon analogs was replacement of the Pro at position 7 with a D-aromatic amino acid residue. This generalization has held true for all bradykinin antagonists synthesized to the present time. Table 1 lists structures and activities of a large

Table 1 Bradykinin Analogs[a]

Number[b] NPC "B"	Structure	Contraction RUT	Contraction GPI	Blood Pressure IA	Blood Pressure IV	Blood Pressure Dest	Binding RUT	Binding GPI	Ref.
	A. Reference Agonists								
	Arg-Pro-Pro-Gly-Phe-Ser-Pro-Phe-Arg (BK)	100	100	100	100	99%	*0.3*	*0.1*	
	Lys-BK	167	93	81	293	90%	*0.1*	*0.5*	
588	DLys-BK	123	114	105	408	85%		99%	38
587	DArg-BK	143	103	66	218	92%		99%	13,39
	Lys-Lys-BK	188	19	640	2058	0%			13
589	DLys-Lys-BK	126	9	158	309	42%		96%	38
	[Thi^{5}]-BK	200	40	10	200	95%			5
	[Thi^{8}]-BK	500	40	10	200	95%			5
	[Thi^{5,8}]-BK	1000	200	15	300	95%			5
	Lys-Lys[Thi^{5,8}]-BK	34	19	36	3606	0%			
	[Hyp^{2}]-BK	200	100	90	500	90%			8
	[Hyp^{3}]-BK	100	35	85	300	94%			8,40
14332	Lys[Hyp^{3}]-BK	145	26	77	327	88%		*14*	
14333	[Hyp^{3},Thi^{5,8}]-BK	106	15	26	123	80%		*2*	
14334	DArg[Hyp^{3},Thi^{5,8}]-BK	237	7	27	263	54%		*32*	
14335	Lys[Hyp^{3},Thi^{5,8}]-BK	109	10	33	213	88%		*67*	
14336	Lys-Lys[Hyp^{3},Thi5^{,8}]-BK	70	7	132	6420	0%		*76*	
	[Tyr^{8}]-BK							*0.8*	
	B. Position 6 Analogs								
	[Gly^{6}]-BK	29	61	17	13	97%			3,46
	[Phe^{6}]-BK	0.1		0.3		94%			1,46
	[PCF^{6}]-BK	0.2	1	0					

Table 1 (continues)

Table 1 Continued

Number[b] NPC "B"	Structure	Contraction RUT	Contraction GPI	Blood Pressure IA	Blood Pressure IV	Blood Pressure Dest	Binding RUT	Binding GPI	Ref.
	[NMF[6]]-BK	0.1	0	0	0				
	[Thi[6]]-BK	0.1	0.8	0	0				
	[His[6]]-BK	0.2	0.5	0.2	4	53%			
	[Trp[6]]-BK	0.2	0.7	0					
13757	[Lys[6]]-BK	0	0	0	0			13%	
13759	[Arg[6]]-BK	0	0	DPR	DPR			53%	
	[Glu[6]]-BK	0.3	0.3	0.7	7	69%			
	[Asp[6]]-BK	0	0	0	0				
	[Pro[6]]-BK	0.3	0	0	0				
	[Asn[6]]-BK	1.6	4	3	15	87%			
	[Gln[6]]-BK	0.1	0.4	0.5	16	11%			
	[desSer[6]]-BK	0	0	0	0				
	[DPhe[6]]-BK	6	11	0.2	8	35%			39
	[DSer[6]]-BK	5	10	1	22	36%			42
	[CDF[6]]-BK	52	159	14	336	2%			39
	[DTrp[6]]-BK	29	47	3	60	44%			39
13758	[DLys[6]]-BK	0	0	0	0			1[illegible]%	
13760	[DArg[6]]-BK	0	0	0	0			5[illegible]%	
	[DAla[6]]-BK	0.3	3	0.3	5	65%			
	[DAsp[6]]-BK	0.05	0	0.1	0.9	69%			
	[DGlu[6]]-BK	0	0	0	0				
	[DPro[6]]-BK	0	0	0	0				

		C. Position 7 Analogs								
590		[Gly^7]-BK	0.2	0.07	0.6	0.07	95%		39%	38
13810		[Phe^7]-BK	0.1	0.1	0	0			86%	
		[Aib^7]-BK	55	418	32	530	49%			39
591		[DAla^7]-BK	0.3	0	0.03	2	0%		44%	4,38,39
383		[DVal^7]-BK	5	0	0.3	8	9%		6%	4,38,39
357		[DNal^7]-BK	0.9	0.2	0.2	14	0%		84%	4,38
425		[MDY^7]-BK	AG	0	0	0			30%	4,38
356		[DHis^7]-BK	2	0	19	29	95%		20%	4,38
380		[DTrp^7]-BK	4	0	0.4	5	50%		55%	4,38
377		[DPhg^7]-BK	0	0	0	0			3%	4,38
359		[DhF^7]-BK	8	0.7	1.3	27	54%		83%	38
382		[DTyr^7]-BK	0.2	0	0	0			14%	4,38
361	3374 3600	[DPhe^7]-BK	4	5.9*	2	4	36%	*22*	73%	4,12,13
331		[CDF^7]-BK	3	5.4*	1	14	50%	*13*	84%	12,38,43
809	4318	[FDF^7]-BK	2.6	5.4*	0.3	7	38%	*11*	97%	14
358	3632 BKA-02	[DPal^7]-BK	0.1	5.3*	0	0		*123*	74%	12,38,43
379	3618	[DThi^7]-BK	0.1	6.4*	0	0		*47*	65%	12,38,43
404		Lys-Lys[DPhe^7]-BK	0.3	5.6*	1				93%	38,13,12,43
405		Lys-Lys[DPhg^7]-BK	0	0					56%	38
403		Lys-Lys[DhF^7]-BK	12	0	AG	AG			79%	38
407		Lys-Lys[DTrp^7]-BK	0.3	0	0.2	4	44%		61%	38
408		Lys-Lys[DTyr^7]-BK	0.1	0					32%	38
402		Lys-Lys[DHis^7]-BK	0.1	0					55%	38

Table 1 (continues)

Table 1 Continued

Number[b] NPC "B"	Structure	Contraction RUT	Contraction GPI	Blood Pressure IA	Blood Pressure IV	Blood Pressure Dest	Binding RUT	Binding GPI	Ref.
341	DArg[DPhe^7]-BK	0.1	6.3*	I	I		*1.4*	97%	38,13,12,43
592	DArg[DAla^7]-BK	0	0	0	0			52%	38
343	DArg[DPhg^7]-BK	0	0					70%	38
340	DArg[DhF^7]-BK	8	0.2	1	36	19%		94%	38
352	DArg[DTrp^7]-BK	0.3	0	0.1	0.3	0%		[illegible]6%	38
355	DArg[DTyr^7]-BK	0.1	0	I	I			64%	38
339	DArg[DHis^7]-BK	0	0					70%	38
813 432	DArg[FDF^7]-BK	2	6.1*	I	I		*1.5*	90%	14
431 3592 3926 4144 4145 BKA-03	[Thi^{5,8},DPhe^7]-BK	MXD	6.3*	I	I			75%	5,13,38,39
436	[Thi^{5,8},DThi^7]-BK	4.2*	0	0	0		*11*	*212*	12,38,43
430	[Thi^{5,8},DPal^7]-BK	4.2*	5.3*	0	0		*114*	42%	12,38,43
434	[Thi^{5,8},DPro^7]-BK	0	0	0	0			17%	38
429	[Thi^{5,8},DNal^7]-BK	0	0	2	89	57%		85%	38
426	[Thi^{5,8},CDF^7]-BK	2	5.3*	0.5	13	47%		82%	12,13,38,43
440	[Thi^{5,8},DTyr^7]-BK	9	0					10%	
441	[Thi^{5,8},DVal^7]-BK	1	0					12%	
428	[Thi^{5,8},DIle^7]-BK	AG	0	0.3	18	0%		25%	
581	[Thi^{5,8},DTrp^7]-BK	2	0					6[illegible]%	
582	[Thi^{5,8},DPhg^7]-BK	0.2	0	0	I			18%	
443	[Thi^{5,8},MDY^7]-BK	0						30%	

569		[Thi^{5,8},DhF^{7}]-BK	15	0.1	5	88	50%		86%	
15889		[DPro^{2},DPhe^{7}]-BK							*654*	
390		[Hyp^{2},DPhe^{7}]-BK	0.8	5.8*	I	I		*46*	74%	12,38,43
392	3852	[Hyp^{3},DPhe^{7}]-BK	0.4	5.6*	I	I			35%	12,38,43
	4416									
	4436									
391		[Hyp^{2,3},DPhe^{7}]-BK	0.4	5.3*	I	I		*11*	32%	12,38,43
15644[b]		[Ala^{2},DPhe^{7}]-BK							*497*	
15645[b]		[Ala^{3},DPhe^{7}]-BK							*352*	
810		[Hyp^{2},FDF^{7}]-BK	0.5	5.9*	I	I		*16*	96%	14
811		[Hyp^{3},FDF^{7}]-BK	4.4*	5.2*	0.1	3	50%	*5*	80%	14
812		[Hyp^{2,3},FDF^{7}]-BK	1.8	5.5*	0.1	4	53%	*7*	79%	14
393		[Hyp^{2},Thi^{5,8},DPhe^{7}]-BK	MXD	6.0*	I	I		*250*	*78*	38,44
394	3820	[Hyp^{3},Thi^{5,8},DPhe^{7}]-BK	0.1	5.7*	I	I			41%	38,44
	4146									
	4147									
	4208									
	BKA-04									
395		[Hyp^{2,3},Thi^{5,8},DPhe^{7}]-BK	6.0*	5.9*	I	I			38%	38,44
804		[Hyp^{3},Thi^{5,8},CDF^{7}]-BK	3	5.1*	0.2	11	0%	*4*	76%	14
805		[Hyp^{2,3},Thi^{5,8},CDF^{7}]-BK	0.4	5.3*	0.4	43	0%	*9*	72%	14
566	4202	DArg[Hyp^{2},DPhe^{7}]-BK	0.5	6.3*	I	I			*11*	43
567	3824	DArg[Hyp^{3},DPhe^{7}]-BK	6.5*	5.9*	I	I		*3*	*30*	43
	4801									
568		DArg[Hyp^{2,3},DPhe^{7}]-BK	6.5*	6.3*	I	I		*6*	*28*	43
347	3816	DArg[Hyp^{2},Thi^{5,8},DPhe^{7}]-BK	5.4*	6.5*	I	I			96%	12,43,44

Table 1 **(continues)**

Table 1 Continued

Number[b] NPC "B"	Structure	Contraction RUT	Contraction GPI	Blood Pressure IA	Blood Pressure IV	Blood Pressure Dest	Binding RUT	Binding GPI	Ref.
349 3824 4162 4307 4881 5630 6572 BKA-06	DArg[Hyp^3,Thi^{5,8},DPhe^7]-BK	6.9*	6.3*	I	I		*2*	*20*	12,43,44
348 3832 4662	DArg[Hyp^{2,3},Thi^{5,8},DPhe^7]-BK	6.9*	6.0*	I	I			39%	12,43,44
14510	DArg[Hyp^2,FDF^7]-BK	1.1	5.6*	I	I			89%	14
814 4360	DArg[Hyp^3,FDF^7]-BK	2.1	6.0*	I	I			96%	14
815	DArg[Hyp^{2,3},FDF^7]-BK	0.5	5.7*	I	I			93%	14
351	DArg[Thi^{5,8},DPhe^7]-BK	5.5*	6.1*	I	I			96%	12,14,38,43
	DArg[Thi^{5,8},DhF^7]-BK	8	0	1	25	13%			38
806 4280	DArg[Thi^{5,8},CDF^7]-BK	0.6	6.1*	0.8	15	52%		96%	14
807	DArg[Hyp^3,Thi^{5,8},CDF^7]-BK	4.8*	5.8*	0.1	3	40%		94%	14
808	DArg[Hyp^{2,3},Thi^{5,8},CDF^7],BK	0.2	5.7*	I	I			90%	14
420 3878 3726	Lys-Lys[Thi^{5,8},DPhe^7]-BK	5.5*	6.1*	I	I		*2*	93%	12,13,38,43
423	Lys-Lys[Thi^{5,8},DThi^7]-BK	5.1*	0	0.3	4	70%	*14*	72%	38
419 3724	Lys-Lys[Thi^{5,8},DPal^7]-BK	0.5	0					19%	38
410	Lys-Lys[Hyp^2,DPhe^7]-BK	0.1	5.7*	I	I			85%	12,38,43
412 3854 4802	Lys-Lys[Hyp^3,DPhe^7]-BK	0.1	5.7*	I	I			87%	12,38,43

411		Lys-Lys[Hyp^{2,3},DPhe^{7}]-BK	0.2	5.4*	I	I			81%	12,38,43
413	3814	Lys-Lys[Hyp^{2},Thi^{5,8},DPhe^{7}]-BK	0.2	6.6*	I	I			83%	38,44
	4148									
	BKA-05									
415	3822	Lys-Lys[Hyp^{3},Thi^{5,8},DPhe^{7}]-BK	MXD	5.5*	I	I		*7*	*77*	38,44
	4310									
	4662									
414	3836	Lys-Lys[Hyp^{2,3},Thi^{5,8},DPhe^{7}]-BK	MXD	5.6*	0.2	0.5	82%	*3*	*85*	38,44
	4308									
13815	4160	DTyr-DArg[Thi^{5,8},DPhe^{7}]-BK	6.3*	5.4*	I	I		*27*	*16*	
		D. Position 4, 7 Analogs								
15646[b]		[Ala^{4},DPhe^{7}]-BK							28%	
15950[b]		[DAla^{4},DPhe^{7}]-BK							*4940*	
13788		[Hyp^{3},DAla^{4},DPhe^{7}]-BK	0	0	I	I			13%	
13790		[Hyp^{3},DPro^{4},DPhe^{7}]-BK	0	0	0	0			5%	
13791		[Hyp^{3},DPhe^{4,7}]-BK	0	0	I	I			15%	
14520		[Hyp^{3},DThi^{4},DPhe^{7}]-BK	0	0	0	0			5%	
13794		[Hyp^{3},DArg^{4},DPhe^{7}]-BK	0	0	0	0			15%	
13789		DArg[Hyp^{3},DAla^{4},DPhe^{7}]-BK	0	MXD	I	I			48%	
14519		DArg[Hyp^{3},DPro^{4},DPhe^{7}]-BK	0	0	I	I			15%	
13792		DArg[Hyp^{3},DPhe^{4,7}]-BK	0	0	I	I			14%	
13793		DArg[Hyp^{3},DThi^{4},DPhe^{7}]-BK	0	0	MXD	MXD			34%	
13795		DArg[Hyp^{3},DArg^{4},DPhe^{7}]BK	0	0	0	0			24%	
		E. Position 5,7 Analogs								
15688[b]		[Ala^{5},DPhe^{7}]-BK							39%	
13801		[DPhe^{5},Aib^{7}]-BK	0.1	0.6	0	0			62%	

Table 1 (continues)

Table 1 Continued

Number[b] NPC	"B"	Structure	Contraction RUT	Contraction GPI	Blood Pressure IA	Blood Pressure IV	Blood Pressure Dest	Binding RUT	Binding GPI	Ref.
13802		[CDF^5,Aib^7]-BK	0	0	0	0			[illegible]3%	
13799		[DPhe^5,DAla^7]-BK	0	0	0	0			0%	39
13800		[CDF^5,DAla^7]-BK	0	0.1	0	0			2%	
15979[b]		[DPhe^{5,7}]-BK	5.9*						129	
		F. Position 6,7 Analogs								
		[Gly^6,Aib^7]-BK	2	4	0.3	6				39
		[DPhe^6,Aib^7]-BK	124	426	117	1473	67%			
		[CDF^6,Aib^7]-BK	97	321	244	2944	61%			
		[DTrp^6,Aib^7]-BK	100	226	170	1753	71%			
	365	[DPhe^6,DPro^7]-BK	0.7	0	AG	AG			8%	38
	332	[CDF^6,DAla^7]-BK	111	120	57	1151	77%		97%	38,39
	334	[CDF^6,DPro^7]-BK	1	0.3					46%	38
	362	[DPhe^6,DAla^7]-BK	11	6	0.6	18	0%		83%	38
	381	[DTrp^6,DAla^7]-BK	31	18	2	52	45%		96%	39
	360	[DPhe^{6,7}]-BK	0.1	0	PRS	PRS			55%	38
	333	[CDF^6,DPhe^7]-BK	0.1	0	0	0			49%	38,39
	336	[CDF^6,DVal^7]-BK	2	0.2	0.9	14	35%		74%	38,39
	368	[DPhe^6,DVal^7]-BK	0.3	0	MXD	MXD			28%	38,39
	330	[CDF^{6,7}]-BK	0.2	0	PRS	PRS			47%	38,39
	388	[Gly^6,DPhe^7]-BK	31	0.3	2	22	20%		71%	39
	387	[Gly^6,CDF^7]-BK	117	5	73	349	79%		94%	39
		[Gly^6,DVal^7]-BK	6	0.2	MXD	MXD				39
	386	[Gly^{6,7}]-BK	0.1	0.04	0	0			21%	
	369	[DPhe^6,Gly^7]-BK	1	1	7	36	81%		97%	38
	335	[CDF^6,Gly^7]-BK	45	139	114	326	87%		99%	38

366		[DPhe^{6},DThi^{7}]-BK	0.1	0	0	0			60%	38
367	3390 BKA-01	[DPhe^{6},CDF^{7}]BK	0.6	5.9*	1	9	68%	*21*	65%	12,38,43
378		[DThi^{6,7}]-BK	0.4	0	I	0			38%	
363		[DPhe^{6},DNal^{7}]-BK	0.02	0	0.1	0.5	77%		69%	38
370		[DPhe^{6},MDY^{7}]-BK	0.1	0	0	0			28%	38
364		[DPhe^{6},DPal^{7}]-BK	0.1	I	0	0			8%	38
15844		[Pro^{6},DPhe^{7}]-BK	1						58%	
15535[b]		[Ala^{6},DPhe^{7}]-BK							*58*	
15546		[Hyp^{6},DPhe^{7}]-BK	0.3	0	0	0			32%	
15845		[Thr^{6},DPhe^{7}]-BK	0.2	5.8*	I	I			*34*	
13761		[DArg^{6},DPhe^{7}]-BK	0	0	0.1	1.3	66%		17%	
15977[b]		[DSer^{6},DPhe^{7}]-BK							*1100*	
15543		DArg[Pro^{6},DPhe^{7}]-BK	0.4	0	0.1	1	50%		*110*	
15547		[DArg[Hyp^{6},DPhe^{7}]-BK	0.1	MXD	0	0			65%	
13762		DArg[DArg^{6},DPhe^{7}]-BK	0	0	I	I			30%	
15846		DArg[Thr^{6},DPhe^{7}]-BK	0.3	5.8*	I				*8*	
342		DArg[DPhe^{6},DAla^{7}]-BK	12	0.7	0.1	3	0%		94%	39
337		DArg[CDF^{6},DAla^{7}]-BK	153	51	12	340	8%		99%	39
354		DArg[DTrp^{6},DAla^{7}]-BK	15	3	3	76	54%		98%	39
432		[Thi^{5,8},DPhe^{6},CDF^{7}]-BK	0.03	5.5*	0	0		*131*	58%	12,43
421		Lys-Lys[Thi^{5,8},DPhe^{6},CDF^{7}]-BK	0.1	5.7*	I	I		*118*	67%	
396		[Hyp^{2},Thi^{5,8},DPhe^{6},CDF^{7}]-BK	0.005	5.6*	I	I		*334*	56%	
398		[Hyp^{3},Thi^{5,8},DPhe^{6},CDF^{7}]-BK	0.1	5.7*	I	I		*159*	34%	
397		[Hyp^{2,3},Thi^{5,8},DPhe^{6},CDF^{7}]-BK	0.01	5.4*	I	I		*1000*	*54*	12,43
416		Lys-Lys[Hyp^{2},Thi^{5,8},DPhe^{6},CDF^{7}]-BK	0.1	5.9*	I	I		*18*	70%	
418		Lys-Lys[Hyp^{3},Thi^{5,8},DPhe^{6},CDF^{7}]-BK	0.1	5.6*	0.03	MXD		*10*	58%	

Table 1 (continues)

Table 1 Continued

Number[b] NPC "B"	Structure	Contraction		Blood Pressure			Binding		Ref.
		RUT	GPI	IA	IV	Dest	RUT	GPI	
417	Lys-Lys[Hyp^{2,3}Thi^{5,8},DPhe^{6}, CDF^{7}]-BK	0.1	5.3*	MXD	I		*13*	[illegible]8%	12,43
	[Thi^{5,8},Gly^{6},DhF^{7}]-BK	56	2						38
	DArg[Thi^{5,8},Gly^{6},DhF^{7}]-BK	52	2						38
15847	[Hyp^{3},Thr^{6},DPhe^{7}]-BK	0.08	0	I(P)	I(P)			*51*	
15848	DArg[Hyp^{3},Thr^{6},DPhe^{7}]-BK	5.9*	5.8*	I	I			*11*	
15544	[Hyp^{3},Pro^{6},DPhe^{7}]-BK	0.8	0	0.1	5	0%		*1563*	
15545	DArg[Hyp^{3},Pro^{6},DPhe^{7}]-BK	0.2	0	0.1	2	53%		*255*	
15548	[Hyp^{3},6,DPhe^{7}]-BK	1	0	0.1	3	75%		3[illegible]%	
15549	DArg[Hyp^{3,6},DPhe^{7}]-BK	0.4	0	I	I			7[illegible]%	
15550	[Hyp^{3},cHyp^{6},DPhe^{7}]-BK	0.1	0	0	0			1[illegible]%	
15551	DArg[Hyp^{3},cHyp^{6},DPhe^{7}]-BK	0	0	0	0			6[illegible]%	
	G. Position 5,6,7 Analogs								
13804	[DPhe^{5,6},Aib^{7}]-BK	15	72	0.8	11	28%		9[illegible]%	
13044	[DPhe^{5},CDF^{6},Aib^{7}]-BK	97	AG	48	71	93%		90%	
13805	[CDF^{5},DPhe^{6},Aib^{7}]-BK	0.1	0.3	PRS	PRS			66%	
13045	[CDF^{5,6},Aib^{7}]-BK	4	3	DPR	DPR			97%	
13046	[DPhe^{5,6},DAla^{7}]-BK	0.02	0	0.1	0			97%	
13803	[DPhe^{5},CDF^{6},DAla^{7}]-BK	2	0.6	0	0			81%	
13047	[CDF^{5},DPhe^{6},DAla^{7}]-BK	0	0	0	0			74%	
13048	[CDF^{5,6},DAla^{7}]-BK	0.04	0	0.1	0.8	58%		68%	
13049	[Thi^{5},DThi^{6,7}]-BK	0	0	0.1	1	85%		75%	
13806	[DPhe^{5},CDF^{6},DPhe^{7}]-BK	0.02	0	AG	AG	89%		20%	
13808	[DPro^{5},CDF^{6},DPhe^{7}]-BK	0	0	0	0			54%	
13807	DArg[DPhe^{5},CDF^{6},DPhe^{7}]-BK	0	I	I				72%	

		H. Position 6,7,8 Analogs							
13037		[Gly^6,DPhe^7,OMT^8]-BK	8	1.2	1	30	68%	96%	
13038		[Gly^6,DThi^7,OMT^8]-BK	2	0.7	0.2	30	0%	93%	
13039		[Gly^6,DPal^7,OMT^8]-BK	2	0	0.2	3	85%		
		[Gly^6,CDF^7,OMT^8]-BK	10	13	14	223	73%		
		I. Position 6,7,9 Analogs							
14360		[Hyp^3,Thi^{5,8},DArg^6,DPhe^7,Phe^9]-BK	0	0	0.1	3	50%	14%	
14361		DArg[Hyp^3,Thi^{5,8},DArg^6,DPhe^7, Phe^9]-BK	0	MXD	0.2	6	49%	31%	
14362		[DPhe^1,Hyp^3,Thi^{5,8},DArg^6, DPhe^7,Phe^9]-BK	0	0	0	0		1%	
14363		[DNal^1,Hyp^3,Thi^{5,8},DArg^6, Phe^7,Phe^9]-BK	MXD	0	0	0		0%	
		J. Position 7,8 Analogs							
13811		[Phe^7,DPro^8]-BK	0	0	0	0		34%	
13090		[DPhe^7,Pro^8]-BK	MXD	6.2*	0	0		44%	45
15689^b		[DPhe^7,Ala^8]-BK						*459*	
13751	5092	[DPhe^7,Hyp^8]-BK	0	5.2*	0	0		42%	45
13786		[DPhe^7,cHyp^8]-BK	MXD	0	0	0		18%	
14511		[DPhe^{7,8}]-BK	0	0	0	0		*1630*	
13812		DArg[Phe^7,DPro^8]-BK	0	MXD	0	0		50%	
13091		DArg[DPhe^7,Pro^8]-BK	5.9*	6.6*	I	I		*25*	45
13752		DArg[DPhe^7,Hyp^8]-BK	0	5.6*	I	I		84%	
13787		DArg[DPhe^7,cHyp^8]-BK	5.7	5.3*	I	I		71%	
14512		DArg[DPhe^7,DPhe^{7,8}]-BK	0	0	0	0		22%	
13749		[Thi^5,DPhe^7,Pro^8]-BK	0	5.8*	I	I		75%	
15347		[Thi^5,Phe^7,Pro^8]-BK	0	0	0	0		2%	

Table 1 **(continues)**

Table 1 Continued

Number[b] NPC "B"	Structure	Contraction		Blood Pressure			Binding		Ref.
		RUT	GPI	IA	IV	Dest	RUT	GPI	
13813	[Hyp^3,Phe^7,DPro^8]-BK	0	0	0	0			26%	
13797	[Hyp^3,DPhe^7,DPro^8]-BK	0	0	0	0			1%	
13092	[Hyp^3,DPhe^7,Pro^8]-BK	5.7*	5.6*	I	I		*457*	*525*	45
13753	[Hyp^3,DPhe^7,Hyp^8]-BK	5.1*	0	0	0			25%	45
14513	[Hyp^3,DPhe^{7,8}]-BK	MXD	0	0	0			22%	
13784	[cHyp^3,DPhe^7,Pro^8]-BK	0	I	MXD	MXD	96%		56%	
15349	[Hyp^1,Thi^5,Phe^7,Pro^8]-BK	0	0	0	0			2%	
13814	DArg[Hyp^3,Phe^7,DPro^8]-BK	0	MXD	0	0			13%	
13798	DArg[Hyp^3,DPhe^7,DPro^8]-BK	0	0	0	0			3%	
13093	DArg[Hyp^3,DPhe^7,Pro^8]-BK	6.3*	6.0*	I	I		*24*	*4[illegible]*	45
13750	DArg[Thi^5,DPhe^7,Pro^8]-BK	5.9*	6.6*	0	0			96%	
	DArg[Hyp^3,DPhe^7,Hyp^8]-BK	5.8*	5.3*						45
14514	DArg[Hyp^3,DPhe^{7,8}]-BK	0	0	I	I			15%	
13785	DArg[cHyp^3,DPhe^7,Pro^8]-BK	5.6*	5.7*	I	I			90%	
15348	DArg[Thi^5,Phe^7,Pro^8]-BK	0	0	0	0			10%	
15350	DArg[Hyp^3,Thi^5,Phe^7,Pro^8]-BK	0	0	0	0			10%	
	K. Position 7,9 Analogs								
15534[b]	[DPhe^7,Ala^9]-BK							10%	
15694[b]	[DPhe^7]-BK-Ala							16%	
15351	[DPhe^7,Lys^9]-BK	AG	MXD	0	0			*211*	
15353	DArg[DPhe^7,Lys^9]-BK	5.4*	5.3*	I	I			*22*	
15353	Lys[DPhe^7,Lys^9]-BK	0	0					*354*	
15354	Lys-Lys[DPhe^7,Lys^9]-BK	0	0	0	0			*169*	
15355	[Hyp^3,DPhe^7,Lys^9]-BK	5.1*	MXD	0	0			*388*	

13120	[Hyp^{3},DPhe^{7},Phe^{9}]-BK	0	MXD	0	0			7%	45,48
13754	[Thi^{5,8},DPhe^{7},Pro^{9}]-BK	0	MXD	0	0			1%	
816	[Thi^{5,8},DPhe^{7},DArg^{9}]-BK	0.01	0	0.1	0.6	77%		30%	45
13755	DArg[Thi^{5,8},DPhe^{7},Pro^{9}]-BK	0	0	0	0			26%	
818	DArg[Thi^{5,8},DPhe^{7},DArg^{9}]-BK	0	0	I	I			62%	45
819	Lys-Lys[Thi^{5,8},DPhe^{7},DArg^{9}]-BK	0	0	0.2	14	0%		38%	45
817	Ac[Thi^{5,8},DPhe^{7},DArg^{9}]-BK	0	0	0	0			2%	45
15981[b]	[DPhe^{7},DArg^{9}]-BK							*1650*	
13121	DArg[Hyp^{3},DPhe^{7},Lys^{9}]-BK	5.5*	5.5*	0	0		*64*	*326*	
15357	Lys[Hyp^{3},DPhe^{7},Lys^{9}]-BK	I	I	I	I			*139*	
15358	Lys-Lys[Hyp^{3},DPhe^{7},Lys^{9}]-BK	I		I	I			*182*	
15356	DArg[Hyp^{3},DPhe^{7},Phe^{9}]-BK	6.1*	5.2*	I	I			*19*	45,48
13756	DArg[Hyp^{3},Thi^{5,8},DPhe^{7}, Pro^{9}]-BK	0	MXD	0	0			21%	
	L. Position 7,8,9 Analogs								
15359	[DPhe^{7},Pro^{8},Lys^{9}]-BK	0	MXD	0	0			50%	
15396	[DPhe^{7},Pro^{8},DArg^{9}]-BK	0	0	0	0			35%	
15397	DArg[DPhe^{7},Pro^{8},DArg^{9}]-BK	0	5.8*	0	0			*138*	
15398	[Hyp^{3},DPhe^{7},Pro^{8},DArg^{9}]-BK	0	5.5*	0	0			19%	
15399	DArg[Hyp^{3},DPhe^{7},Pro^{8},DArg^{9}]-BK	MXD	5.4*	0	0			*127*	
15361	DArg[DPhe^{7},Pro^{8},Lys^{9}]-BK	0	MXD	0	0			*60*	
	M. Position 5,8 Analogs								
15343	[Thi^{5},Pro^{8}]-BK	0	0	0	0			10%	
15344	DArg[Thi^{5},Pro^{8}]-BK	0	0	0	0			14%	
15345	[Hyp^{3},Thi^{5},Pro^{8}]-BK	0	0	0	0			3%	
15346	DArg[Hyp^{3},Thi^{5},Pro^{8}]-BK	0	0	0.1	4	78%		4%	

Table 1 (continues)

Table 1 Continued

Number[b] NPC "B"	Structure	Contraction		Blood Pressure			Binding		Ref.
		RUT	GPI	IA	IV	Dest	RUT	GPI	
	N. Position 5/8,6 Analogs								
	[Gly^{6},Pro^{5,8}]-BK	0	0	0.1	0.8	82%			
	DArg[Gly^{6},Pro^{5,8}]-BK	0	AG	AG		80%			
	O. Posotion 5/8,7 Analogs								
13085	[Pro^{5,8},DPhe^{7}]-BK	0	0	0	0			15%	
13086	DArg[Pro^{5,8},DPhe^{7}]-BK	0	0	0	0			5%	
13087	[Hyp^{3},Pro^{5,8},DPhe^{7}]-BK	0	0	0	0			1%	
13088	DArg[Hyp^{3},Pro^{5,8},DPhe^{7}]-BK	0	0	0	0			2%	
	[OMT^{5,8},DPhe^{7}]-BK	0.2	5.0*	0	0				
13034	[OMT^{5,8},DThi^{7}]-BK	0.3	0.2	0	0			95%	
13035	[OMT^{5,8},DPal^{7}]-BK	0	0	0	0			71%	
13036	[OMT^{5,8},CDF^{7}]-BK	4.4*	0	0.1	6	8%		81%	
577	[His^{5,8},DPhe^{7}]-BK	0.01	0	0	0			7%	
578	DArg[His^{5,8},DPhe^{7}]-BK	0	0	0	0				
579	[Hyp^{3},His^{5,8},DPhe^{7}]-BK	0	0	0.04	0.7	31%		12%	
580	DArg[Hyp^{3},His^{5,8},DPhe^{7}]-BK	0	0	0	0			10%	
	P. Position 5/8,6,7 Analogs								
	[Gly^{6},Pro^{5,8},DPhe^{7}]-BK	0	0	0	0				
13089	DArg[Gly^{6},Pro^{5,8},DPhe^{7}]-BK	0	0	0	0			4%	
13040	[Gly^{6},OMT^{5,8},DPhe^{7}]-BK	0.1	0	0	0			73%	
13042	[Gly^{6},OMT^{5,8},CDF^{7}]-BK	1	0	0.6	14	41%		61%	
13041	[Gly^{6},OMT^{5,8},DPal^{7}]-BK	0	0	0	0				
	[Gly^{6},OMT^{5,8},DThi^{7}]-BK	0.02	0	0	0				

722	4642	[Gly^{6},Lys^{5,8},DPhe^{7}]-BK	0.2	5.9*	0.1	12	0%		*54*	
		DArg[Gly^{6},Lys^{5,8},DPhe^{7}]-BK	0.8	6.5*	I	I				
		Lys-Lys[Gly^{6},Lys^{5,8},DPhe^{7}]-BK	0.2	6.2*	I	I				
		Q. Position 2/3,7 Analogs								
13782		[cHyp^{3},DPhe^{7}]-BK	5	5.3*	0.6	6	64%		75%	
13043		DArg[DHP^{2},Hyp^{3},DPhe^{7}]-BK	6.5*	6.3*	I	I		*5*	*14*	
13783		DArg[cHyp^{3},DPhe^{7}]-BK	2	5.6*	0	0			96%	
13020		[DPhe^{2}]-BK	0.1	0	0.1	0.8	35%		77%	
13021		[DPhe^{3}]-BK	0	0	0.02	0			54%	
13022		[DPhe^{2,3}]-BK	0	0	0.1	0	34%			46
13023	4404	[DPhe^{2,7}]-BK	5.5*	0	0	0		*183*	44%	46
13024		[DPhe^{3,7}]-BK	5.5*	0	I	I		*1529*	25%	46
13025		[DPhe^{2,3,7}]-BK	0	0	I	I			21%	46
13026	4772	[Phe^{2},DPhe^{7}]-BK	0	0	I	I			49%	46
13030		DArg[Phe^{2},DPhe^{7}]-BK	0.4	0	I	I			77%	46
13027		[Phe^{3},DPhe^{7}]-BK	0.1	0	MXD	MXD			11%	46
13031		DArg[Phe^{3},DPhe^{7}]-BK	5.9*	0	I	I			54%	46
13028		[Phe^{2},^{3},DPhe^{7}]-BK	0	0	I	I			16%	46
13032		DArg[Phe^{2,3},DPhe^{7}]-BK	0	0	0.2	4	28%		28%	46
13029		[Phe^{2},Hyp^{3},DPhe^{7}]-BK	0	0	I	I			40%	46
13033		DArg[Phe^{2},Hyp^{3},DPhe^{7}]-BK	6.5*	0	I	I		*8*	69%	46
15849		[Ser^{2},DPhe^{7}]-BK	0	0	0.01	0			64%	
15851		[Ser^{3},DPhe^{7}]-BK	0	0	I(P)	I(P)			67%	
15853		[Ser^{2,3},DPhe^{7}]-BK	0	0	I	I			23%	
15855		[Ser^{2},Hyp^{3},DPhe^{7}]-BK	0	0	0	0			24%	
15857		[Thr^{2},Hyp^{3},DPhe^{7}]-BK	0	0	0	0			32%	

Table 1 (continues)

Table 1 Continued

Number[b] NPC "B"	Structure	Contraction		Blood Pressure			Binding		Ref.
		RUT	GPI	IA	IV	Dest	RUT	GPI	
15850	DArg[Ser^2,$DPhe^7$]-BK	0	0	I(P)	I(P)			73%	
15852	DArg[Ser^3,$DPhe^7$]-BK	I(P)	0	0	0			45	
15854	DArg[$Ser^{2,3}$,$DPhe^7$]-BK	0	0	0	0			44%	
15856	DArg[Ser^2,Hyp^3,$DPhe^7$]-BK	5.4*	I(P)	I	I			55%	
15858	DArg[Thr^2,Hyp^3,$DPhe^7$]-BK	5.3*	I(P)	I	I			65%	
444	[Thz^2,$Thi^{5,8}$,$DPhe^7$]-BK	0.8	5.6*	0	0		*58*	67%	49
	[Thz^3,$Thi^{5,8}$,$DPhe^7$]-BK	0.2	5.4*	I	I				49
	[$Thz^{2,3}$,$Thi^{5,8}$,$DPhe^7$]-BK	0.5	5.5*	0	0				49
327	[Aib^2,$Thi^{5,8}$,$DPhe^7$]-BK	0	0	I	I			3%	49
328	[Aib^3,$Thi^{5,8}$,$DPhe^7$]-BK	0	0	MXD	MXD			14%	49
329	[Azt^2,$Thi^{5,8}$,$DPhe^7$]-BK	0.01	5.6*	0	0		*74*	51%	49
	[$Inip^2$,$Thi^{5,8}$,$DPhe^7$]-BK	0	0	MXD	MXD				
400	[$Inip^3$,$Thi^{5,8}$,$DPhe^7$]-BK	0	0	0	0			11%	49
399	[$Inip^{2,3}$,$Thi^{5,8}$,$DPhe^7$]-BK	0	0	0	0			7%	49
	R. Position 2/3,7/9 Analogs								
15400	[Phe^2,Hyp^3,$DPhe^7$,Phe^9]-BK	0	0	0	0			11%	
15402	[$DPhe^2$,Hyp^3,$DPhe^7$,Phe^9]-BK	0	0	0	0			5%	
15404	[Nal^2,Hyp^3,$DPhe^7$,Phe^9]-BK	0	0	0	0			7%	
15406	[$DNal^2$,Hyp^3,$DPhe^7$,Phe^9]-BK	0	MXD	MXD	MXD			4%	
15401	DArg[Phe^2,Hyp^3,$DPhe^7$,Phe^9]-BK	0	0	I	I			38%	
15403	DArg[$DPhe^2$,Hyp^3,$DPhe^7$,Phe^9]-BK	0	0	0	0			9%	
15405	DArg[Nal^2,Hyp^3,$DPhe^7$,Phe^9]-BK	0	0	0	0			17%	
15407	DArg[$DNal^2$,Hyp^3,$DPhe^7$,Phe^9]-BK	0	0	0	0			11%	

	S. Position 1 Analogs								
13774	[DPhe^{1},Hyp^{3}]-BK	0	0	0	0			0%	45
13775	DArg[DPhe^{1},Hyp^{3}]-BK	0.01	0	0.03	2	50%		20%	45
13776	[DTyr^{1},Hyp^{3}]-BK	0.1	0	0	0			3%	45
13777	DArg[DTyr^{1},Hyp^{3}]-BK	0.1	0	0.1	2	53%		31%	45
13778	[CDF^{1},Hyp^{3}]-BK	0	0	0.03	3	61%		3%	45
13779	DArg[CDF^{1},Hyp^{3}]-BK	0.02	0	0.04	1	13%		22%	45
13780	[DNal^{1},Hyp^{3}]-BK	0.1	0	0	0			10%	45
13781	DArg[DNal^{1},Hyp^{3}]-BK	0.6	0	0	0			28%	
14517	[Bz^{1},Hyp^{3}]-BK	0	0	0	0			10%	45
14518	[Pba^{1},Hyp^{3}]-BK	0	0	0	0			12%	45
14337	[DNal^{1},Hyp^{3},Thi^{5,8}]-BK	0.1	0	0.04	5	0%		9%	
14338	DArg[DNal^{1},Hyp^{3},Thi^{5,8}]-BK	0.1	0	0	0			16%	
	T. Position 1,7 Analogs								
15690[b]	[Ala^{1},DPhe^{7}]-BK							23%	
15888[b]	[DArg^{1},DPhe^{7}]-BK							*614*	
13059	[DNal^{1},DPhe^{7}]-BK	5.4*	0	I	I		8%	5%	45,48
13061	DArg[DNal^{1},DPhe^{7}]-BK	5.6*	0	I	I		*305*	38%	45,48
13060	[DNal^{1},Hyp^{3},DPhe^{7}]-BK	0	0.1	0	0			44%	45,48
13062	DArg[DNal^{1},Hyp^{3},DPhe^{7}]-BK	5.9*	0	I	I		*90*	*583*	45,48
13063	[DThi^{1,7}]-BK	0	0	0	0			3%	
13065	DArg[DThi^{1,7}]-BK	0	0	I	I			43%	
13064	[DThi^{1,7},Hyp^{3}]-BK	0	MXD	I	I			0%	
13066	DArg[DThi^{1,7},Hyp^{3}]-BK	5.5*	0	I	I		*353*	28%	
13067	[DNal^{1},DThi^{7}]-BK	0	0	I	I			19%	
13069	DArg[DNal^{1},DThi^{7}]-BK	5.4*	0	0	0		*731*	40%	
13077	[DTyr^{1},Hyp^{3},DPhe^{7}]-BK	5.1*	0	I	I		21%	14%	45,48
13078	DArg[DTyr^{1},Hyp^{3},DPhe^{7}]-BK	6.1*	MXD	I	I			43%	45,48

Table 1 (continues)

Table 1 Continued

Number[b] NPC "B"	Structure	Contraction RUT	Contraction GPI	Blood Pressure IA	Blood Pressure IV	Blood Pressure Dest	Binding RUT	Binding GPI	Ref.
13079	[FDF^1, Hyp^3, DPhe^7]-BK	MXD	0	I	I			5%	45,48
13080	DArg[FDF^1,Hyp^3,DPhe^7]-BK	5.7*	0	I	I		*74*	38%	45,48
14515	[DTrp^1,Hyp^3,DPhe^7]-BK	MXD	0	MXD	MXD			9%	
14516	DArg[DTrp^1,Hyp^3,DPhe^7]-BK	5.9*	0	0	0			15%	
13081	[DVal^1,Hyp^3,DPhe^7]-BK	5.7*	0	0	0			2%	45,48
13082	DArg[DVal^1,Hyp^3,DPhe^7]-BK	5.4*	0	0	0		*452*	33%	45,48
13083	[DIle^1,Hyp^3,DPhe^7]-BK	5.0*	0	0	0		7%	[illegible]%	45,48
13084	DArg[DIle^1,Hyp^3,DPhe^7]-BK	5.1*	0	0	0		*500*	23%	45,48
13068	[DNal^1,Hyp^3,DThi^7]-BK	0	0	I	I			25%	
13070	DArg[DNal^1,Hyp^3,DThi^7]-BK	5.6*	0	I	I		*700*	36%	
	[DArg^1,Hyp^3,DPhe^7]-BK	0	5.3*	0	0				
	DArg[DArg^1,Hyp^3,DPhe^7]-BK	I	0	I	I				
13071	[CDF^1,DPhe^7]-BK	5.0*	0	I	I		12%	8%	45,48
13073	DArg[CDF^1,DPhe^7]-BK	5.4*	MXD	I	I		*272*	44%	45,48
13072	[CDF^1,Hyp^3,DPhe^7]-BK	5.2*	0	I	I			6%	45,48
13074	DArg[CDF^1,Hyp^3,DPhe^7]-BK	5.8*	0	I	I		*97*	39%	45,48
13075	[CDF^1,DThi^7]-BK	0	0	0	0			2%	
13076	DArg[CDF^1,DThi^7]-BK	0	MXD	0	0			47%	
576 4158	[DPhe^1,Thi^{5,8},DPhe^7]-BK	0	0	I	I			1%	45,48
575	[DThi^1,Thi^{5,8},DPhe^7]-BK	0	0	0	0			19%	45,48
574	[DPal^1,Thi^{5,8},DPhe^7]-BK	0	0	0	0			6%	45,48
573 4152	[DNal^1,Thi^{5,8},DPhe^7]-BK	5.6*	0	I	I		*248*	3%	45,48
13053	Lys-Lys[DNal^1,Thi^{5,8},DPhe^7]-BK	0	0	MXD	MXD			34%	48
13052	DArg[DNal^1,Thi^{5,8},DPhe^7]-BK	5.8*	0	I	I		*506*	*792*	48

13054	DNal[DNal^{1},Thi^{5,8},DPhe^{7}]-BK	5.6*	0	ins	ins		*841*	8%	48
13055	[DNal^{1},Hyp^{2,3},Thi^{5,8},DPhe^{7}]-BK	0	0	I	I			6%	
13056	DArg[DNal^{1},Hyp^{2,3},Thi^{5,8}, DPhe^{7}]-BK	5.3*	0	I	I		*190*	50%	
13057	Lys-Lys[DNal^{1},Hyp^{2,3},Thi^{5,8}, DPhe^{7}]-BK	0	0	MXD	MXD			34%	
13117	[Bz^{1},Hyp^{3},DPhe^{7}]-BK	0	5.4*	0	0			14%	45,47,48
13118	[Pba^{1},Hyp^{3},DPhe^{7}]-BK	0	0	0	0			17%	45,47,48
	U. Position 1,6,7 Analogs								
13818	[Bz^{1},Hyp^{3},DArg^{6},DPhe^{7}]-BK	6.3*	0	0	0		11%	42%	
13819	[Pba^{1},Hyp^{3},DArg^{6},DPhe^{7}]-BK	0	0	0	0			20%	
13816	[Bz^{1},DArg^{6},DPhe^{7}]-BK	0	0	0	0			6%	
13817	[Pba^{1},DArg^{6},DPhe^{7}]-BK	0	4.9*	0.1	0.7	74%		64%	
	V. Position 1,7,8 Analogs								
13747	[DArg^{1},Thi^{5},DPhe^{7},Pro^{8}]-BK	0	5.0*	0	0			31%	
13748	DArg[DArg^{1},Thi^{5},DPhe^{7},Pro^{8}]-BK	5.9*	5.3*	I	I			68%	
13744	[DNal^{1},DPhe^{7},Pro^{8}]-BK	0	0	0	0			3%	45
13745	[DPhe^{1},DPhe^{7},Pro^{8}]-BK	0	0	0	0			2%	45
13746	[DThi^{1},DPhe^{7},Pro^{8}]-BK	0	0	0	0			2%	45
	W. Position 1,7,9 Analogs								
13122	[DArg^{1},Hyp^{3},DPhe^{7},Phe^{9}]-BK	0	0	0	0			9%	45
13123	DArg[DArg^{1},Hyp^{3},DPhe^{7},Phe^{9}]-BK	6.3*	5.0*	I	I		*379*	66%	45
13742	[DNal^{1},Hyp^{3},DPhe^{7},Phe^{9}]-BK	0	0	ins	ins			2%	45
13743	DArg[DNal^{1},Hyp^{3},DPhe^{7},Phe^{9}]-BK	5.1*	0	I	I			13%	45

Table 1 (continues)

Table 1 Continued

Number[b] NPC "B"	Structure	Contraction RUT	Contraction GPI	Blood Pressure IA	Blood Pressure IV	Blood Pressure Dest	Binding RUT	Binding GPI	Ref.
	X. N-Terminal Analogs								
	Ac-BK	50		40		95%			
	Bz-BK	2	2	9	2	97%			
	Pba-BK	19	15	18	56	90%			
	Oct-BK	13	6	10	26	87%			
	Sta-BK	0.1	0.1	0.7	<10				
	Cys-BK	123	30	11	139	90%			
13959	Eac-BK	36	25	13	82	94%		9[illegible]%	
13960	Eac-Eac-BK	26	16	4	94	92%		10[illegible]%	
	Sta-Eac-BK	30	19	9	80	79%			
	OMT-Lys-BK	42	46	38	190	90%			
	Lys-OMT-Lys-BK	21	13	26	1308	0%			
13962	Eac[DPhe^7]-BK	0.5	4.8*	I	I			74%	
	Eac-Eac[DPhe^7]-BK	0	5.5*	0	0				
385	Eac[Thi^{5,8},DPhe^7]-BK	0.1	5.5*	I	I		*6*	33%	
384 4046	Eac-Eac[Thi^{5,8},DPhe^7]-BK	0.8	5.8*	I	I		*138*	32%	
	Ac[Hyp^3,DPhe^7]-BK	5.3*	MXD	I	I				
	AcDArg[Hyp^3,DPhe^7]-BK	5.9*	MXD	I	I				
15337	Ac[Hyp^3,Thi^{5,8},DPhe^7]-BK	5.2*	5.1*	I	I			32%	
15338	AcDArg[Hyp^3,Thi^{5,8},DPhe^7]-BK	6.5*	5.0*	I	I			77%	
	Y. T-Kinin Analogs								
13763	Ile-Ser-BK	66	52	90	158	95%	*0.3*	*0.[illegible]*	
13764	Ile-DSer-BK	112	11	2	11	90%		97%	45
13765	DIle-Ser-BK	271	11	10	48	82%		99%	45

13773	DIle-DSer[Hyp^{3},DPhe^{7}]-BK	0	0	I	I			44%	45
13766	Ile-Ser[DPhe^{7}]-BK	1.5	6.3*	0	0			85%	45
13767	DIle-Ser[DPhe^{7}]-BK	5.8*	5.6*	I	I			76%	45
13768	Ile-DSer[DPhe^{7}]-BK	0	5.2*	I	I			65%	45
13769	DIle-DSer[DPhe^{7}]-BK	MXD	5.1*	I	I			66%	45
13770	Ile-Ser[Hyp^{3},DPhe^{7}]-BK	1.1	6.2*	I	I			62%	45
13772	Ile-DSer[Hyp^{3},DPhe^{7}]-BK	5.9*	0	I	I			44%	45
13771	DIle-Ser[Hyp^{3},DPhe^{7}]-BK	6.5*	5.2*	I	I			58%	45
	Z. C-Terminal Analogs								
820	[Thi^{5,8},DPhe^{7}]-BK-NH_2	0.02	0	0.1	1.5	52%		75%	45
821	Ac[Thi^{5,8},DPhe^{7}]-BK-NH_2	0	0	I	I			18%	45
822	DArg[Thi^{5,8},DPhe^{7}]-BK-NH_2	0	0	MXD	MXD			90%	45
823	Lys-Lys[Thi^{5,8},DPhe^{7}]-BK-NH_2	0.02	0	DPR	DPR			61%	45
824	[Thi^{5,8},DPhe^{7},DArg^{9}]-BK-NH_2	0.01	0	0.1	0.9	61%		25%	45
825	Ac[Thi^{5,8},DPhe^{7},DArg^{9}]-BK-NH_2	0	0	I	I			6%	45
826	DArg[Thi^{5,8},DPhe^{7},DArg^{9}]-BK-NH_2	0.003	0	O/I	O/I			32%	45
827	Lys-Lys[Thi^{5,8},DPhe^{7},DArg^{9}]-BK-NH_2	0.002	0	0.2	3	60%		14%	45
	AA. C-Terminal Ile-Tyr Analogs								
594	BK-Ile-Tyr	26	21	6	103	61%		93%	45
595	DArg-BK-Ile-Tyr	25	34	12	189	47%		95%	45
596	Lys-Lys-BK-Ile-Tyr	18	21	9	497	0%		89%	45
597	DLys-Lys-BK-Ile-Tyr	5	1	5	165	0%		82%	45
598	[DPhe^{7}]-BK-Ile-Tyr	0.6	5.0*	0.2	1.6	70%		52%	45
599	DArg[DPhe^{7}[-BK-Ile-Tyr	0.7	6.2*	MXD	MXD		*11*	67%	45
602	[Hyp^{3},Thi^{5,8},DPhe^{7}]-BK-Ile-Tyr	0.1	0	0	0			32%	45

Table 1 (continues)

Table 1 Continued

Number[b] NPC "B"	Structure	Contraction RUT	Contraction GPI	Blood Pressure IA	Blood Pressure IV	Blood Pressure Dest	Binding RUT	Binding GPI	Ref.
13602	[Hyp³,Thi⁵,⁸,DPhe⁷]-BK-Ile-Tyr	0.1	0	0	0			32%	45
603	DArg[Hyp³,Thi⁵,⁸,DPhe⁷]-BK-Ile-Tyr	0.02	6.7*	I	I		*5*	48%	45
600	[Thi⁵,⁸,DPhe⁷]-BK-Ile-Tyr	0.5	MXD	0.1	8	0%		44%	45
601	DArg[Thi⁵,⁸,DPhe⁷]-BK-Ile-Tyr	0.3	5.8*	I	I		*16*	52%	45
13107	[DPhe⁷]-BK-DIle-Tyr	0	0	0.3	2	75%		10%	45
13108	DArg[DPhe⁷]-BK-DIle-Tyr	0	0	0	0			31%	45
13109	[Thi⁵,⁸DPhe⁷]-BK-DIle-Tyr	0	0	0.2	2	55%		5%	45
13110	DArg[Thi⁵,⁸,DPhe⁷]-BK-DIle-Tyr	0	0	0	0			26%	45
13111	[Hyp³,Thi⁵,⁸,DPhe⁷]-BK-DIle-Tyr	0.03	0	0	0			4%	
13112	DArg[Hyp³,Thi⁵,⁸,DPhe⁷]-BK-DIle-Tyr	0	0	I	I			34%	
13113	[DNal¹,Thi⁵,⁸,DPhe⁷⁸]-BK-DIle-Tyr	0	5.2*	ins/0	ins/0			4%	
13114	DArg[DNal¹,Thi⁵,⁸,DPhe⁷]-BK-DIle-Tyr	0	0	0	0			5%	
13115	[DNal¹,Hyp³,Thi⁵,⁸,DPhe⁷]-BK-DIle-Tyr	0	0	ins/0	ins/0			8%	
13116	DArg[DNal¹,Hyp³,Thi⁵,⁸,DPhe⁷]-BK-DIle-Tyr	I	0	MXD	MXD			8%	
	BB. C-Terminal DTyr Analogs								
15408	[Hyp³,DPhe⁷]-BK-DTyr	0	0	0	0			10%	
15409	DArg[Hyp³,DPhe⁷]-BK-DTyr	I	MXD	0	0			43%	
15410	[DNal¹,Hyp³,DPhe⁷]-BK-DTyr	0	0	0	0			5%	

15411	DArg[DNal^{1},Hyp^{3},DPhe^{7}]-BK-DTyr	0	0	0	0		31%
15566	[Hyp^{3},Thi^{5,8},DPhe^{7}]-BK-DTyr	0	0	AG	AG	54%	9%
	DArg[Hyp^{3},Thi^{5,8},DPhe^{7}]-BK-DTyr	0	0	0	0		
15567	[DNal^{1},Hyp^{3},Thi^{5,8},DPhe^{7}]-BK-DTyr	0	MXD	0.1	5	0%	4%
15825	[DNal^{1},Hyp^{3},Thi^{5,8},DPhe^{7}]-BK-DTyr	0.4	0				7%
15826	[Phe^{3,9},DPhe^{7}]-BK-DTyr	0	0				7%
15827	DArg[Phe^{3,9},DPhe^{7}]-BK-DTyr	0	0				6%
15568	[Hyp^{3},DPhe^{7},Phe^{9}]-BK-DTyr	MXD	0	0	0		11%
15828	DArg[Hyp^{3},DPhe^{7},Phe^{9}]-BK-DTyr	0	0				23%
15829	[Phe^{2,9},Hyp^{3},DPhe^{7}]-BK-DTyr	0	0				1%
	Arg[Phe^{2,9},Hyp^{3},DPhe^{7}]-BK-DTyr	0	0				
	CC. BPP5a Analogs at C-Terminal						
14370	BK-KWAP	2	33	22	231	75%	*0.92*
14535	Lys-BK-KWAP	4	9	2	254	0%	70%
14371	Lys-Lys-BK-KWAP	3	14	9	763	0%	*24*
14536	DArg-BK-KWAP	6	19	3	178	28%	82%
14537	BK-WAP	24	4	0.2	5	71%	89%
14538	DArg-BK-WAP	11	1	0.2	9	20%	78%
15340	[Lys^{9}]-BK-WAP	0.1	0.1	0	0		71%
15342	Lys-Lys-BK-WAP	0	AG	AG	AG	0%	28%
15341	DArg[Lys^{9}]-BK-WAP	0	0	AG	AG	76%	68%

Table 1 (continues)

Table 1 Continued

Number[b] NPC "B"	Structure	Contraction RUT	Contraction GPI	Blood Pressure IA	Blood Pressure IV	Blood Pressure Dest	Binding RUT	Binding GPI	Ref.
14532	[DPhe⁷]-BK-KWAP	1	0	0	0			43%	
14533	Lys[DPhe⁷]-BK-KWAP	0.8	0	0.3	34	0%		38%	
14372	Lys-Lys[DPhe⁷]-BK-KWAP	0.3	0	0.3	10	3%		35%	
14534	DArg[DPhe⁷]-BK-KWAP	1	0	0.4	26	11%		47%	
14539	DArg[DPhe⁷]-BK-WAP	0.2	0	0.1	0.9	80%		45%	
15339	Lys-Lys[DPhe⁷]-BK-WAP	0.1	0	0	0			18%	
	DD. Analogs with Single Deletions								
14717	desArg¹[Hyp³,DPhe⁷]-BK	0	0	0	0			7%	
14716	desArg¹[DPhe⁷]-BK	0	0					5%	
14715	desArg¹-BK	0	0	0	0			21%	
13097	desPro²[Hyp³,DPhe⁷]-BK	0	0	0	0			4%	45,47
13098	DArg-desPro²[Hyp³,DPhe⁷]-BK	5.4*	0	I	I			29%	45,47
	desGly⁴[Hyp³,DPhe⁷]-BK	0	0	0	0				45
	DArg-desGly⁴[Hyp³,DPhe⁷]-BK	0	0	0	0				45
13095	desPro³[bAla²,DPhe⁷]-BK	0	0	0	0			2%	
13096	DArg-desPro³[bAla²,DPhe⁷]-BK	0.1	5.4*	0	0			89%	
13102	desPro³[Phe²,DPhe⁷]-BK	0	0	0	0				45
13103	DArg-desPro³[Phe²,DPhe⁷]-BK	5.6*	0	PRS	PRS			27%	45
13104	desPro²[DPhe¹,Hyp³,DPhe⁷]-BK	0	0	0	0			3%	45,48
13105	desPro²[DNal¹,Hyp³,DPhe⁷]-BK	0	0	0	0			3%	45,48
13106	desPro²[DArg¹,Hyp³,DPhe⁷]-BK	0	0	I	I			6%	45,48
13124	desPro²[Hyp³,DPhe⁷,Phe⁹]-BK	0	0	0	0			13%	

13125	DArg-desPro^{2}[Hyp^{3},DPhe^{7}, Phe^{9}]-BK	0	0	MXD	MXD	8%	
13126	desPro^{2}[DArg^{1},Hyp^{3},DPhe^{7}, Phe^{9}]-BK	0	0	0	0	15%	
13127	DArg-desPro^{2}[DArg^{1},Hyp^{3}, DPhe^{7},Phe^{9}]-BK	0	0	0	0	3%	
	EE. Analogs with Multiple Deletions/Truncations						
	des(Pro^{2},Gly^{4})[Hyp^{3},DPhe^{7}]-BK	0	0	0	0		45,47
	DArg-des(Pro^{2},Gly^{4})[Hyp^{3},DPhe^{7}]-BK	0	0	0	0		45,47
13099	desPro^{2,3}[DPhe^{7}]-BK	0	0	0	0		45,47
	DArg-desPro^{2,3}[DPhe^{7}]-BK	I	5.3*	MXD	MXD		45,47
13822	desPro^{2,3}[DArg^{1},DPhe^{7}]-BK	0	MXD	0	0	12%	
13823	desPro^{2,3}[DNal^{1},DPhe^{7}]-BK	0	0	0	0	26%	
13824	desPro^{2,3}[DPhe^{1},DPhe^{7}]-BK	0	0	0	0	18%	
13825	desPro^{2,3}[DPal^{1},DPhe^{7}]-BK	0	0	0	0	16%	
13826	desPro^{2,3}[DArg^{1},Thi^{5,8}, Phe^{7}]-BK	0	0	I	I	32%	
13827	desPro^{2,3}[DNal^{1},Thi^{5,8}, DPhe^{7}]-BK	0	0	0	0	18%	
13828	desPro^{2,3}[DPhe,Thi^{5,8},DPhe^{7}]-BK	0	0	0	0	20%	
13119	desPro^{2}[Pba^{1},Hyp^{3},DPhe^{7}]-BK	0	5.2*	ins	ins	1%	45,47
13820	desPro^{2}[Bz^{1},Hyp^{3},DArg^{6},DPhe^{7}]-BK	0	0	0	0	18%	
13821	desPro^{2}[Pba^{1},Hyp^{3},DArg^{6}, DPhe^{7}]-BK	4.9*	0	0	0	5%	

Table 1 (continues)

Table 1 Continued

Number[b] NPC "B"	Structure	Contraction RUT	Contraction GPI	Blood Pressure IA	Blood Pressure IV	Blood Pressure Dest	Binding RUT	Binding GPI	Ref.
14712	Pro-Gly-Phe-Ser-Pro-Phe-Arg	0	0					[illegible]	
14714	Hyp-Gly-Phe-Ser-DPhe-Phe-Arg	0	MXD	MXD	MXD			4%	
14713	Pro-Gly-Phe-Ser-DPhe-Phe-Arg	0	0	0	0			4%	
14711	Gly-Phe-Ser-DPhe-Phe-Arg	0	0	0	0			5%	
14710	Gly-Phe-Ser-Pro-Phe-Arg	0	0	0	0			6%	
	Gly-Thi-Ser-DPhe-Thi-Arg	0	0	0	0				
14000	Ppa-Gly-Phe-Ser-DPhe-Phe-Arg	0	MXD	MXD	MXD			6%	
13999	Paa-Gly-Phe-Ser-DPhe-Phe-Arg	0	4.9*	0	0			4%	
14001	Pba-Gly-Phe-Ser-DPHe-Phe-Arg	0	4.9*	0	0			7%	50
14318	Aaa-Gly-Phe-Ser-DPhe-Phe-Arg	0	I	ins	ins			3%	
14007	Ppa-Gly-Thi-Ser-DPhe-Thi-Arg	0	4.9*	0	0			4%	
14008	Aaa-Gly-Thi-Ser-DPhe-Thi-Arg	5.0*	5.0*	0	0			5%	
14321	Pba-Gly-Thi-Ser-DPhe-Thi-Arg	0	0	ins	ins			2%	
14009	Paa-DAla-Phe-Ser-DPhe-Phe-Arg	0	I	0	0			2%	
14010	Ppa-DAla-Phe-Ser-DPhe-Phe-Arg	0	MXD	ins	ins			1%	
14319	Paa-DIle-Phe-Ser-DPhe-Phe-Arg	0	9	MXD	0			4%	
14322	Lau-Gly-Thi-Ser-DPhe-Thi-Arg	0	I	ins	ins			2%	
14320	Aaa-DIle-Phe-Ser-DPhe-Phe-Arg	0	0	ins	ins			2%	
14323	Tba-Gly-Thi-Ser-DPhe-Thi-Arg	0	0	0	0			3%	
14324	Nba-Gly-Thi-Ser-DPhe-Thi-Arg	0	MXD	0	0			9%	50
14325	Cpa-Gly-Thi-Ser-DPhe-Thi-Arg	0	I	0	0			2%	
14326	Cha-Gly-Thi-Ser-DPhe-Thi-Arg	0	4.9*	I	0			0%	
14004	Bz-Gly-Phe-DArg-DPhe-Phe-Arg	0	0	0	0			4%	

14005	Pba-Gly-Phe-DArg-DPhe-Phe-Arg	0	0	0.1	0.7	80%	5%
14708	Phe-Ser-Pro-Phe-Arg	0	0	0	0		2%
	Thi-Ser-DPhe-Thi-Arg	0	0	AG	AG	84%	
14709	Phe-Ser-DPHe-Phe-Arg	0	0	0	0		5%
14015	Aaa-Thi-Ser-DPhe-Thi-Arg	0	4.8	ins	ins		4%
14011	Ac-Thi-Ser-DPhe-Thi-Arg	0	0	0	0		3%
14012	Paa-Thi-Ser-DPhe-Thi-Arg	0	4.9	0	0		3%
14013	Ppa-Thi-Ser-DPhe-Thi-Arg	0	MXD	0	0		4%
14016	Ac-Thi-Ser-DPhe-Pro-Arg	0	0	0	0		30%
14017	Paa-Thi-Ser-DPhe-Pro-Arg	0	MXD	0	0		0%
14018	Ppa-Thi-Ser-DPhe-Pro-Arg	0	0	0	0		0%
14019	Pba-Thi-Ser-DPhe-Pro-Arg	0	0	0	0		0%
14020	Aaa-Thi-Ser-DPhe-Pro-Arg	0	MXD	0	0		0%
14706	Ser-Pro-Phe-Arg	0	0				5%
14707	Ser-DPhe-Phe-Arg	0	0	0	0		3%
14021	Ppa-Ser-DPhe-Thi-Arg	0.5	4.9*	0.3	0.7	94%	37%
14022	Pba-Ser-DPhe-Thi-Arg	0	4.8*	0	MXD		1%
14023	Aaa-Ser-DPhe-Thi-Arg	0	5.0*	3	0.5	99%	2%
14024	Ppa-Ser-DPhe-Pro-Arg	0	MXD	0	0		6%
14025	Pba-Ser-DPhe-Pro-Arg	0	0	0	0		7%
14704	Pro-Phe-Arg	0	MXD	0	0		8%
14705	DPhe-Phe-Arg	0	MXD	0	0		7%
14028	Ppa-DPhe-Thi-Arg	0	0	0	0		3%
14029	Pba-DPhe-Thi-Arg	0	4.7*	0	0		9%
14310	Aaa-DPhe-Thi-Arg	0	4.9*	ins	ins		8%
14026	Ppa-DPhe-Pro-Arg	0	0	0	0		5%
14027	Pba-DPhe-Pro-Arg	0	0	0	0		4%
14703	Phe-Arg	0	0	0	0		0%

Table 1 (continues)

Table 1 Continued

Number[b] NPC "B"	Structure	Contraction RUT	Contraction GPI	Blood Pressure IA	Blood Pressure IV	Blood Pressure Dest	Binding RUT	Binding GPI	Ref.
15371	Pba-Phe-Arg	0	0.04	0.8	0				
15372	Pba-Thi-Arg	0	0	0.2	7	34%		0%	
15373	Pba-Pro-Arg	0	0	0	0			2%	

[a]Biological activities of BK analogs on rat uterus (RUT) and guinea pig ileum (GPI), and on rat blood pressure (RBP) by intraarterial (IA) or intravenous (IV) administration. Percent apparent pulmonary destruction (Dest) for RBP agonist analogs is calculated from the IA and IV potencies. Agonist potency is relative to BK = 100%. AG indicates agonist activity not precisely determined. Antagonist activity on smooth muscle is indicated by pA_2 values (followed by asterisks) or by I where antagonist potency was not precisely determined. Antagonist activity in RBP is indicated by I, where a reduction of the response of an ED_{25mm} dose of BK was produced following bolus administration of BK plus antagonist. PRS indicates pressor effect; DPR indicates depressor effect. MXD indicates mixed agonist/antagonist activity; INS indicates that the peptide is insoluble at required concentrations. Competition for BK binding was in membranes from RUT or GPI (see Ref. 30 for methods). Presented are K_i values in nM (*in italics*), or percent inhibition at antagonist concentration of 1 μM.

[b]All compounds were synthesized by Vavrek and Stewart except those marked with superscript b, which were synthesized by Douglas Kalvin at Nova Pharmaceutical Corp. All biological data are from John Stewart and Ray Vavrek. All binding data are from Ronald M. Burch and represent means from at least three separate experiments.

Abbreviations: Aaa = adamantylacetyl; Ac = acetyl; Aib = α-aminoisobutyric acid; Azt = azetine-carboxylic acid; bAla = β-Ala; Bz = benzoyl; CDF = p-chloro-DPhe; Cha = cyclohexyl-Ala; cHyp = *cis*-4-hydroxy-Pro; Cpa = cyclopropyl-Ala; DHP = 3,4-dehydro-Pro; FDF = *p*-fluoro-DPhe; hPhe = homo-Phe; Hyp = *trans*-4-hydroxy-Pro; Inip = isonipecotic acid; Lau = lauroyl; KWAP = Lys-Trp-Ala-Pro; MDY = O-methyl-DTyr; Nal = β-2-naphthyl-Ala; Nba = norbornyl; NMF = N-methyl-Phe; Oct = octanoyl; OMT = O-methyl-Tyr; Paa = phenylacetyl; Pal = β-3-pyridyl-Ala; Pba = phenylbutyryl; PCF = *p*-chloro-Phe; Phg = phenyl-Gly; Ppa = phenylpropionyl; Sta = stearoyl; Tba = *t*-butylacetyl; Thi = β-2-thienyl-Ala; and Thz = thiazolidine carboxylic acid; WAP = Trp-Ala-Pro.

Structures are indicated as follows: A residue appended to the beginning of a compound is added to the N-terminus of BK. Thus, Lys-BK is *Lys*-Arg-Pro-Pro-Gly-Phe-Ser-Pro-Phe-Arg. Residues inside brackets replace the numbered natural residue in BK. Thus, [Thi^5]-BK is Arg-Pro-Pro-Gly-*Thi*-Ser-Pro-Phe-Arg. Residues appended after BK are added to the C-terminus. Thus, BK-Ile-Tyr is Arg-Pro-Pro-Gly-Phe-Ser-Pro-Phe-Arg-*Ile-Tyr*. The term "des" indicates that the named residue has been deleted from the structure. Thus, desPro$_2$-BK is Arg-Pro-Gly-Phe-Ser-Pro-Phe-Arg.

number of bradykinin analogs synthesized in this laboratory with the aim of increasing the potency, selectivity, and lifetime of action of bradykinin antagonists. This table does not include B1 receptor antagonists, which are discussed in Chapter 2. Methods for synthesis of these peptides have been described (4,10).

II. STRUCTURE-ACTIVITY RELATIONSHIPS IN ANTAGONISTS

A. Substitution at Position 7

During the course of structure-activity studies of bradykinin analogs many modifications of the Pro residue at position 7 were investigated. Replacement of Pro at position 7 by Ala or by D-Pro destroyed biological activity, as did most other substitutions (Table 1, Section C). A striking difference in this pattern came with the introduction of α-aminoisobutyric acid (Aib) in position 7. [Aib^7]bradykinin proved to be a superagonist in the guinea pig ileum assay and had very good potency in the other assay systems (11). Since this unnatural, symmetrical amino acid is not optically active, its interaction with bradykinin receptors could be in a conformation that resembles either a D- or a L-amino acid residue. This observation prompted examination of a large number of bradykinin analogs having D-amino acid residues in position 7. Among these analogs, [DPhe^7]-bradykinin proved to be the first bradykinin analog showing competitive antagonist activity on any classical kinin assay system. This antagonist activity was seen only in assays on isolated guinea pig ileum, and this analog showed weak agonist activity in the other two assays performed routinely in this laboratory, isolated rat uterus and rat blood pressure (4). Acting on the assumption that modifications previously found to enhance receptor affinity might increase the potency of this very weak antagonist, Thi was placed in positions 5 and 8, Hyp was placed in positions 2 and 3, and basic residues or dipeptides were added to the amino end of the molecule. These manipulations were successful in converting the weak partial antagonist of action of [DPhe^7]-bradykinin to that of a much more potent analog with antagonist activity on all the standard assay tissues (12-14). Among these antagonists DArg[Hyp^3,DPhe^7]bradykinin (NPC 567), DArg[Hyp^3,Thi^{5,8},DPhe^7]bradykinin (NPC 349), and Lys-Lys[Hyp^3,Thi^{5,8},DPhe^7]bradykinin (NPC 415), have been widely used by different investigators (15-17). NPC 567 is in clinical trials for use as an antibradykinin drug in several pathological states.

Only a narrow range of D-amino acid residues appears to be acceptable at position 7 for production of bradykinin antagonist activity. D-Phe has been most widely used and appears to be acceptable in analogs having a wide variety of additional structure modifications. The phenyl ring in [DPhe[7]]bradykinin (NPC 361) can be halogenated in the *para* position (NPC 331, NPC 809) with retention of activity, but a hydroxy ([D-Tyr[7]]-bradykinin, NPC 382) or methoxy group (NPC 425) is not acceptable. The more polar thiophene (NPC 379) and pyridine (NPC 358) rings are acceptable, but imidazole (NPC 356) is not; neither are the larger rings naphthalene (NPC 357) and indole (NPC 380). The distance between the phenyl ring and the peptide backbone at this position is apparently critical as well. Neither phenylglycine (NPC 377) nor homophenylalanine (NPC 359) in position 7 yields an antagonist.

Lacking any knowledge of the three-dimensional hormone-combining surface of the bradykinin receptor, one can only speculate as to the reason for antagonist activity of bradykinin analogs containing a D-aromatic amino acid residue at position 7. Proline residues in peptides, because of their cyclic structure, exert a major influence on peptide conformation. Proteins frequently contain beta-turns at Pro residues, and bradykinin in solution does show a beta- or gamma-turn at position 7 (18). The presence of this Pro can be expected to have a significant effect on the conformation of bradykinin in the receptor-bound position, and replacement of this Pro by a noncyclic α-amino acid can be expected to cause a significant change. However, such a replacement is not sufficient for formation of antagonists, as has been amply demonstrated; it generally leads only to inactive analogs, which cannot bind to bradykinin receptors. This is the case with [Phe[7]]bradykinin (NPC 13810). However, in the case of the D-isomer the aromatic side chain being in the opposite configuration possibly fits into a hydrophobic pocket of restricted size and accessibility on the receptor. This interaction, then, apparently allows strong binding to the receptor, but prevents combination of the peptide with the receptor in a way that causes activation of the second-messenger systems coupled to the receptor.

Another function of Pro residues in peptides and proteins is to regulate the conformation of the peptide bond itself. Except for X-Pro bonds, peptide bonds are stabilized by resonance in a planar, *trans* conformation. The *trans* designation means that in the peptide group, -C = O-NH-, the oxygen of the carbonyl group and the hydrogen on the nitrogen are on opposite sides of the peptide backbone. In the *cis* conformation these two atoms are on the same side of the backbone, but this conformation is prohibited by steric interaction in non-Pro peptides. In X-Pro peptide bonds the hydrogen atom normally on the nitrogen is replaced by C-5 of the Pro ring. With carbon chains in both positions on the nitrogen, there is much less energy difference between *cis* and *trans* conformations, and *cis* X-Pro bonds are found in many proteins (19). Interconversion between the two forms is slow, and may have a half-time of the order of minutes. Nuclear magnetic resonance (NMR) studies showed that there is about 10% *cis* conformation of the Ser-Pro bond of bradykinin, while the bonds to the prolines in positions two and three were in the normal *trans* conformation. In [Gly^6]bradykinin there appeared to be about 30% *cis* conformation at the 6-7 position (20). The fact that [Gly^6]bradykinin has about 30% the agonist potency of bradykinin on smooth muscles suggested that the Ser-Pro bond may need to be in the *trans* conformation for combination with receptors, although there is surely no firm evidence for this. It is also not clear at this time what implications this *cis-trans* ratio may have for bradykinin antagonist action.

B. Substitution at Position 6

Studies with bradykinin agonists suggested that the Ser residue in position 6 served principally as a "spacer" to hold more important amino acid residues in the proper conformation for combination with the receptor. The finding, mentioned above, that the serine residue appeared to prevent *cis*-Pro structure at the 6-7 bond suggested that the role of this residue might be more important, and prompted investigation of a number of position 6 analogs (see Table 1, Section B). Among those analogs, only the peptides having *p*-chloro-D-Phe and D-Trp at position 6 showed significant agonist activity. Following discovery of the D-aromatic 7 antagonists, a series of analogs having D-aromatic residues in both positions 6 and 7 was synthesized (Table 1, Section F). Several of these showed good antagonist activity on guinea pig ileum and blood pressure, but in some cases retained slight agonist activity on rat uterus.

C. Substitutions at Positions 5 and 8

The two Phe residues at positions 5 and 8 in bradykinin have generally been found to be essential for kinin agonist activity (1,2). The finding that replacement of these Phe residues in bradykinin by Thi gave superagonists (Table 1, Section A) and the later observation that this potency was probably due to increased receptor affinity prompted incorporation of Thi into the initial [DPhe^7]bradykinin antagonist (4). This modification increased the potency of [DPhe^7]bradykinin antagonism on guinea pig ileum and broadened the spectrum of antagonism to include rat uterus and rat blood pressure. Consequently, this modification has been used in a wide variety of subsequent bradykinin antagonists (Table 1, Section C and others).

The discovery that replacement of the Phe residue at position 8 of bradykinin antagonist analogs by Pro yielded effective antagonists was surprising (Table 1, Section J), especially since slight modification of the residue at position 8 had not seemed to be acceptable (Table 1, Section O). Antagonist activity was also found when Hyp was present at position 8, but D-Pro at position 8 destroyed activity.

D. Substitutions at Positions 2 and 3

The Pro residues at positions 2 and 3 of bradykinin, like that at position 7, cause turns in the solution conformation of the peptide chain. For significant agonist activity, the Pro at position 2 is essential, and cannot be replaced by Ala or D-Pro with retention of significant activity (1). In contrast, the Pro at position 3 can be replaced by Ala with retention of full agonist potency. Replacement of either of these Pro residues by Hyp yields superagonists, especially with respect to potency on rat uterus (8).

Similar modifications at positions 2 and 3 were tried in antagonist analogs. Hyp at position 2 or 3 was found to yield very good antagonists (14), and this type of modification was used extensively throughout all the work in the search for more potent and more selective bradykinin antagonists. Among other substitutions in positions 2 and 3 (Table 1, Section Q), the acceptability of D- or L-Phe in antagonists was remarkable. These antagonists, in contrast to most bradykinin antagonists, were inactive on guinea pig ileum, but showed antagonist activity on rat uterus and blood pressure. Thiazolidine carboxylic acid was acceptable in either position, or both simultaneously (NPC 444 and the following compounds in the table), but changing the size of the heterocyclic ring did not yield potent antagonists (NPC 329 and following compounds in table). Ser and Thr were also acceptable at position 2 of antagonists (NPC 15856 and NPC 15858).

E. Substitution at Positions 1 and 9

A basic amino acid residue is necessary in both positions 1 and 9 of analogs for agonist activity on all kinin receptors except those of the B1 class, which recognize desArg^9-bradykinin. With many biologically active peptides it has been found that more extensive structural alterations are possible in antagonists than in agonists (21), and the kinins are no exception to this generalization. Significant bradykinin antagonist activity has been found in analogs in which either one of the basic residues has been replaced, and in one case (NPC 13743, Table 1, Section W), both Arg residues were replaced by aromatic amino acids with retention of some antagonist activity. D-aromatic amino acids appear to be generally acceptable in position 1 of bradykinin antagonists (Table 1, Section 7). Most of these show antagonist activity on rat uterus and blood pressure without any activity on guinea pig ileum. Replacement of the amino acid in position 1 by a simple acyl group has yielded an interesting antagonist in one case (NPC 13818). This analog, with a benzoic acid residue in position 1, is a good antagonist selective for rat uterus.

Several antagonists were found among analogs with modifications at position 9 (Table 1, Sections K,L). Presence of a D-amino acid residue or nonbasic residue at this position should make the peptide stable against aminopeptidase N (kininase 1) of plasma, a major inactivating enzyme for kinins. D-Arg in position 9 of bradykinin destroys agonist activity (1), but when used in conjunction with D-Phe at position 7 and Pro at position 8, several antagonists were found (Table 1, Section L). These were selective for guinea pig ileum, without activity in the other assays. One analog having Phe in position 9 (NPC 15356) was found to be an effective antagonist in all assays. This modification probably deserves further investigation.

F. Antagonists with N-Terminal Modifications

Since the discovery that Lys-Lys-bradykinin was completely stable on passage through the pulmonary circulation in rats and was not degraded by isolated angiotensin converting enzyme (ACE) (6), addition of basic amino acid residues to the N-terminus of bradykinin analogs has become a valuable tool (Table 1, Section A). The addition of a single Lys residue, or of a D-Lys or D-Arg residue, to bradykinin confers some resistance to degradation by pulmonary enzymes, although not so impressive as the Lys-Lys modification. These bradykinin agonists with N-terminal basic extensions have high affinity for receptors and show superagonist biological activity in most systems. It was logical to apply these same modifications to the newly discovered antagonists, and indeed, these N-extended antagonists were found to have enhanced potency. Most of the practically useful bradykinin antagonists possess modifications of this type. The D-Arg modification seems to give better potency to most antagonists than does the Lys-Lys modification, even though DArg-bradykinin is less stable to pulmonary degradation than is Lys-Lys-bradykinin (Table 1, Section A). Ile-Ser-bradykinin is produced by treatment of rat plasma with trypsin. It is the major kinin in the rat and has been called "T-kinin" (22). Several analogs of bradykinin antagonists were synthesized incorporating various modifications of this Ile-Ser extension (Table 1, Section Y). These proved generally to be broad-spectrum antagonists with quite good potency in some cases.

N-terminal acylation of bradykinin has long been known to be consistent with agonist activity (2). Several analogs of bradykinin with large aliphatic acyl groups were explored in the hope of obtaining membrane-selective analogs with extended life (Table 1, Section X). Several acetylated antagonists were synthesized (NPC 15337 and following compounds in the table) and were found to have potencies not grossly different from the same antagonists lacking the acetyl group. It has been suggested that N-terminal acetylation of antagonists may prevent release of histamine from mast cells by these compounds (23).

G. Antagonists With C-Terminal Modifications

A free carboxyl group of the C-terminal arginine of bradykinin has long been considered essential for significant agonist activity. The only exception to this generalization comes with phyllokinin and its analogs, in which bradykinin is extended at the C-terminus with the sulfated dipeptide -Ile-Tyr(SO_4) (2). Although bradykinin amide has no agonist activity, amides of several antagonist sequences were synthesized to see if this same rule carried over into the antagonists (Table 1, Section Z). With the exception of two analogs, which had antagonist activity on blood pressure (NPC 821, NPC 825), the other amides were inactive. Substituted amides of C-terminal fragments of bradykinin had earlier been reported (24) to be bradykinin antagonists in smooth muscles, but they were not specific for kinins and evidently did not act at kinin receptors.

Since the nonsulfated form of phyllokinin has good agonist potency (NPC 594), several antagonist sequences were modified with C-terminal extensions related to phyllokinin (Table 1, Sections AA and BB). Two of these (NPC 599 and NPC 603) had quite good antagonist potency on guinea pig ileum and were also active on rat blood pressure. The simple addition of -Ile-Tyr to the C-terminus of [DPhe^7]bradykinin (NPC 598) yielded an antagonist with essentially the same potency and pattern of activities as [DPhe^7]-bradykinin itself.

Antagonist analogs extended at the C-terminus with -DIle-Tyr should be particularly useful, if good potency could be obtained. Such peptides should not be degraded by either ACE or plasma carboxypeptidase N. Unfortunately, with the exception of one antagonist active on blood pressure (NPC 13112), these peptides were not interesting. The analogs with a single D-Tyr addition at the C-terminus (Table 1, Section BB) were disappointing.

The bradykinin-potentiating peptides from *Bothrops jararaca* are excellent inhibitors of ACE. These peptides served as models for the currently widely used converting enzyme inhibitors captopril and enalapril. The simplest of the bradykinin-potentiating peptides from *Bothrops* venom has the structure Pyroglu-Lys-Trp-Ala-Pro (25). With the aim of incorporating a converting enzyme inhibitor into a bradykinin antagonist, several analogs having C-terminal extensions related to this bradykinin potentiating peptide were synthesized (Table 1, Section CC). Several of these bradykinin derivatives had significant agonist potency (NPC 14370 and following compounds in the table), but addition of this extension to antagonist-like sequences did not yield active compounds.

H. Analogs Lacking the Full Kinin Chain

As was mentioned above, more severe structural modification is possible in bradykinin antagonists than in agonists. This observation was pursued further by synthesis of a group of analogs having deletion of one or more amino acid residues from within the kinin sequence or from the N-terminus of the chain (Table 1, Sections DD and EE). The chain of bradykinin itself modified in these ways does not show any agonist activity. Although most of these shortened analogs were totally inactive, a few instances of antagonist—and even agonist—activity were found. In the shortened analogs, antagonist activity was most commonly found among peptides in which the N-terminus was blocked with a large acyl group.

III. SPECIFICITY OF BRADYKININ ANTAGONISTS

The bradykinin antagonists which possess the full kinin sequence with a basic residue in positions 1 and 9 are quite specific for antagonism of bradykinin and related kinins. They do not antagonize the responses of tissues to other peptides such as angiotensin II and substance P on guinea pig ileum or of angiotensin II or vasopressin on rat uterus. The competitive nature of the antagonism has been demonstrated both in biological responses and in binding to receptors (or binding sites) on cells, tissues, and membranes (see Chapter 1). When the structure is modified more extensively, however, such as by replacement of one of the basic residues or shortening of the peptide chain, the resulting peptide may antagonize biological responses to other peptides as well as to bradykinin. NPC 573, [DNal^{1},Thi^{5,8},DPhe^{7}]bradykinin, which antagonized the action of bradykinin on rat uterus and blood pressure, but not on guinea pig ileum, was found to antagonize the action of vasopressin on rat uterus (26). Remarkably, this peptide did not appear to bind to bradykinin receptors in ileum or uterus or to vasopressin receptors. The investigators suggested that the antagonism shown by this peptide is probably mediated through nonreceptor mechanisms. Several analogs shorted at the N-terminus and acylated with aromatic acid groups were found to antagonize substance P on ileum and angiotensin II on ileum or uterus. For example, antagonism of substance P action on ileum was seen with NPCs 13119, 14000, 13999, 14318, 14007, 14321, 14012, 14013, 14022, 14023, and 14028 (Table 1, Section EE). Action of angiotensin II on ileum was antagonized by NPCs 13119, 14000, 13999, 14008, 14022, 14024, and 14026. Contractions evoked by angiotensin II on rat uterus were inhibited by NPCs 13119, 14000, 14008, and 14019. It is not known at this time whether or not these peptides actually bind to receptors for substance P and angiotensin II. While most of these peptides also showed bradykinin antagonist action, NPCs 14321 and 14028 did not.

IV. SELECTIVITY OF BRADYKININ ANTAGONISTS

Until the description of the bradykinin B1 system of Regoli, it had been assumed that all actions of bradykinin were mediated through a single relatively homogeneous class of receptors. Even then, the remaining actions of bradykinin were thought to be mediated by a single class of B2 receptors. With the discovery of the full-chain bradykinin B2 antagonists in this laboratory and application of them to a wide variety of biological systems by various investigators, it has become increasingly clear that there are several subclasses of bradykinin receptors which recognize and require the entire nonapeptide chain for agonist action. This information was not apparent from studies with agonist analogs, since the differences found in potency of various analogs on various tissues was thought to be due to relative abundance of bradykinin-degrading enzymes in the different tissues.

Work with the initial bradykinin antagonist [DPhe^{7}]bradykinin already suggested heterogeneity of bradykinin receptors on smooth muscle, since it was an antagonist on guinea pig ileum, but a weak agonist on rat uterus and rat blood pressure. The more potent antagonists (such as NPCs 567, 349, and 415) developed by further modification of the [DPhe^7]bradykinin structure were found to be broad-spectrum antagonists. In addition to being good antagonists on the three classical assay systems used in this laboratory, these compounds have proved to be effective bradykinin antagonists in a wide variety of systems.

Inspection of Table 1 will reveal several antagonists having different spectra of antagonist activity. Some antagonists have been found to be effective against two of the assays without activity on the third. Among these, NPC 13750 (Section J) and NPC 13121 (Section K) are active on the isolated smooth muscle assays (rat uterus and guinea pig ileum), but not on rat blood pressure. Antagonists active on rat uterus and blood pressure, but not on guinea pig ileum, are NPCs 13024, 13031, 13033 (Section O), 13062, and 13074 (Section T). Antagonists active on ileum and blood pressure, but not on rat uterus, are NPC 13752 and NPC 13749 (Section J). Antagonists quite specific for only one tissue have also been found. Among those specific for rat uterus are NPCs 13023 (Section O), 14516, 13084 (Section J), and 13818 (Section U). Among those specific for guinea pig ileum are NPC 15397 and NPC 15398 (Section L). Among those active only on rat blood pressure are NPCs 14514 (Section J), 13025, 13026 (Section O), and 821 (Section Z).

Among other biological systems, neuronal and smooth-muscle bradykinin receptors in rat vas deferens were differentiated by use of bradykinin antagonists. [Thi^{5,8},DPhe^7]bradykinin (NPC 431) is an antagonist on smooth muscle receptors in this tissue, but is an agonist for neuronal receptors. In contrast, DArg[Hyp^3,Thi^{5,8},DPhe^7]bradykinin (NPC 349) is an antagonist on both receptors (27). Comparing action of these two antagonists in this tissue with their actions on other smooth muscles, Table 1 shows that while both compounds have the same pA_2 on guinea pig ileum, NPC 349 is a far better antagonist on rat uterus than is NPC 431. NPC 431 was also an agonist for stimulation of phosphatidyl inositol turnover in the neuronal cell line N1E-115 (28). A further dissociation of neuronal and tissue kinin receptors is seen with use of NPC 573. As noted above, this analog antagonized bradykinin and vasopressin action on uterus but did not combine with uterus receptors. This analog was unable to block kinin-evoked vascular pain, but blocked the hyperalgesia due to bradykinin- or urate-evoked tissue inflammation (29).

Although bradykinin is a potent agonist for bronchoconstriction, several of the potent D-aromatic 7 antagonists were unable to block the action of bradykinin in guinea pig trachea. Farmer and coworkers have concluded that the bradykinin receptors in this tissue are of a different class and have suggested the designation "B3" for these kinin receptors (30). In contrast, bradykinin-evoked ciliary movement in rabbit trachea epithelial cells was blocked by a B2 antagonist (31). In another tissue, opossum esophagus, Goyal has found that all the D-aromatic 7 antagonists are agonists, suggesting that this tissue contains an even further class of kinin receptors (32).

In various tissues, kinins produce their effects through activation of every known second-messenger system, and potent B2 bradykinin antagonists have been able to block the effects of bradykinin in all these types of responses. In some other hormone and neurotransmitter systems, receptors have been classified on the basis of the second-messenger system involved, and it has been possible to correlate the mechanism with agonist or antagonist structures. At the moment it does not seem possible to categorize bradykinin receptors on the basis of second messengers. The present working system, based on agonist and antagonist effectiveness, remains the working model as our understanding of kinin biology evolves.

V. ANTAGONIST STRUCTURE AND METABOLIC STABILITY

In order to preserve the role of bradykinin as a "local hormone," this peptide is degraded rapidly in vivo by several enzymes. The principal kininases studied have been carboxypeptidase N (CPN, kininase I) and ACE (Kininase II). CPN, a plasma enzyme, requires a C-terminal basic amino acid residue in substrates and causes the half-life of bradykinin in plasma to be about 15 seconds. ACE is localized to vascular membranes, principally in the pulmonary circulation, and destroys about 99% of the bradykinin in blood on a single pass through the pulmonary circulation. More recently, degradation by metalloendopeptidase EC 3.4.24.11, which cleaves bradykinin at the Gly4-Phe5 and Pro7-Phe8 bonds, and aminopeptidase P, EC 3.4.11.9, which removes the N-terminal residue from bradykinin, have been described (33). Evidence for some of these activities in blood-free rat pulmonary circulation has long been available (34). Rat lung has a very impressive hydrolytic activity; at least 100 mg of kinin analog can evidently be processed in a single passage through the pulmonary circulation (35).

The true relative potencies of kinin agonists in the blood pressure assay can be determined only from intraarterial administration of the peptide;

by this route of administration the peptide is not subjected to pulmonary enzymes before it reaches the peripheral circulation. Potency of kinin agonist analogs determined by intravenous administration is thus a reflection of pulmonary destruction as well as actual inherent agonist potency of the peptide. Intravenous potencies of agonists reported in Table 1 are relative to that of bradykinin, which is destroyed 98-99% upon passage through the pulmonary circulation. Pulmonary destruction of kinin agonist analogs is normally determined by comparison of the depressor potency of the peptide by intravenous and intraarterial administration (35). Apparent pulmonary destruction of all agonist analogs, determined in this way, is reported in Table 1. Further information on kininases can be found in Chapter 6 of this volume.

A major goal of bradykinin antagonist design in this laboratory is to incorporate into antagonist structures those features necessary to make the peptides resistant to the actions of all these enzymes. Analogs not susceptible to rapid degradation are particularly valuable for in vivo studies and for drug design. Although much progress has been made in this direction, the best antagonists now available do not have very long activity in vivo, suggesting the need for further improvement. The essential structure modification which gives rise to antagonist activity, incorporation of a D-amino acid in position 7, confers resistance to the action of ACE (36). Addition of a D-amino acid residue to the N-terminus should confer resistance to the action of aminopeptidase P. Designing resistance to CPN has been more difficult, due to the importance of the free carboxyl group of the basic C-terminal arginine residue. The C-terminus-extended analogs (Table 1, Sections AA-CC), which should overcome this problem, were disappointing. Other types of structural modification (37) may provide the necessary metabolic stability. Structure modifications designed to block cleavage of antagonists by the endopeptidase 24.11 are also in progress.

An antagonist such as DArg[DArg^{1},Hyp^{3},DPhe^{7},Phe^{9}]bradykinin (NPC 13123) should be resistant to the action of aminopeptidase P, ACE, and CPN. Persistence of the bradykinin antagonist action of this analog (and several others) in the rat in vivo has been examined. When this antagonist is infused at the rate necessary to cause a 50% inhibition of the depressor response to a bolus of bradykinin, and the infusion is stopped, the normal response to bradykinin returns in 10-15 minutes. Results with NPC 349 were similar. These results suggest that the antagonists are much more resistant to kininase action than is bradykinin, but that some enzyme susceptibility remains. Modifications to decrease renal clearance of these small peptides may also be necessary. In any event, the goal of a long-acting antagonist has not yet been achieved.

VI. CROSS-REFERENCES TO ANTAGONIST LITERATURE

Bradykinin antagonists synthesized in this laboratory have been used by a large number of investigators throughout the world. Due to the particular system of numbering peptides in this laboratory, there has been some duplication and confusion of numbers referring to a given peptide structure, especially for those most widely used. In addition, other investigators have assigned their numbers to the same peptides. In order to clarify this situation, Table 1 contains both "B" numbers provided by this laboratory, and NPC numbers provided by Nova Pharmaceutical Corp., as well as the actual peptide structure.

ACKNOWLEDGMENTS

Bradykinin antagonist studies at the University of Colorado were supported by grants from the United States National Institutes of Health (HL-26284) and Nova Pharmaceutical Corp.

REFERENCES

1. Schröder, E. Structure-activity relationships of kinins, in: *Bradykinin, Kallidin and Kallikrein* (*Handbuch Experimentellen Pharmakologie*), Vol. 25 (E. G. Erdos, ed.). Springer-Verlag, Heidelberg, pp. 324-350 (1970).
2. Stewart, J. M. Chemistry and biological activity of peptides related to bradykin, in: *Bradykinin, Kallidin and Kallikrein* (*Handbook of Experimental Pharmacology*), Vol. 25 (suppl) (E. G. Erdos, ed.). Springer, Heidelberg, pp. 227-272 (1979).
3. Regoli, D., and J. Barabé. Pharmacology of bradykinin and related kinins. *Pharmacol. Rev.* **32**:1-46 (1980).
4. Vavrek, R. J., and J. M. Stewart. Competitive antagonists of bradykinin. *Peptides* **6**:161-164 (1985).
5. Dunn, F. W., and J. M. Stewart. Analogs of bradykinin containing beta-2-thienyl-L-alanine. *J. Med. Chem.* **14**:779 (1971).
6. Dorer, F. E., J. M. Stewart, and J. W. Ryan. Studies on the hydrolysis of bradykinin by angiotensin converting enzyme (kininase II). *Experientia* **34**:1436 (1978).
7. Dorer, F. E., J. W. Ryan, and J. M. Stewart. Hydrolysis of bradykinin and its higher homologues by angiotensin converting enzyme. *Biochem. J.* **14**:915 (1974).

8. Stewart, J. M., J. W. Ryan, and A. H. Brady. Hydroxyproline analogs of bradykinin. *J. Med. Chem.* **17**:537 (1974).
9. Fredrick, M. J., R. J. Vavrek, J. M. Stewart, and C. E. Odya. Further studies of myometrial bradykinin receptor-like binding. *Biochem. Pharmacol.* **33**:2887-2892 (1984).
10. Stewart, J. M., and J. D. Young. *Solid Phase Peptide Synthesis.* Pierce Chemical Co., Rockford, IL (1984).
11. Vavrek, R. J., and J. M. Stewart. Bradykinin analogs containing alpha-aminoisobutyric acid. *Peptides* **1**:231-235 (1980).
12. Stewart, J. M., and R. J. Vavrek. Bradykinin competitive antagonists: design and applications, in: *Protides of the Biological Fluids*, Vol. 34 (H. Peeters, ed.). Pergamon, New York, pp. 473-476 (1986).
13. Stewart, J. M., and R. J. Vavrek. Bradykinin competitive antagonists for classical kinin systems, in: *Kinins IV* (*Adv. Exp. Med. Biol.* 198A) (L. M. Greenbaum and H. S. Margolius, eds.). Plenum, New York, pp. 537-542 (1986).
14. Vavrek, R. J., and J. M. Stewart. Bradykinin antagonists containing hydroxyproline, in: *Peptides 1986* (D. Theodoropoulos, ed.). deGruyter, Berlin, pp. 655-658 (1987).
15. Abe, K., H. Moriya, and S. Fujii (Eds.). *Kinins V*, parts A and B (*Adv. Exp. Med. Biol.* 247A and B). Plenum Press, New York (1989).
16. Griesbacher, T., and F. Lembeck. Effect of bradykinin antagonists on bradykinin-induced plasma extravasation, venoconstriction, prostaglandin E_2 release, nociceptor stimulation and contraction of the iris sphincter muscle in the rabbit. *Br. J. Pharmacol.* **92**:333-340 (1987).
17. Steranka, L. R., D. C. Manning, C. J. DeHaas, J. W. Ferkany, S. A. Borosky, J. R. Connor, R. J. Vavrek, J. M. Stewart, and S. H. Snyder. Bradykinin as a pain mediator: receptors localized to sensory neurons and antagonists have analgesic actions. *Proc. Natl. Acad. Sci. USA* **85**:3245-3249 (1988).
18. Cann, J. R., R. E. London, N. A. Matwiyoff, and J. M. Stewart. A combined spectroscopic study of the solution conformation of bradykinin, in: *Kinins-III*, Pt. A. (H. Fritz, N. Back, G. Dietze, and G. Haberland, eds.). Plenum Press, New York, pp. 495-500 (1982).
19. Takahashi, N., T. Hayano, and M. Suzuki. Peptidyl-prolyl *cis-trans* isomerase is the cyclosporine A-binding protein cyclophilin. *Nature* **337**:473-478 (1989).
20. London, R. E., J. M. Stewart, R. Williams, J. R. Cann, and N. A. Matwiyoff. Carbon-13 NMR spectroscopy of [20%-1,2-^{13}C2-Gly^{6}]-bradykinin. The role of serine in reducing structural heterogeneity. *J. Am. Chem. Soc.* **101**:2455-2462 (1979).
21. Manning, M., A. Misicka, A. Olma, W. A. Klis, K. Bankowski, E. Nawrocka, M. Kruszynski, A. Kolodziejczyk, L-L. Cheng, J. Seto, N. C. Wo, and W. H. Sawyer. C-terminal deletions in agonistic and antagonistic analogues of vasopressin that improve their specificities for antidiuretic (V2) and vasopressor (VI) receptors. *J. Med. Chem.* **30**:2245-2251 (1987).

22. Okamoto, H., and L. M. Greenbaum. Isolation and structure of T-kinin. *Biochem. Biophys. Res. Comm.* **112**:701-708 (1983).
23. Barabe, J., and D. Regoli. Kinin antagonists. *Methods Enzymol.* **163**:282-292 (1988).
24. Claeson, G., J. Fareed, C. Larsson, G. Kindel, S. Arielly, R. Simnonsson, H. L. Messmore, and J. U. Balis. Inhibition of the contractile action of bradykinin on isolated smooth muscle preparations by derivatives of low molecular weight peptides, in: *Kinins II* (S. Fujii, H. Moriya, and T. Suzuki, eds.). (*Adv. Exp. Med. Biol.* 120B). Plenum Press, New York, pp. 691-713 (1979).
25. Stewart, J. M., L. J. Greene, and S. H. Ferreira. Bradykinin potentiating peptide PCA-Lys-Trp-Ala-Pro: An inhibitor of the pulmonary inactivation of bradykinin and conversion of angiotensin I to II. *Biochem. Pharmacol.* **20**:1557 (1971).
26. Farmer, S. G., R. M. Burch, C. J. Dehaas, J. Togo, and L. R. Steranka. [Arg^1-D-Phe^7]-substituted bradykinin alalogs inhibit bradykinin- and vasopressin-induced contractions of uterine smooth muscle. *J. Pharmacol. Exp. Therap.* **248**:677-681 (1989).
27. Rifo, J., M. Pourrat, R. J. Vavrek, J. M. Stewart, and J. P. Huidobro-Toro. Bradykinin receptor antagonists used to characterize the heterogeneity of bradykinin-induced responses in rat vas deferens. *Eur. J. Pharmacol.* **142**: 305-312 (1987).
28. Braas, K. M., D. C. Manning, D. C. Perry, and S. H. Snyder. Bradykinin and analogues: Differential agonist and antagonist activities suggesting multiple receptors. *Br. J. Pharmacol.* **94**:3-5 (1988).
29. Steranka, L. L., R. M. Burch, R. J. Vavrek, J. M. Stewart, and S. J. Enna. Multiple bradykinin receptors: Results of studies using a novel class of receptor antagonists, in: *Neuroreceptors and Signal Transduction* (S. Kito, T. Segawa, K. Kuriyama, M. Tohyama, and R. Olsen, eds.). Plenum, New York, pp. 111-127 (1988).
30. Farmer, S. G., R. M. Burch, S. A. Meeker, and D. E. Wilkins. Evidence for a pulmonary B3 bradykinin receptor. *Molec. Pharmacol.* **36**:1-8 (1989).
31. Tamaoki, J., K. Kobayashi, N. Sakai, A. Chiyotani, T. Kanemura, and T. Takizawa. Effect of bradykinin on airway ciliary motility and its modulation by neutral endopeptidase. *Amer. Rev. Resp. Dis.* **140**:430-435 (1989).
32. Saha, J. K., J. N. Sengupta, and R. K. Goyal. *Gastroenterology* **96**:A434 (1989).
33. Orawski, A. T., J. P. Susz, and W. H. Simmons. Metabolism of bradykinin by multiple coexisting membrane-bound peptidases in lung: techniques for investigating the role of each peptidase using specific inhibitors. *Kinins V, Adv. Exp. Med. Biol.* **247B**:355-364 (1989).
34. Ryan, J. W., J. Roblero, and J. M. Stewart. Inactivation of bradykinin in the pulmonary circulation. *Biochem. J.* **110**:795 (1968).
35. Roblero, J., J. W. Ryan, and J. M. Stewart. Assay of kinins by their effects on blood pressure. *Res. Commun. Chem. Path. Pharmacol.* **6**:207 (1973).

36. Togo, J., R. M. Burch, C. J. DeHaas, J. R. Connor, and L. R. Steranka. D-Phe7-substituted peptide bradykinin antagonists are not substrates for kininase II. *Peptides* **10**:109-112 (1989).
37. Drapeau, G., N-E., Rhaleb, S. Dion, D. Jukic, and D. Regoli. [Phe-pseudo-(CH_2-NH)Arg^9]-bradykinin, a B_2 receptor selective agonist which is not broken down by either kininase I or kininase II. *Eur. J. Pharmacol.* **155**:193-195 (1988).
38. Stewart, J. M., and R. J. Vavrek. Bradykinin competitive antagonists: Design and activities. in: *Enzyme Inhibitors* (A. Barth and R. L. Schowen, eds.). Pergamon, Oxford, pp. 73-80 (1987).
39. Vavrek, R. J., and J. M. Stewart. Smooth muscle selectivity in bradykinin analogs with multiple D-amino acid substitutions, in: *Kinins IV* (*Adv. Exp. Med. Biol.* 198A) (L. M. Greenbaum and H. S. Margolius, eds.). Plenum, New York, pp. 543-547 (1986).
40. Felix, A. M., M. H. Jiminez, R. Vergona, and M. R. Cohen. Synthesis and biological activity of novel bradykinin analogs. *Int. J. Prot. Peptide Res.* **5**: 201-206 (1973).
41. Stewart, J. M., and D. W. Woolley. The search for peptides with specific antibradykinin activity, in: *Hypotensive Peptides* (E. G. Erdos, N. Back, and F. Sicuteri, eds.). Springer-Verlag, New York, pp. 23-33 (1966).
42. Nicolaides, E. D., and M. K. Craft. The synthesis of kinin analogs. *Ann. N.Y. Acad. Sci.* **104**:15 (1963).
42b. DeWald, H. A., M. K. Craft, and E. D. Nicolaides. The synthesis of 6-carbamoyl-L-serine, 6-D-serine and 6-L-threonine bradykinin. *J. Med. Chem.* **6**:741 (1963).
43. Stewart, J. M., and R. J. Vavrek. Bradykinin antagonists and their possible application for therapy of inflammation. *Atemew.-Lungenkrkh.* **144**: 593-596 (1988).
44. Vavrek, R. J., and J. M. Stewart. Development and modification of competitive antagonists of bradykinin, in: *Peptides, Structure and Function* (*Proc. 9th Amer. Peptide Symp.*) (C. M. Deber, V. J. Hruby, and K. D. Kopple, eds.). Pierce Chemical Co., Rockford, IL, pp. 655-658 (1985).
45. Vavrek, R. J., and J. M. Stewart. New bradykinin antagonist peptides as tools for the study of the kallikrein-kinin system, in: *Renal Function, Hypertension and Kallikrein-Kinin System* (O. Iimura and H. S. Margolius, eds.). Univ. of Tokyo Press, Tokyo, pp. 85-89 (1988).
46. Stewart, J. M., and R. J. Vavrek. Design of bradykinin antagonists, in: *Peptides 1987* (G. R. Marshall, ed.). ESCOM Science Publishers, Leiden, pp. 433-437 (1988).
47. Vavrek, R. J., and J. M. Stewart. Desamino and deletion analogs of bradykinin antagonists: A full nonapeptide sequence is not necessary for antagonist activity, in: *Second Forum on Peptides* (A. Aubry, M. Marraud, and B. Vitoux, eds.). John Libbey Eurotext, London, pp. 453-456 (1989).

48. Vavrek, R. J., and J. M. Stewart. Bradykinin antagonists with modifications at positions one and nine (the arginine positions): Is arginine necessary in bradykinin antagonists? in: *Peptides* (*Proc. 20th Euro. Peptide Symp.*) (G. Jung and E. Bayer, eds.), Walter de Gruyter, Berlin, pp. 565-567 (1989).
49. Vavrek, R. J., and J. M. Stewart. Bradykinin antagonists modified at the proline positions: Heterocyclic residues at positions two and three, in: *Peptides* (B. Penke and A. Torok, eds.), W. de Gruyter, Berlin, pp. 423-426 (1988).
50. Vavrek, R. J., and J. M. Stewart. Minimum structure bradykinin antagonists, in: *Proc. 11th Amer. Peptide Symp.* (J. Rivier, ed.). ESCOM, Leiden, The Netherlands, pp. 157-158 (1990).

4

Nonpeptide Bradykinin Antagonists

João B. Calixto, Rosendo A. Yunes, Giles A. Rae, and Yara S. Medeiros
Universidade Federal de Santa Catarina
Florianópolis, Santa Catarina, Brazil

I. INTRODUCTION

Recent years have exhibited a substantial improvement in our knowledge of the pathophysiological roles and mechanisms of action of bradykinin (BK) and closely related kinins. Formed during tissue injury or trauma, these peptides constitute an important class of inflammatory mediators. Indeed, Rocha e Silva et al. (1), in their pioneer study in 1949, suggested that BK could be one of the main mediators of shock. Besides their ability to dilate blood vessels and increase vascular permeability leading to edema, BK and related kinins are powerful nociceptive agents, which can contract or relax the smooth muscle of several tissues and modulate secretory functions of the gastrointestinal mucosa. It is not surprising, therefore, that BK has been implicated in the etiology of several inflammatory diseases including arthritis, allergic rhinitis, asthma, anaphylaxis, pancreatitis, myocardial infarction, and inflammatory bowel disease (for review, see Refs. 2-8).

Studies on the structure-activity relationships of several BK analogs in isolated tissues led Regoli and Barabé (6) to propose the existence of B1 and B2 BK receptor types. According to this classification, virtually all of the most relevant physiological BK receptors known were characterized as being of the B2 type. The lack of selective antagonists at B2 BK receptors precluded for a long time a more detailed insight into whether they constitute a homogeneous entity. Most of the research on BK receptor antagonists conducted thus far has relied on the systematic examination of kinin analogs for blocking activity and has provided several peptide BK antagonists, the characteristics of which are reviewed in depth in Chapters 2 and 3. Another approach, the search for BK receptor antagonists of nonpeptide nature, will be dealt with in the present chapter.

The mechanisms by which BK brings about its actions appear to be very complex and to involve multiple second messenger transduction pathways depending on the tissue and animal species considered. Thus, BK has been shown to activate both phospholipase A_2, leading to synthesis of cyclooxygenase- and lipoxygenase-derived eicosanoids, and phospholipase(s) C with consequent formation of phosphoinositides and diacylglycerol, activation of protein kinasse C, and increased intracellular concentration of calcium (see Fig. 1). Furthermore, it has been suggested that BK can modify cyclic nucleotide levels and that its effects may also involve guanine nucleotide-binding regulatory (G) protein-mediated mechanisms. Such a multiplicity of effector mechanisms would alone be sufficient to suggest the existence of several BK receptors.

Although it should be borne in mind that nonpeptide compounds stand a greater chance of being active following oral administration, this should not preclude the therapeutic potential of peptide BK receptor antagonists. This is adequately illustrated by the design of orally active inhibitors of kininase II, such as captopril, based on the molecular structure of bradykinin-potentiating peptides isolated from *Bothrops jararaca* venom (9). Thus, the rational development of nonpeptide BK receptor antagonists, which retain the pharmacological profile of active peptide compounds, would seem to be a feasible approach to providing useful new therapeutic agents.

There are many examples of nonpeptide compounds which specifically bind with high affinity to peptide receptors. Perhaps the most outstanding example of this is provided by the opiate antagonists. Designed to antagonize the action of morphine and other opiate analgesics, these antagonists truly block receptors for the endogenous opioid peptides enkephalins, endorphins, and dynorphins. Indeed, the most selective and potent opioid receptor antagonists are of nonpeptide nature (10). Recently, Chiu et al. (11) reported on the first selective nonpeptide angiotensin II receptor antagonist, S-8308, an imidazoleacetic acid derivative which, unlike the

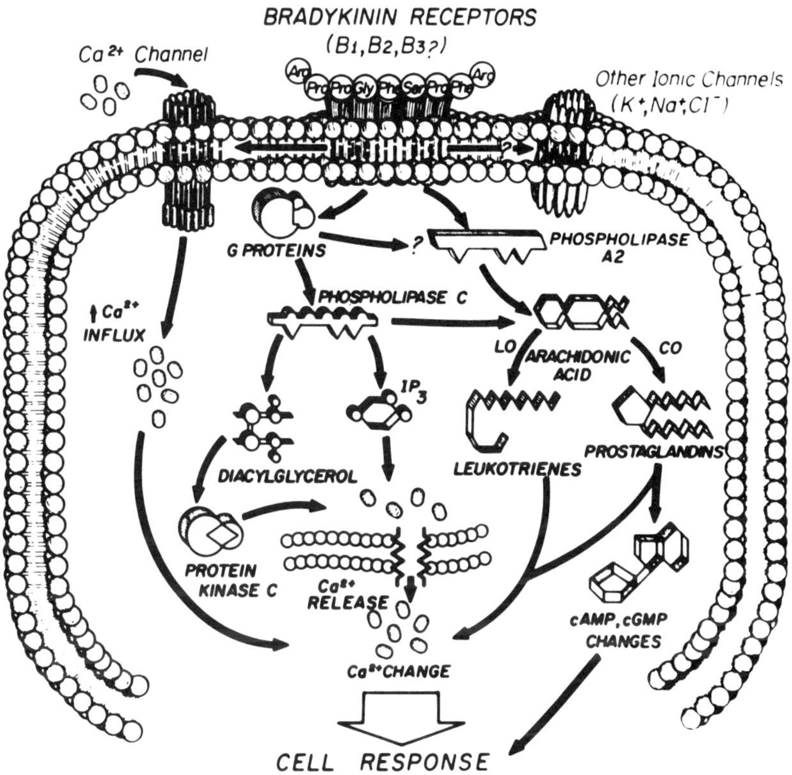

Figure 1 Schematic representation of the possible signal transduction mechanisms coupled to bradykinin receptors. Bradykinin receptor activation in the plasma membrane presumably promotes the activation of membrane ion channels and/or of putative G proteins which stimulate either phospholipase A_2 or different types of phospholipase C. Activation of these pathways triggers either the generation of arachidonic acid metabolites or hydrolysis of phosphatidylinositol. Thus, lipoxygenase (LO) or cyclooxygenase (CO) arachidonic acid metabolites and/or diacylglycerol or protein kinase C activation will contribute to further increase intracellular free calcium levels. The extension of the contribution of each pathway depends on the type of cell and/or animal species considered. Also, the correlation between these transduction mechanisms and the different types of bradykinin receptors are not fully established.

peptide antagonist saralasin, is also active following oral administration. Other examples of nonpeptide antagonists of peptide receptors include the potent and selective cholecystokinin receptor antagonists, MK-329 and L-365260, the benzodiazepine tifluadom, which blocks receptors for thyrotropin releasing hormone, and the fungicide ketoconazole, which binds to gonadotropin releasing hormone receptors (10).

II. NONPEPTIDE ANTAGONISTS OF BRADYKININ

Mariani (12) examined a variety of compounds for activity against BK-induced contraction in the isolated guinea pig ileum and detected significant antagonism using chlorpromazine. Subsequently, Rocha e Silva and colleagues screened a large number of synthetic compounds in the guinea pig ileum, including many phenothiazine derivatives (13-15; for review see Ref. 16). The majority of these compounds acted as noncompetitive BK antagonists and, in some cases, the inhibition proved to be irreversible and nonselective. However, some dibenzocycloheptadine derivatives, such as cyproheptadine and imipramine, presented functional BK antagonistic activity, as evaluated by their pK_i values, determined by means of Lineweaver-Burk plots. Unfortunately, these compounds were only weak antagonists and were not submitted to Schild analysis to assess possible competitive BK antagonism. Moreover, both substances also exert other actions apparently unrelated to BK antagonism. Cyproheptadine is also a serotonin receptor blocker, whereas imipramine is an antidepressant drug which also inhibits neuronal uptake of catecholamines.

Mention must be made of some nonsteroidal anti-inflammatory aspirin-like drugs which inhibit BK-induced bronchoconstriction and pain (for review see 17, 18; see also Chapter 7). These actions are not selective for kinins and are almost certainly mediated by inhibition of eicosanoid synthesis.

Another study reported that pyridinol carbamate blocks BK-induced constriction of rabbit isolated veins (19). Again, however, the selectivity of anti-BK action was limited. Gieldanowski et al. (20) reported that *p-bis*-(2-benzylaminopropyl)-benzene effectively antagonizes BK-induced contractions of the rat isolated uterus and enhances vascular permeability in rat skin. This compound, however, does not block responses of the guinea pig ileum to BK (8). Furthermore, ethanolamine compounds derived from 2-bromo-2-phenylethyldimethylamine hydrobromide potentiated, while its amine or carbonium derivatives antagonized, responses to BK in the guinea pig vas deferens (21). These effects, however, were not selective. Finally, an analog of the diuretic drug amiloride has been shown to compete with bradykinin's actions, and binding to its receptor, in a kidney-derived cell line (21a).

Several compounds of plant origin have also been screened for potential BK antagonistic activity. Thus, the anti-BK actions of the flavonoids apiin and hesperitin and the related bronchodilator and antispasmodic furanochromone khellin were tested in the guinea pig isolated ileum and in rat paw edema models (22,23). Although the three compounds antagonized BK action in the ileum, only khellin exerted a competitive type of inhibition. In addition, all three compounds affected responses to angiotensin II and/or eledoisin. When tested against carrageenan- or BK-induced paw edema, khellin and apiin, given systemically, exhibited greater anti-inflammatory activity than hesperitin. Other flavonoids including quercetin, rhamnetin, homoeriodictyol, and, to a lesser extent, morin and esculin (24), as well as the biflavonoids amentoflavone from *Ginko biloba* and cupressuflavone from *Cupressus tarubosa* (25), have also been shown to antagonize BK action on the guinea pig ileum. Another flavonoid, O-(β-hydroxyethyl)-rutin, exhibits anti-BK activity in the rat uterus at high concentrations (26). Vitexin, a flavone glycoside isolated from the flowers of *Ochrocarpus longifolius L* and *Arneba hispidissimica Dc*, also inhibited BK-induced contraction in the guinea pig ileum and exhibited anti-inflammatory activity (27). The functional antagonism of BK-induced responses by all these compounds must, however, be analyzed with caution, because data regarding their selectivity and nature of action are still largely lacking. Indeed, we have found that acetylation of eucryphin and the flavonoid glycoside astilbin, isolated from the bark of *Hymenaea martiana*, results in compounds with apparently competitive BK antagonist properties in rat isolated uterus, but which are also capable of affecting responses to nonkinin agonists (28).

Vitamin K_3 (menadione) and streptomycin have also been found to antagonize BK-induced contractions of the guinea pig ileum in a concentration-dependent and noncompetitive fashion, but these compounds also depressed responses to acetylcholine and histamine (29). It was also shown that both substances blocked BK-induced bronchoconstriction in guinea pigs but enhanced responses to histamine (30). We have recently shown that jatrophone, a diterpene from *Jatropha elliptica*, exhibits some selectivity against BK-induced contractions of the rat uterus and guinea pig ileum in a noncompetitive manner (31). Also, the saponin, aescin, from horse chestnut exhibits functional antagonistic activity against BK-induced increase of vascular permeability and has a lymphopenic action (32).

Another interesting study reported that tiaramide, an anti-inflammatory compound that does not inhibit prostaglandin synthesis, effectively antagonizes BK-induced contractions of the guinea pig isolated bladder detrusor muscle in an apparently competitive fashion (33). This action was also accompanied by antagonism of BK-triggered prostaglandin release, phosphoinositide accumulation, and elevation of intracellular calcium. The authors suggest that the inhibition on BK action may occur at the level of phospholipase A_2.

Recently, Burch et al. (8) have assessed the ability of several of these putative anti-BK compounds to displace radiolabeled BK from guinea pig ileum membranes. At high concentrations (100 μM), cyproheptadine, pyridinol carbamate, *p-bis* (2-benzylamino)-benzene, and vitamin K_3 all failed to displace selectively radiolabeled BK in guinea pig ileum membranes, whereas imipramine was only marginally effective (about 30% displacement). This important finding strongly suggests that the functional antagonism of responses to BK exerted by such compounds is not mediated at the level of the receptor recognition sites.

Considering that several intracellular transduction mechanisms are involved in the manifestation of BK-triggered effects (see above and Fig. 1), the anti-BK activity of some nonpeptide BK antagonists may reflect interference with such processes. Possible mechanisms of anti-BK action may include inhibition of eicosanoid formation via reduction of cyclooxygenase/lipoxygenase and/or phospholipase A_2 activities, blockade of phospholipase(s) C-mediated phosphatidylinositol pathways, inositol-trisphosphate and diacylglycerol accumulation, protein kinase C activation, or calcium mobilization. In this regard, it has been demonstrated that the flavonoid quercetin is capable of modulating protein kinase C activation in rat brain and pig thyroid (34). Additionally, the protein kinase C inhibitor, staurosporine, inhibits BK- and phorbol ester-induced activation of peripheral capsaicin-sensitive nociceptors. The effect of BK was reversibly antagonized by the peptide B2 BK receptor antagonists indicating that B2 receptors on nociceptors are coupled to protein kinase C (35). Further biochemical studies are needed to clarify the cellular mechanisms of anti-BK action of these compounds. Interference with second messenger transduction mechanisms may explain their limited selectivity towards the blockade of BK-induced effects.

III. NONPEPTIDE BRADYKININ ANTAGONISTS FROM *MANDEVILLA VELUTINA*

Mandevilla velutina (Apocinaceae) is a plant native to central Brazil which is frequently used in the form of infusion or alcoholic extract as a folk medicine to treat poisonous snake bites, especially those caused by *Both-*

rops jararaca, and as an anti-inflammatory preparation. The demonstration of BK-releasing (1) and BK-potentiating (36) properties of *B. jararaca* venom prompted us to investigate whether hydroalcoholic extracts of the rhizome of this plant display anti-BK activity. In the following sections we shall present some of our recent results obtained with the crude extract of and some pure nonpeptide compounds isolated from *M. velutina*.

A. Effects on Nonvascular Smooth Muscle Preparations

The crude extract of *M. velutina* (0.5-4.0 mg/ml) was found to antagonize BK-induced contractions of the rat isolated uterus in a competitive and concentration-related manner (37). This pharmacological effect appeared to be quite selective since, within the same concentration range, the extract did not inhibit contractions evoked by angiotensin II, acetylcholine, oxytocin, or barium chloride (Table 1). Paradoxically, the highest extract concentration increased the sensitivity to prostaglandin $F_{2\alpha}$ slightly (2-fold), but significantly (37).

Subsequent studies revealed that the extract also antagonized uterine responses to Lys-BK (kallidin) and contractions of the guinea pig ileum and urinary bladder caused by BK, kallidin and Met, Lys-BK (38,39). In all three preparations the functional antagonistic activity was of rapid onset (equilibrium within 10 minutes), selective, reversible upon washout and characterized by parallel rightward shifts of the concentration-response curves to the kinins. Although Schild analysis of these data revealed strong linear relationships between extract concentration and inhibition of kinin responses (correlation coefficient close to 1), the slopes of the Schild plots were significantly higher than unity (see Table 1). This implies that either the extract contains multiple compounds with varying affinities for the BK receptors and/or that the active compound it contains may not exhibit strictly competitive receptor kinetics. Despite this, the nominal pA_2 values (as g/ml) for the extract determined in each preparation were similar, suggesting that these tissues possess closely related BK receptors (Table 1).

In addition to its direct contractile effect on the guinea pig urinary bladder, BK also potentiated nerve-mediated responses evoked by electrical stimulation. Both effects appeared to be mediated by B2 receptors, since they were not caused by the selective B1 receptor agonist desArg^9-BK, and were similarly inhibited by a low concentration (0.4 mg/ml) of *M. velutina* extract (39). However, in the rat isolated vas deferens the extract antagonized the direct contractile effect of BK, but not the potentiation of electrically evoked nerve-mediated responses (M. Nicolau, unpublished

Table 1 Mean pA_2 Values for Antagonistic Effects of the Crude Extract and Several Compounds from *Mandevilla velutina* Against Kinin-Induced Contractions in Isolated Smooth Muscle Preparations

		Rat uterus[a]		Guinea pig ileum[a]		Guinea pig urinary bladder[a]	
Antagonist	Agonist	pA_2	Slope	pA_2	Slope	pA_2	Slope
Crude extract	BK	3.2	1.8*	3.2	1.5*	3.5	2.2*
	Kal	3.5	1.7*	3.8	1.1	3.7	2.4*
	ACh	no effect		—		no effect	
	OT	no effect		—		—	
	His	—		—		no effect	
	AII	no effect		—		—	
MV8608	BK	5.3	1.8*	4.9	[b]	not tested	
	Kal	5.0	1.1	—			
	ACh	no effect		no effect			
	OT	no effect		—			
	His	—		[c]			
MV8609	BK	5.3	1.3	5.2	[b]	not tested	
	Kal	—		—			
	ACh	no effect		no effect			
	OT	no effect		—			
	His	no effect		[c]			
MV8610	BK	5.3	1.4	5.2	[b]	not tested	
	ACh	no effect		no effect			
	OT	no effect		—			
	His	—		[c]			
MV8611	BK	5.3	1.2	5.3	[b]	not tested	
	Kal	5.8	1.0	—			
	ACh	no effect		no effect			
	OT	no effect		—			
	His	—		[c]			
MV8612	BK	5.4	1.3	5.2	1.0	not tested	
	Kal	5.2	0.8	—			
	ACh	no effect		no effect			
	OT	no effect		—			
	His	—		no effect			

Each group represents the mean of 4 to 8 experiments.

[a]pA_2 values (-log of antagonist concentration which caused a 2-fold displacement to the right of the agonist concentration-response curves) are in molar basis, except for the crude extract (as g/ml).

[b]The slope could not be calculated, since maximal response was inhibited.

[c]Compound at 20 μg/ml affected histamine response.

*Significantly different from unity ($p<0.05$).

Bradykinin (BK), kallidin (Kal), acetylcholine (ACh), oxytocin (OT), histamine (His), angiotensin II (AII).

Source: From Refs. 37-39, 44.

results). This finding reinforces the view that in this latter preparation, both effects are mediated through distinct BK receptors (40, 41).

The cat isolated ileum is a more selective bioassay preparation for kinins than the rat uterus or guinea pig ileum (6, 42). In this preparation, *M. velutina* extract was again found to antagonize responses to BK in a concentration-dependent fashion, leaving responses to acetylcholine and histamine largely unaffected (38). Similar selective BK antagonistic activity of the extract was also detected in the rat stomach strip (M. Nicolau, unpublished results).

The isolation of the compounds responsible for the anti-BK activity of *M. velutina* rhizome extract proved to be a difficult task due, mainly, to the multiplicity of compounds in the material and especially to their high affinity to lipids of the extract. Nevertheless, we were able to obtain two semipurified fractions following chromatography on silica gel columns (fractions 11 and 12) which retained the anti-BK action of the crude extract (43). These fractions were 80- to 160-fold more potent than the crude extract in inhibiting selectively responses of the rat isolated uterus to BK. Moreover, in contrast to the rhizome extract, these fractions exhibited a strictly competitive mechanism of action against the peptide, since the slopes of the Schild plots did not differ from unity. Further purification of the active fractions has led to the isolation of five distinct nonpeptide compounds which antagonize BK actions in the rat uterus (44). Four of these compounds have been characterized as steroidal glycosides (MV8609, MV8610, MV8611, and MV8612, with molecular weights ranging from 527 to 1182), and the fifth (MV8608) is an aglycone steroid (MW 362; R.A. Yunes and J. B. Calixto, unpublished results). All of them present similar selective antagonistic potencies against BK-induced uterine responses (dissociation constants, K_b values, ranging between 2 and 14 μM) and, with the exception of MV8608, yield Schild plots with slopes not different from unity (Table 1).

The compounds purified from *M. velutina* were also found to inhibit BK-induced contractions of the guinea pig ileum. However, the pharmacological profile of this activity was markedly different from that observed in the rat uterus (44). Although inhibition was quite selective against BK, all compounds, except MV8612, depressed maximal responses to BK in addition to causing rightward shifts of the concentration-response curve to the peptide. Thus, only MV8612 behaved as a simple competitive and selective BK antagonist (Table 1). Although the pA_2 values determined for MV8612 against BK-induced contractions of the rat uterus and guinea pig ileum were similar, the different patterns of activity of the other four compounds in both preparations suggest that the B2 BK receptors in these tissues may not be identical.

Interestingly, functional and binding studies conducted with some peptide BK antagonists in these preparations have led to similar conclusions. In such studies, some BK analogs were found to be effective blockers solely in the rat uterus or in the guinea pig ileum, whereas others interacted selectively with BK receptors in both tissues (8, 45-47).

We have also analyzed the influence of the crude extract of *M. velutina* and some of its anti-BK compounds on the rat isolated duodenum. This preparation exhibits a diphasic response to BK characterized by a relaxation which is followed by contraction (48). It has been suggested that BK-induced relaxation and contraction are mediated through activation of B1 and B2 BK receptors, respectively (49, 50). However, the same dose of the extract which antagonized BK actions in other preparations dose-dependently inhibited the manifestation of both effects of BK in the duodenum, leaving qualitatively similar responses evoked by adrenaline relatively unaffected (51, 52). The antagonistic effect against BK could be overcome by raising the concentration of peptide and was reversible upon washout. Compounds MV8608 and MV8612 were also found to antagonize both effects of BK at micromolar concentrations. Although compound MV8612 was more potent than MV8608, it did not discriminate between the two components. In contrast, compound MV8608 was found to be more effective in blocking the contractile response than relaxation and slightly affected the diphasic response to potassium (52). It is difficult to draw firm conclusions from these experiments as to the nature of the antagonism exerted by the *M. velutina* compounds in the rat duodenum. Its responses to kinins show great variability between preparations and the contractile responses increase in magnitude with time, rendering the construction of reliable consecutive full concentration-response curves to BK very difficult to accomplish. Nevertheless, it would seem that these anti-BK compounds do not detect a clear-cut BK receptor heterogeneity in the rat duodenum. This view is also supported by a report showing that in this tissue, radiolabeled BK binds to a single class of high affinity sites (53).

As with the rat duodenum, in preparations of the circular muscle of guinea pig isolated ileum, BK induces a diphasic concentration-dependent effect consisting of contraction followed by relaxation. While relaxation is an indirect effect mediated presumably by release of prostaglandin E_2, contraction seems to be a direct BK action. The active anti-BK compounds from *M. velutina* MV8612, MV8610, and MV8608 (8.0, 11.0, and 27.0 μM, respectively) antagonized both effects of BK but were more effective blockers of the relaxant component of the response (J. B. Calixto, unpublished results).

Recently, a novel BK receptor has been proposed to mediate BK-induced contractions of guinea pig airways (54). This putative B3 BK receptor has been characterized on the basis of functional and radioligand data. We have preliminary evidence in deepithelialized tracheal strips isolated from guinea pigs, that the three *M. velutina* compounds (8.0-27.0 μM) each displace the BK concentration-response curve to the right about 2-to 3-fold. However, the evidence is still insufficient to conclude that this action reflects a selective and competitive antagonism. It is important to mention that, in contrast to many peptide BK receptor antagonists, none of the anti-BK compounds from *M. velutina* displayed agonistic activity in any of the preparations tested.

Finally, we have conducted some experiments on the anti-BK activity of the crude extract of rhizomes of *Mandevilla illustris*, another plant of the same genus as *M. velutina*, which is also used in Brazil as a folk medicine against snake bites. Although the crude extract antagonized BK-induced responses of the rat uterus in a competitive manner in the same concentration range as seen with the *M. velutina* extract, this action was nonselective, since responses to acetylcholine, angiotensin II, and oxytocin were also partially affected. Similar nonselective inhibitory actions were observed in rat uterus with low concentrations (20-40 μg/ml) of three compounds recently purified from the crude *M. illustris* extract (J. B. Calixto and R. A. Yunes, unpublished results).

B. Effects on Vascular Smooth Muscle Preparations

Extensive functional studies on the structure-activity relationships of several peptide kinin analogs have established that the biological effects of kinins on blood vessels are mediated by at least two distinct receptors: the B1 and B2 BK receptors (6). The anti-BK activity of crude *M. velutina* extract has been tested in smooth muscle preparations of rabbit aorta and mesenteric artery, which contain B1 receptors, and the jugular vein, which expresses only B2 receptors. The crude extract was found to antagonize contractions induced by the B1-selective agonist desArg^9-BK in the first two preparations, and by BK in all tissues (55). The action appeared to be competitive in that the inhibition was surmounted by increasing agonist concentration in the bath 10- to 30-fold and was not accompanied by changes in reactivity of the preparations to noradrenaline. Thus, it appears that the anti-BK compounds in this extract do not discriminate B1 from B2 receptors in these tissues.

The vascular endothelium plays a key role in regulating the tone of blood vessels via the production of vasodilators such as prostacyclin and endothelium-derived relaxing factor (EDRF, recently characterized as nitric oxide) and vasoconstrictors such as endothelin (56,57). Among the several substances which trigger EDRF release is BK, and this action has been proposed to be the major vasodilator mechanism of BK in vitro (58). We have assessed the influence of *M. velutina* extract and of some of the anti-BK compounds on endothelium-mediated relaxation of several ring preparations.

In dog femoral and mesenteric artery rings precontracted with noradrenaline, the crude extract, at concentrations which did not affect established tone, fully reversed BK-induced, endothelium-dependent relaxations (51). The antagonistic activity was not, however, selective against BK, since the extract also reversed vasorelaxation caused by acetylcholine in 20% of the preparations tested. In rabbit aortic rings, the extract failed to modify relaxation caused by BK but markedly inhibited dilation triggered by acetylcholine and the calcium ionophore A23187. Also in rat aortic rings, the extract markedly antagonized histamine-mediated relaxation but caused little reversal of that stimulated by acetylcholine or A23187 (J. B. Calixto, unpublished results).

Only two anti-BK *M. velutina* compounds have been tested in these preparations so far. The first, MV8608, selectively antagonized BK-induced dilation of rabbit aortic rings, without affecting responses to acetylcholine or A23187 at concentrations up to 50 μM and reversed responses to the two other vasodilators in rat aortic rings. The second compound tested, MV8612, which is the most potent and selective BK antagonist in nonvascular smooth muscle preparations, was found to be completely inactive up to 20 μM against all endothelium-dependent vasodilators in both rabbit and rat isolated blood vessels (J. B. Calixto, unpublished results). Neither the extract nor the pure compounds modified the magnitude of responses to endothelium-independent vasodilators such as papaverine and sodium nitroprusside in any of the preparations tested.

It is difficult, at present, to reconcile the lack of selective anti-BK activity seen in isolated vessels with the results obtained in nonvascular preparations. The complete absence of activity of MV8612 in isolated blood vessels may be even more surprising in view of recent evidence showing that both B1 and B2 receptors mediate EDRF release from cultured endothelial cells and that these receptors can be competitively blocked by some peptide BK antagonists (59, 60). However, these discrepancies may be ascribed partly to an oxidant effect of the *M. velutina* extract or compounds and/or to the fact that, unlike most EDRF releasers, BK also stimulates endothelial cells to release prostacyclin. In addition, responses of endothelial cells to drugs are known to exhibit tissue and species variation (58).

C. Anti-Inflammatory Effects

There is substantial evidence supporting important roles for BK and related kinins as inflammatory mediators in several acute and chronic diseases. These substances are potent vasodilators and enhancers of vascular permeability (and hence induce edema), cause pain, and activate leukocytes (5, 7, 61-64). Thus, in an attempt to characterize the pharmacological profile of *M. velutina* extract and its anti-BK compounds, we have analyzed their effects in some models of inflammation and pain. In the following sections we shall present some of our recent results obtained in such studies.

1. Influence on Edematogenic Responses

Pretreatment of rats by gavage with the crude extract of *M. velutina* (50-200 mg/kg) 1 hour before the intraplantar injection of different phlogistic agents into a hind paw resulted in significant and long-lasting inhibition of edematogenic responses. The results summarized in Table 2 show that the anti-inflammatory effect of the extract was most evident against edema

Table 2 Effect of Crude Extract from *Mandevilla velutina* on Paw Edema and Pleurisy Induced by Various Phlogistic Agents in the Rat

Phlogistic agent	(mg/kg/p. o.)	Edema (μl)	Percent inhibition	Pleural exudate (μl)	Percent inhibition
Bradykinin	Saline	750.0 ± 45.0	—	533.3 ± 36.6	—
(50 nmol/site)	50	640.0 ± 35.0	14.6*	366.6 ± 20.0	31.2*
	100	390.0 ± 60.0	48.0**	353.3 ± 23.3	33.7*
	200	310.0 ± 30.0	58.6**	360.0 ± 27.2	32.4*
Cellulose	Saline	255.0 ± 26.2	—	335.5 ± 17.5	—
sulfate	50	225.0 ± 20.6	11.7	275.8 ± 15.3	17.8*
(0.5 mg/site)	100	150.3 ± 18.7	41.0**	185.2 ± 12.5	44.8**
	200	86.2 ± 15.5	66.2*	200.6 ± 17.5	40.2*
Platelet	Saline	118.4 ± 9.8	—	532.2 ± 64.4	—
activating factor	50	84.2 ± 6.5	28.8*	352.4 ± 32.7	33.8*
(2.0 nmol/site)	200	64.4 ± 6.2	45.7**	483.6 ± 49.1	9.2
Carrageenan	Saline	526.6 ± 30.0	—	not tested	—
(100 μg/site)	50	380.2 ± 40.5	27.7*	not tested	—
	100	302.5 ± 31.5	42.6*	not tested	—
B. jararaca	Saline	732.5 ± 72.3	—	not tested	—
venom	200	696.8 ± 70.4	4.8	not tested	—
(10 μg/site)	400	828.5 ± 31.5	0.0	not tested	—

Data are reported as mean ±SEM (n = 5 to 8 for each group) of the peak values of edema and pleural exudate. *$p < 0.05$; **$p < 0.01$ (ANOVA and Dunnett's test). The extract was administered p.o. 60 minutes before phlogistic agent injection.
Source: Henriques et al., unpublished data.

induced by BK and cellulose sulfate (ED_{50}s of 70 and 86 mg/kg, respectively). However, significant effects were also observed against edema caused by carrageenan, platelet activating factor, zymosan, dextran, and serotonin, but not by histamine (Table 2 and M. G. Henriques, unpublished observations). The extract was also ineffective in blocking edema triggered by *B. jararaca* venom, even at high doses (400 mg/kg). This was a somewhat surprising finding in view of the BK-releasing and BK-potentiating properties of the venom. Despite such properties, we have recently shown that paw edema caused by *B. jararaca* venom is mediated mainly by cyclooxygenase-derived eicosanoids and activation of both α_1 and α_2-adrenoceptors, whereas histamine, platelet activating factor, and serotonin play only minor roles in the genesis of this edema (65). In addition, no evidence was found for a participation of kinins in the mediation of *B. jararaca* venom-induced paw edema.

Some of the compounds purified from *M. velutina* were injected intraplantarly in captopril-pretreated rats in combination with BK (3 nmol/paw). In such experiments, compound MV8610 (60-240 nmol/paw) and, to a greater extent, MV8612 (40-170 nmol/paw) significantly antagonized the edematogenic response to BK (Table 3). Both MV8612 and MV8610 (5-10 μmol/kg, i.p.), but not MV8608, were also effective inhibitors of BK-induced rat paw edema (Table 3).

Significant anti-edematogenic activity of *M. velutina* extract was also detected in models of paw edema in mice. In this species, the edema caused by intraplantar injection of carrageenan is quite distinct from that observed in rats in that it presents 2 peaks: one between 4 and 24 hours and another between 48 and 72 hours after administration (66). Oral administration of the extract (50 mg/kg) 1 hour before and 12 hours after injection of carrageenan significantly antagonized the development of paw edema measured 4, 48, and 72 hours later (67). Higher oral doses of the extract (100 and 200 mg/kg) were all also effective against mouse paw edema triggered by BK, cellulose sulfate, platelet activating factor, and serotonin (M. G. Henriques, unpublished results).

Compound MV8612 (40-170 nmol/paw), injected intradermally, dose-dependently antagonized BK (50 nmol/site)- and carrageenan (100 μg/paw)-induced mouse paw edema (Table 3). Compound MV8608 was less active, while MV8610 had no effect. At the same dose, compound MV8612 failed to affect mouse paw edema caused by platelet activating factor and serotonin (68).

These studies indicate that the extract of *M. velutina* and compounds MV8610 and MV8612, which selectively antagonize BK actions in vitro, exhibit potent and long-lasting anti-inflammatory activities in rats and

Table 3 Influence of Compounds from *Mandevilla velutina* on Bradykinin- and Carrageenan-Induced Paw Edema in the Rat and Mouse

Phlogistic agent	Treatment	Dose: nmol/paw	Dose: μmol/kg/i.p.	Paw edema (μl): Rat	Percent inhibition	Mouse	Percent inhibition
Bradykinin	Saline	—		380.0 ± 23.2		61.5 ± 4.2	—
	MV8612	40.0		338.0 ± 38.8	11.1	33.6 ± 3.8	45.3**
		80.0		208.3 ± 36.4	45.3**	20.8 ± 2.8	66.1**
		160.0		259.0 ± 73.4	32.0*	7.8 ± 3.2	87.3**
	MV8610	60.0		299.2 ± 11.6	21.4*	59.5 ± 3.8	3.2
		120.0		244.1 ± 33.4	36.6**	62.3 ± 4.1	0
		240.0		185.0 ± 21.1	51.3**	55.8 ± 3.0	9.3
	MV8608	140.0		not tested		50.4 ± 3.4	18.0*
		280.0				43.3 ± 4.1	29.4*
		560.0				44.6 ± 3.0	27.4*
	Saline	—	—	277.6 ± 49.0		not tested	
	MV8612		2.5	310.4 ± 49.5	0		
			4.0	152.2 ± 57.8	45.2**		
			9.0	105.1 ± 15.9	62.0**		
	MV8610		3.5	244.4 ± 30.0	12.1		
			5.5	247.8 ± 24.2	10.7	not tested	
			11.0	157.2 ± 22.8	43.4**		
	MV8608		14.0	282.8 ± 28.3	0	not tested	
			28.0	319.8 ± 36.3	0		
Carrageenan	saline	—		not tested		63.5 ± 5.3	—
(300 μg/paw)	MV8612	40.0				35.8 ± 3.1	43.6**
		80.0				18.4 ± 3.4	71.0**
		160.0				20.8 ± 2.7	67.2**

Bradykinin was injected at doses of 50 and 3 nmol/paw in rats and mice, respectively. Data are reported as mean ±SEM (n = 6 to 8 animals) of the peak values of edema. *$P < 0.05$. **$P \oplus 0.01$. (ANOVA and Dunnett's test).
Source: From Ref. 68.

mice. Indeed, the extract was a more potent inhibitor of edema caused by BK and cellulose sulfate, which appears to be largely mediated by generated BK (69). However, its efficacy and that of the purified compounds against edema caused by other phlogistic agents may indicate that either this anti-inflammatory activity is nonselective or that part of the responses to such agents is mediated by kinin formation. This issue can only be resolved by further studies. Moreover, the efficacy of the crude *M. velutina* extract and of compound MV8612, against platelet activating factor-induced paw edema and pleurisy, does not seem related to the blockade of platelet activating factor receptors. Compounds MV8612 and MV8610, at concentrations 100-fold greater than those necessary to antagonize BK responses of smooth muscle, both failed to inhibit platelet aggregation triggered by platelet activating factor, ADP or thrombin in human, rabbit, or guinea pig platelet-rich plasma (70). However, MV8608 did antagonize the aggregatory actions of platelet activating factor and ADP (but not thrombin), albeit at exceedingly high concentrations (ED_{50} ca. 1 mM).

In recent years, new simple models have been developed for studying the topical and systemic anti-edematogenic activity of anti-inflammatory drugs, such as the ear edema induced in mice by topical application of arachidonic acid (AA) or croton oil. Edema triggered by AA is mediated mainly by local formation of lipoxygenase products such as leukotrienes C_4 and D_4, while cyclooxygenase products (prostaglandin E_2), serotonin, and histamine participate to a much lesser extent (71-73). On the other hand, ear edema caused by croton oil or by its active constituent, the tumor promoter phorbol myristate acetate, appears to be mediated mainly by cyclooxygenase metabolites, including prostaglandin E_2, prostacyclin and thromboxane A_2, and by histamine and serotonin (74,75). An important difference between the models is that, unlike AA-induced ear edema, edema caused by croton oil is very sensitive to inhibition by anti-inflammatory steroid drugs, which act through blockade of phospholipase A_2. The fact that many effects of BK are mediated via local stimulation of eicosanoid synthesis, by activation of phospholipases A_2 and C, and that the anti-BK compounds from *M. velutina* display pregnane structures, led us to assess their efficacy in both models.

Ear edema triggered by AA was significantly and dose-dependently inhibited by treating the mice orally with the crude extract (50-400 mg/kg) 1 hour before AA application (maximal inhibition of 58% at 200 mg/kg) (76). As shown in Table 4, MV8612 was also an effective anti-inflammatory compound in this model. Thus, given topically or intraperitoneally 30 minutes before AA, MV8612 caused a potent and dose-dependent reduction of the edematogenic response. Compound MV8610 also inhibited

Table 4 Influence of Nonpeptide Natural Compounds from *Mandevilla velutina* of Arachidonic Acid-Induced Ear Edema in Mice

Treatment	Dose nmol/ear	Dose μmol/kg, i. p.	Edema (mg)	Percent inhibition
Saline			15.1 ± 0.6	—
MV8612	160	—	8.2 ± 1.7	45.6**
	250	—	5.0 ± 1.5	66.9***
	500	—	6.0 ± 0.9	60.2***
	—	2.5	13.5 ± 0.9	10.6
	—	8.0	10.5 ± 1.1	30.4**
	—	25.0	6.5 ± 0.8	59.6**
MV8610	230	—	14.9 ± 1.5	1.3
	350	—	9.2 ± 2.0	39.0**
	700	—	8.7 ± 0.8	42.3**
	—	3.5	11.1 ± 1.2	26.5**
	—	12.0	11.9 ± 0.9	21.2**
	—	35.0	8.0 ± 1.3	47.0**
MV8608	550	—	10.2 ± 0.7	32.4**
	830	—	10.1 ± 1.3	32.2**
	1660	—	12.6 ± 1.2	16.5
	—	8.0	13.5 ± 0.9	10.5
	—	28.0	11.5 ± 0.7	23.8*
	—	83.0	13.0 ± 0.9	13.9

Values are reported as the mean ± SEM ($n = 6$ for each group). *$p < 0.05$, **$p < 0.01$, and ***$p < 0.001$ (ANOVA and Newmann-Keuls test). The animals were treated with the compounds 30 min before application of arachidonic acid (2 mg/ear).
Source: Calixto et al., unpublished data.

edema development, but was slightly less potent than MV8612, whereas MV8608 was only marginally effective. Compounds MV8612 and, to a lesser extent, MV8608 both exhibited significant anti-inflammatory activity against the slowly developing edema caused by topical croton oil application (Table 5). Thus, edema was substantially inhibited when the compounds were injected intraperitoneally 30 minutes before, but not 3 hours after applying the phlogistic agent. However, only MV8612 was found to be effective upon topical application to the ear 3 hours after croton oil administration (Zanini et al., unpublished observations).

Taken together, such findings demonstrate that the functional anti-BK compounds from *M. velutina* are effective anti-inflammatory agents against ear edema caused by AA and croton oil. Considering that inflammation

Table 5 Influence of Nonpeptide Natural Compounds from *Mandevilla velutina* on Croton Oil-Induced Ear Edema in Mice

Treatment	Dose (nmol/ear)	Dose (μmol/kg, i. p.)	Edema (mg)	Percent inhibition
Control	—	—	15.7 ± 0.9	—
MV8612		2.5	13.0 ± 0.8	17.2*
		8.0	14.5 ± 0.8	7.6
		25.0	7.3 ± 1.1	53.5**
	160		12.5 ± 0.6	20.3**
	250		12.6 ± 0.5	19.7**
	500		11.2 ± 0.7	29.0**
MV8608		8.0	16.4 ± 0.4	0.0
		28.0	16.0 ± 0.6	0.0
		83.0	11.6 ± 1.7	26.2**
	550		14.7 ± 0.6	6.3
	830		16.3 ± 0.7	0.0
	1660		14.7 ± 0.9	0.0

Values are reported as the mean ±SEM ($n = 6$ for each experimental group). *$p < 0.05$ and **$p < 0.01$ (ANOVA and Dunnett's test). Compounds were administered 30 min before (topically) or 3 h after (i.p.) croton oil. Edema was measured 6 h after application of croton oil.
Source: Zanini et al., unpublished data.

in both these models is mediated via eicosanoid synthesis, an inhibitory effect of the compounds on one or more steps of the eicosanoid biosynthetic pathways seems most likely. Among the several possibilities are blockade of phospholipase A_2, lipoxygenase, and/or cyclooxygenase activities. It is well established that some of the actions of BK can involve these enzymatic pathways (see Fig. 1). Which of these mechanisms is (are) ultimately involved in the mediation of the anti-edematogenic activity, as well as the extent to which this action is due to blockade of BK receptors, remain to be established. Interestingly, we have been unable to detect significant cyclooxygenase-blocking activity with these compounds, at concentrations that markedly inhibit BK action, when tested against AA-induced contractions of the rat isolated stomach strip (76).

2. *Influence on Pleurisy, Vascular Permeability, and Pain*

There is also experimental evidence relating the anti-inflammatory action of *M. velutina* extract to inhibition of pleural exudate accumulation and/or leukocyte infiltration. Thus, when administered orally to rats (50-200 mg/kg) or mice (50-100 mg/kg), the extract clearly and markedly reduced exudate accumulation in the pleural cavity stimulated by intrapleural injection of BK or cellulose sulfate (Table 2). Although the extract was found effective in inhibiting paw edema caused by platelet activating factor, serotonin and zymosan, the pleural exudate accumulation induced by these substances was much less affected by the same doses of the extract (M.G. Henriques, unpublished observation).

Similarly, but less markedly, the extract also reduced pleural exudation triggered by BK, carrageenan, serotonin, and platelet activating factor in mice (M. G. Henriques, unpublished results). Interestingly, the extract failed to affect differential leukocyte counts in both species. Experiments are currently underway to assess the efficacy of the extract against the latter phlogistic agents in rats and that of compounds MV8612, MV8610, and MV8608 in this model in both species.

The increases in vascular permeability determined by intradermal injections of BK and *B. jararaca* venom into the backs of rats have been found to be significantly antagonized by intraperitoneal administration of *M. velutina* extract (200-400 mg/kg, i.p.). Since responses to histamine were only partially affected, this result could reflect some selectivity against the actions of BK (77). However, subsequent experiments have failed to detect significant reductions of BK- and *B. jararaca* venom-induced enhanced vascular permeability following intradermal (160-560 nmol/site) or intravenous (0.8-3,0 μmol/kg) injections of MV8612, MV8610, or MV8608 (68). In addition, of the three compounds, only MV8608 slightly reduced the effect of histamine on vascular permeability following intravenous administration, indicating that this action is not selectively mediated via blockade of BK receptors. These findings were somewhat unexpected in view of the efficacy of these compounds against BK-induced paw edema and may suggest that the BK receptors involved in these models are not the same. It has been shown that, in the skin of the rat's back, vascular permeability is increased by BK through a mechanism which involved the release of histamine from mast cells and which is resistant to blockade by selective peptide B2 receptor antagonists (78). However, when the animals are pretreated with mepyramine and cimetidine or with cyproheptadine, several of the peptide BK antagonists effectively antagonize BK-induced plasma extravasation (8, 79).

In a model of inflammatory pain, acetic acid-induced writhing in mice, MV8612 (0.25-8.4 μmol/kg, i.p.) was found to exhibit significant dose-dependent antinociceptive activity with an ED_{50} of 1.2 μmol/kg. In contrast, the inhibition of writhing afforded by MV8608 was much less marked

(J. B. Calixto, unpublished results). Although these are preliminary results, it seems important to note that the analgesic activity of MV8612 was detected within the same range of doses found to inhibit paw or ear edema in response to different phlogistic agents.

D. Influence on Ovalbumin-Induced Anaphylaxis

The anti-inflammatory profile of activity of the *M. velutina* extract and compounds detected in the several above-mentioned models led us to investigate their effects on some parameters of ovalbumin-induced anaphylaxis in guinea pigs actively sensitized to this antigen. Intravenous injection of ovalbumin to anesthetized, mechanically ventilated guinea pigs caused marked bronchoconstriction and hypotension in all animals, which was followed by death within 15 minutes of the injection in 45% of the animals (Fig. 2). Pretreatment with *M. velutina* extract (60 mg/kg, i.v.) 15 min before antigen challenge, which alone did not modify the parameters measured, significantly reduced the hypotensive response to and the mortality caused by ovalbumin (Fig. 2). However, the bronchoconstriction induced by the antigen was not modified by pretreatment with the extract. Pretreatment with MV8612 (0.8 μmol/kg) or MV8608 (3.0 μmol/kg) reduced the mortality and hypotension induced by ovalbumin, as well as slightly, but significantly, inhibiting bronchoconstriction (80) (Fig. 2).

Neither the extract nor the purified compounds affected the bronchoconstrictor and hypotensive responses to acetylcholine, histamine, or serotonin in nonsensitized animals. Although it has been reported that BK causes bronchoconstriction in guinea pigs (17, 54), in our hands the peptide failed to do so. However, BK did induce its well-known hypotensive effect, which was significantly antagonized by pretreatment with the MV8612 (0.8 μmol/kg), but not with MV8608 (3.0 μmol/kg) (80).

In ovalbumin-sensitized guinea pigs, pretreated with pyrilamine and indomethacin, challenge with ovalbumin caused much less bronchoconstriction. These responses are likely to be mediated by synthesis of leukotrienes, release of platelet activating factor and, perhaps, BK (for review see 81). In this experimental model, treatment with MV8612 (0.8 and 3 μmol/kg, i.v.), 15 minutes prior to injection of the antigen, antagonized ovalbumin-induced bronchoconstriction and hypotension. In contrast, MV8610 (up to 7 μmol/kg) and MV8608 (up to 16.5 μmol/kg) failed to affect either parameters (80).

Collectively, these findings indicate that the *M. velutina* extract and some of its components, particularly MV8612, attenuate anaphylaxis

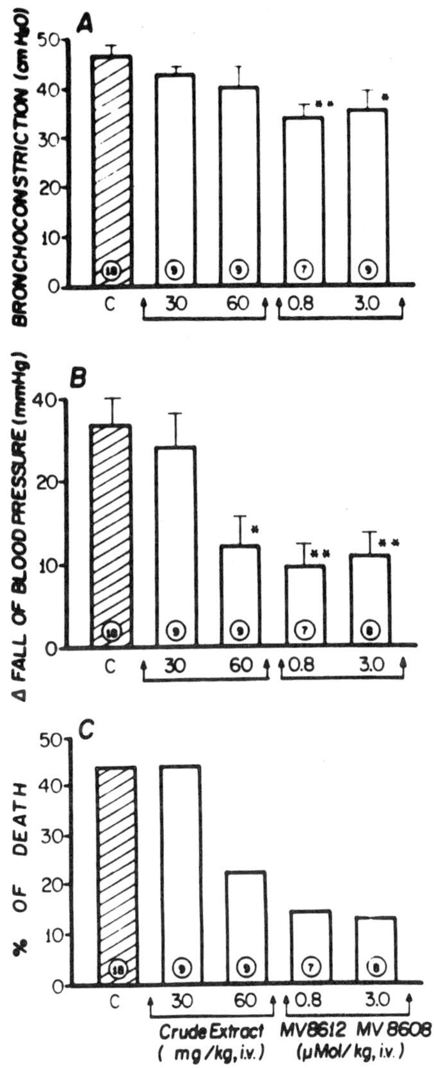

Figure 2 Effect of the crude *Mandevilla velutina* extract and of some of its natural antibradykinin compounds on ovalbumin-induced bronchoconstriction (3 mg/kg i.v.) (A), changes in mean arterial blood pressure (B), and on percentage of death (C) in guinea pigs actively sensitized to ovalbumin. The animals (200-300 g) were previously sensitized by i.p. injection of 10 μg of ovalbumin and 1 mg of $Al(OH)_3$ on days 1 and 14. Between 21 and 28 days later, the animals were anesthetized with pentobarbitone sodium (50 mg/kg, i.p.), treated with pancuronium (2 mg/kg, i.v.), and mechanically ventilated (80 cycles per minute, 2 ml/100 g). The extract and compounds from *M. velutina* were administered via the jugular vein 15 min before antigen challenge and arterial blood pressure was measured from a catheter placed in a carotid artery. Values refer to the peak effects observed within the first 15 minutes following antigen injection. The number of animals per group is indicated at the base of each column. (From Ref. 80).

caused by ovalbumin in guinea pigs actively sensitized to this antigen, mainly by interfering with the cardiovascular components of the reaction. These actions are apparently unrelated to histamine release, since compounds MV8612 (up to 16 μM) and MV8608 (up to 50 μM) failed to inhibit histamine release from rat peritoneal mast cells (80). Further investigations are required to assess whether such effects against anaphylaxis involve inhibition of the release and/or the action of leukotrienes, platelet activating factor or BK, or antagonism of putative B3 BK receptors. In addition, MV8612 was found to antagonize BK (3 nmol/kg)-induced hypotension. The latter finding is in marked contrast to results obtained in conscious or anesthetized rats, in which hypotension induced by intra-arterial injection of BK was blocked neither by the injection of the extract (up to 400 mg/kg, p.o. or i.p.) nor of MV8612 (0.84 mol/kg, i.v.) (M. Nicolau, unpublished results). The reasons for this discrepancy are not clear, but may involve species variability in the actions of BK and/or of the extract and MV8612.

IV. STRUCTURE-ACTIVITY RELATIONSHIP AMONG NONPEPTIDE BRADYKININ ANTAGONISTS

The several nonpeptide compounds with anti-BK activity mentioned in this chapter can be divided into two large groups: flavonoids and nonflavonoids. The first group comprises flavones (vitexin, apiin, cupressoflavone, amentoflavone), flavonols (quercetin, rhamnetin, morin and O-(β-hydroxyethyl)-rutin), flavonones (hesperitin and homoeriodictyol), and flavonols (astilbin), the structures of which are shown in Figure 3. The group of nonflavonoid compounds, the structures of which are shown in Figure 4, includes both natural (khellin, vitamin K_3, esculin, acetylated eucryphin, streptomycin, aescin, jatrophone, and the compounds from *M. velutina*) and synthetic substances (imipramine, cyproheptadine, staurosporine, chlorpromazine, pyridinol carbamate, tiaramide, and *p-bis*-2-benzylaminopropyl-benzene). Although, at first sight, the molecular structures of all those compounds appear markedly diverse, some common chemical features can be detected. Chau and Haley (24) suggested that the anti-BK activities of flavonoids in the guinea pig ileum involve the phenolic hydroxyl groups in positions 5 and 7, since methoxylation of position 7 results in a 10-fold decrease of anti-BK activity (quercetin vs. rhamnetin) and that the hydroxyl groups in the β-ring should also contribute to the anti-BK activity of flavonoids. It was proposed as well that, in coumarin derivatives, the glycoside linkage is an important determinant of anti-BK activity (esculin vs. sculetin and 4-methylsculetin), but

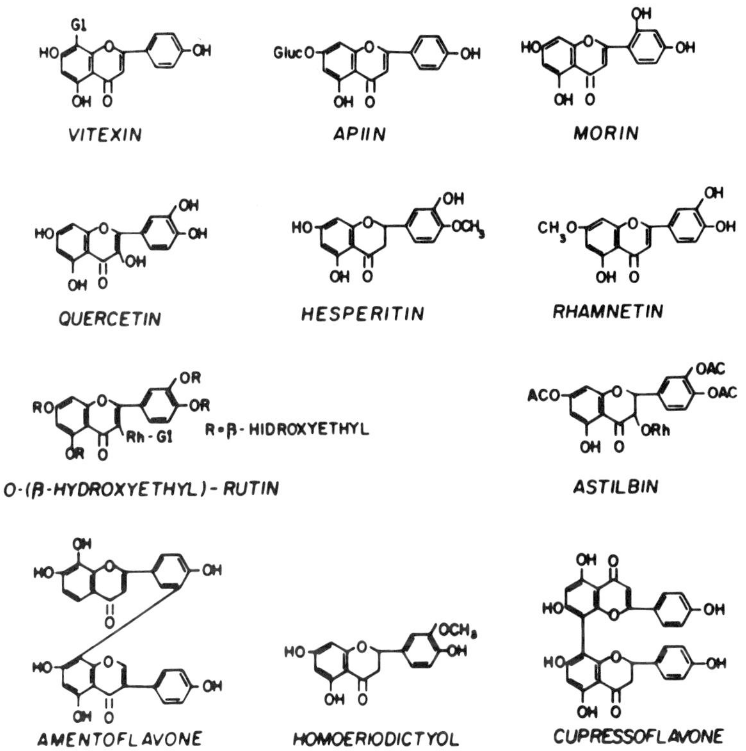

Figure 3 Molecular structures of flavonoids reported to exhibit antibradykinin activities.

that, generally, the aglycones exhibit a greater potency than glycosides (quercetin vs. quercetrin, rhamnetin vs. xantorhamnin). Indeed, this view led us to test the anti-BK action of eucryphin and astilbin, which only exhibited activity when acetylated (28). The activity shown by acetylated eucryphin would indicate that neither the aromatic β-ring nor the hydroxyl at position 7 are basic structural requirements. This view is strengthened by the significant activities of khellin, which has methoxy groups in positions 5 and 8, and of the napthoquinone vitamin K_3, which presents an isosteric structure without hydroxy or methoxy groups. The lower potency of the flavanone homoeriodictyol in the guinea pig ileum when compared to that of the flavonol quercetin (24) would indicate that reduction of the double bond between C2 and C3 with consequent disruption of planarity results in less activity. However, this possibility should be considered with caution because we failed to observe a significant difference between the

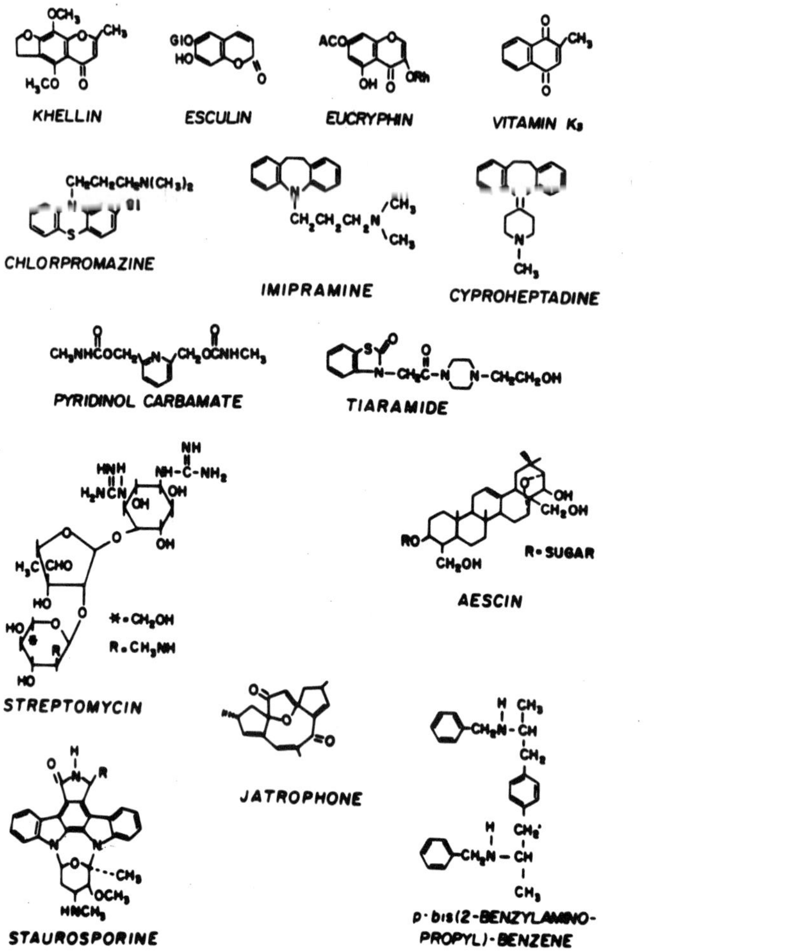

Figure 4 Molecular structures of nonflavonoid compounds reported to exhibit antibradykinin activities.

potencies of acetylated eucryphin and acetylated astilbin, which show a similar structural difference (28).

It is interesting to note that hexaacetylation of the inactive compounds eucryphin and astilbin, leaving a free hydroxyl at position 5, conferred significant anti-BK activity (28). This observation strongly suggests that the effect is related to increased hydrophobicity of the glycoside moiety. This view is further strengthened by the greater anti-BK potency of those

M. velutina glycoside compounds which contain markedly methylated sugars compared to that of the aglycone molecule. Taken together, these results argue against the general prediction that aglycones have greater anti-BK activity than the glycosides (24).

It is evident that all of the flavonoids and the majority of the nonflavonoids exhibiting anti-BK activity present a common structural moiety: a benzene ring conjugated with a double and/or a lone pair of electrons on a nitrogen, oxygen, or sulphur atom belonging to another condensed ring. This may enable us to predict that the benzothiazolinone nucleus of tiaramide is the major determinant of the BK antagonistic activity of this compound. Further studies should be directed to assess the electronic, steric, and hydrophobic effects of other groups introduced to the abovementioned basic structure.

Although the structures of the *M. velutina* compounds cannot yet be presented, they are markedly different from the other anti-BK compounds depicted in Figures 3 and 4. We suggest that they will open an important new perspective in studies on the structure-activity relationships of nonpeptide BK antagonists.

V. CONCLUDING REMARKS

The recent discovery of BK analogs capable of blocking B2 receptors (82) has given new impetus to kinin research by providing pharmacologists with new tools to further characterize the receptors by which BK induces its multiple effects. Thus, the use of these new peptide BK receptor antagonists has begun to detect differences in their ability to antagonize the actions of BK in several models, providing evidence that B2 receptors constitute a heterogenous population and that B2 receptor subtypes may coexist in the same tissue (8, 45, 83). It has also led to the proposal that tracheal smooth muscle contains a B3 BK receptor (54).

Considerable effort has also been expended to discover BK receptor antagonists of nonpeptide nature. Most of these attempts have resulted in compounds which lack the necessary selectivity against BK-induced effects. Among such substances are several synthetic phenothiazine derivatives, vitamin K_3 and several plant-derived flavonoids. However, we have found that the rhizome of *M. velutina* contains some glycoside steroids which are functional selective and competitive BK receptor antagonists in several isolated smooth muscle preparations. Unlike some of the peptide BK receptor antagonists, the compounds from *M. velutina* do not appear to discriminate between B1 and B2 receptors and are also capable of functionally inhibiting the putative B3 receptor. It should be pointed out, however, that some compounds failed to exhibit a strictly competitive type of inhibition in the guinea pig ileum.

In vivo, these nonpeptide BK antagonists exhibit potent and long-lasting anti-inflammatory activity in several models. The most effective compound is MV8612, which significantly antagonizes paw and ear edema and pleurisy induced by several phlogistic agents in rats and mice. This compound also exhibits antinociceptive properties in mice and attenuates the hypotension and bronchoconstriction associated with ovalbumin-induced anaphylaxis in actively sensitized guinea pigs. Also unlike the peptide antagonists, the compounds are active following systemic, and sometimes topical, administration.

Although the evidence accumulated thus far strongly supports the view that compounds from *M. velutina* may constitute a new class of nonpeptide BK antagonists, data showing that such compounds can displace radiolabeled kinins from their receptors must still be provided in order to consider them competitive BK receptor antagonists. An alternative mode of action for these highly lipid/soluble compounds may involve interference with one or more of the intracellular transduction mechanisms responsible for the manifestation of BK-induced responses (see Fig. 1).

Whichever is the ultimate cellular mode of action of the nonpeptide compounds from *M. velutina*, they may constitute useful tools to investigate the several actions and roles of BK and related kinins. Furthermore, they may also provide a basis for the development of a new class of anti-inflammatory therapeutic drugs.

The lack of selectivity of the majority of nonpeptide flavonoid and nonflavonoid compounds against kinin-induced effects in different tissues and experimental conditions may impose great difficulty on the design of orally active BK receptor antagonists. However, it is important to note that virtually all inflammatory states involve multiple and complex interactions between a large number of mediators. As seen with the prostaglandins, it is not unlikely that BK also subserves multiple modulatory roles in inflammation. If this challenging view is correct, and there is ample evidence to suggest that it is, the development of compounds capable of blocking many direct and indirect effects of kinins should provide a novel class of agents with a wide spectrum of anti-inflammatory and analgesic activities.

Since rhizome of the *M. velutina* furnishes low yields of pure active compounds (44), and in view of the difficulty of obtaining large amounts of this plant, we have recently succeeded in obtaining some active anti-BK compounds from this plant through callus culture (84, 85). In addition, recently, Silva et al. (86) have achieved mass in vitro propagation of *M.*

velutina. Together, both approaches may be useful as rapid and efficient methods for large-scale production of these active compounds.

Finally, the results presented in this chapter, concerning the effects of the *M. velutina* compounds, show that studies on the pharmacological properties of extracts and active principles of medicinal plants still constitute an interesting and feasible approach to the discovery of prototypes of new drug classes.

ACKNOWLEDGMENTS

The authors wish to thank Mrs. Elizabet T. Ramos Ganzer for secretarial assistance and Mr. Paulo Cesar Araujo Neves for the graphical work. Research from these laboratories was funded by grants from FINEP and CNPq (Brazil).

REFERENCES

1. Rocha e Silva, M., W. T., Beraldo, and G. Rosenfeld. Bradykinin, a hypotensive and smooth muslce stimulating factor released from plasma by snake venoms and by trypsin. *Am. J. Physiol.* **156**:261-273 (1949).
2. Rocha e Silva, M. The physiological significance of bradykinin. *Ann. N.Y. Acad. Sci.* **104**:190-210 (1963).
3. Kellermeyer, R. W., and R. C. Graham. Kinins—possible physiologic and pathologic roles in man. *New England J. Med.* **279**:754-759 (1968).
4. Kellermeyer, R. W., and R. C. Graham. Kinins—possible physiologic and pathologic roles in man (continued). *New England J. Med.* **279**:802-807 (1968).
5. Colman, R. W., and P. Y. Wong. Kallikrein-kinin system in pathologic conditions, In: *Handbook of Experimental Pharmacology*, vol. XXV (suppl) (E. G. Erdos, ed.). Springer-Verlag, Berlin, pp. 189-185 (1979).
6. Regoli, D., and J. Barabé. Pharmacology of bradykinin and related kinins. *Pharmacol. Rev.* **32**:1-46 (1980).
7. Proud, D., and A. L. Kaplan. Kinin formation: Mechanisms and role in inflammatory disorders. *Ann. Rev. Immunol.* **6**:49-83 (1989).
8. Burch, R. M., S. G. Farmer, and L. R. Steranka. Bradykinin receptor antagonists. *Med. Res. Rev.*, (in press).
9. Ondetti, M. A., N. J. Rubin, and D. W. Cushing. Design of specific inhibitors of angiotensin-converting enzyme: New class of orally active antihypertensive agents. *Science* **196**:441-444 (1977).
10. Fredinger, R. M. Non-peptide ligands for peptide receptors. *Trends Pharmacol. Sci.* **10**:270-274 (1989).
11. Chiu, A. T., D. J. Carni, A. L. Johnson, T. E. McCall, W. A. Price, N. J. N. C. Thoolen, P. C. Wong, R. I. Taber, and P. B. M. W. M. Timmerman. Non-peptide angiotensin II receptor antagonists. II. Pharmacology of S-8308. *Eur. J. Pharmacol.* **157**:13-21 (1988).

12. Mariani, L. Pharmaci antagonisti della bradichinina. *Bol. Soc. Ital. Biol. Sper.* **37**:1481-1484 (1961).
13. Rocha e Silva, M., and J. G. Leme. Antagonists of bradykinin. *J. Med. Exp.* **8**:287-295 (1963).
14. Rocha e Silva, M., and J. G. Leme. On some antagonists of bradykinin. *Naunyn Schmiedberg's Arch. Exp. Pathol. Pharmacol.* **250**:166-170 (1964).
15. Leme, J. G., and M. Rocha e Silva. Competitive and noncompetitive inhibition of bradykinin in the guinea-pig ileum. *Br. J. Pharmacol.* **25**:50-58 (1965).
16. Rocha e Silva, M., and J. G. Leme. Studies on the antagonists of bradykinin, in: *Excerpta Medica Internation Congress,* series 82, pp. 120-133 (1964).
17. Collier, H. O. J. Kinins and ventilation of the lungs, in: *Handbook of Experimental Pharmacology*, vol. XXV (E. G. Erdos, ed.). Springer-Verlag, Berlin, pp. 409-420 (1970).
18. Armstrong, D. Pain, in: *Handbook of Experimental Pharmacology*, vol. XXV (E. G. Erdos, ed.). Springer-Verlag, Berlin, pp. 434-481 (1970).
19. Shimamoto, T. H., H. Maezawa, H. Yamazaki, T. Atsumi, T. Fujita, T. Ishioka, and T. Sunaga. Pyridinolcarbamate, a bradykinin antagonist in veins. *Am. Heart J.* **71**:297-302 (1966).
20. Gieldanowski, J., A. Pelczarska, and J. Patkowski. On the pharmacologic properties of substituted derivatives of *bis*-(aminopropyl)-benzene. *Arch. Immunol. Ther. Exp.* **17**:536-540 (1969).
21. Graham, J. P. P., and H. Al-Katib. The effect of 2-halogenoalkylamines on the biological activity of some peptides. *Br. J. Pharmacol.* **27**:377-386 (1966).
21a. Coyne, D. W., M. Mordhorst, E. J., Cragoe, and A. R. Morrison. Inhibition of bradykinin-induced increases in cytosolic Ca^{++} by a novel amiloride analog. *J. Pharmacol. Exp. Ther.* **250**:795-799 (1989).
22. Leme, J. G., and E. J. Walaszeck. Antagonists of pharmacologically active peptides: Effect on guinea pig ileum and inflammation. *Pharmacologist* **9**:242 (1967).
23. Leme, J. G., and E. J. Walaszeck. Antagonists of pharmacologically active peptides. Effect on guinea pig ileum and inflammation. Pharmacology and the future of man, in: *Proceedings 5th International Congress of Pharmacology*, vol. V, San Francisco, Basel, Karger, pp. 328-335 (1973).
24. Chau, T. T., and T. J. Haley. Flavonoid antagonism of the spasmogenic effect of angiotensin, bradykinin, and eledoisin on guinea pig ileum. *J. Pharm. Sci.* **58**:621-623 (1969).
25. Ramaswamy, A. S. Pharmacological action of the biflavonoids from the gymnosperms with special reference to *Ginko biloba*, L. *J. Ind. Med. Assoc.* **55**:163-165 (1970).
26. Garbor, M. Anti-inflammatory substances of plant origin, in: *Handbook of Experimental Pharmacology*, vol. 50, pt. 2 (J. R. Vane, S. H. Ferreira, eds.). Springer-Verlag, Berlin, pp. 698-739 (1979).

27. Prabhakar, M. C., H. Bano, I. Kumar, M. A. Shamsi, and M. S. Y. Khan. Pharmacological investigations on vitexin. *Planta Medica* **43**:396-403 (1981).
28. Calixto, J. B., J. C. Gomes, E. Carneiro, R. A. Yunes, F. Delle Monache and Y. S. Medeiros. Pharmacological evaluation of fractions and two glycoside flavonoids from the bark of *Hymenaea martiana in vitro*, in: *Brazilian-Sino Symposium on Chemistry and Pharmacology of Natural Products,* Rio de Janeiro, 174P (1989).
29. Altinkurt, O., and I. Kanzik. Non-competitive inhibition of bradykinin, acetylcholine and histamine on guinea-pig ileum with streptomycin and vitamin K_3. *Arzneim. -Forsch./Drug Res.* **30**:41-44 (1980).
30. Altinkurt, O., and I. Kanzik. Effects of vitamin K_3 on the hypotensive and bronchoconstrictor responses to bradykinin and histamine in the guinea pig. *Drug Res.* **30**:286-287 (1980).
31. Calixto, J. B., and A. E. G. Sant'Ana. Pharmacological analysis of the inhibitory effect of jatrophone, a diterpene isolated from *Jatropha elliptica*, on smooth and cardiac muscles. *Phytotherapy Res.* **1**:122-126 (1987).
32. Vogel, G. The effect of drugs of plant origin on capillary permeability and the lymphatic system, in: *Pharmacognosy and Phytochemistry* (H. Wagner, L. Horhammet, eds). Springer-Verlag, Berlin, pp. 370-386 (1971).
33. Nakahata, N., and H. Nakanishi. Bradykinin-induced contraction is inhibited by tiaramide, an anti-inflammatory drug, with an inhibition of increase in intracellular free calcium. *J. Pharmacol. Exp. Ther.* **246**:635-640 (1988).
34. Picq, M., M. Dubois, Y. Munari-Silem, A.-F. Prigent, and H. Pacheco. Flavonoid modulation of protein kinase C. *Life Sci.* **44**:1563-1571 (1989).
35. Dray, A., and M. N. Perkins. Bradykinin activates peripheral capsaicin-sensitive fibers via a second messenger system. *Agents Actions,* **25**:214-215, 1988.
36. Ferreira, S. H. A bradykinin-potentiating factor (BPF) present in the venom of *B. jararaca. Br. J. Pharmacol.* **24**:163-169 (1965).
37. Calixto, J. B., M. Nicolau, and R. A. Yunes. The selective antagonism of bradykinin action on rat isolated uterus by crude *Mandevilla velutina* extract. *Br. J. Pharmacol.* **85**:729-731 (1985).
38. Calixto, J. B., M. Nicolau, and R. A. Yunes. Antagonistic effect of *Mandevilla velutina* extract on kinin-induced contractions of guinea pig and cat ileum longitudinal smooth muscle. *Gen. Pharmacol.* **19**:595-599 (1988).
39. Calixto, J. B., and R. A. Yunes. Blockade of kinin-induced responses of the isolated guinea pig urinary bladder by the extract of *Mandevilla velutina. Gen. Pharmacol.* **21**:285-290 (1990).
40. Llona, I., R. J. Vavrek, J. M. Stewart, and J. P. Huidobro-Toro. Identification of pre- and postsynaptic bradykinin receptor sites in the vas deferens: Evidence for different structural prerequisites. *J. Pharmacol. Exp. Ther.* **241**:608-614 (1987).
41. Rifo, J., M. Pourrat, R. J. Vavrek, J. M. Stewart, and J. P. Huidobro-Toro. Bradykinin receptor antagonists used to characterize the heterogeneity of bradykinin-induced responses in rat vas deferens. *Eur. J. Pharmacol.* **42**:305-312 (1987).

42. Ferreira, S. H., and J. R. Vane. The detection and estimation of bradykinin in the circulating blood. *Br. J. Pharmacol.* **29**:367-377 (1967).
43. Calixto, J. B., M. Nicolau, M. G. Pizzolatti, and R. A. Yunes. Kinin antagonist activity of compounds from *Mandevilla velutina* in the rat isolated uterus. *Br. J. Pharmacol.* **91**:199-204 (1987).
44. Calixto, J. B., M. G. Pizzolatti, and R. A. Yunes. The competitive antagonistic effect of compounds from *Mandevilla velutina* on kinin-induced contractions of rat uterus and guinea pig ileum *in vitro*. *Br. J. Pharmacol.* **94**: 1133-1142 (1988).
45. Steranka, L. R., R. M. Burch, R. J. Vavrek, J. M. Stewart, and S. J. Enna. Multiple bradykinin receptors: Results of studies using a novel class of receptor antagonists, in: *Neuroreceptors and Signal Transduction* (S. Kito, T. Segawa, K. Kuriyama, M. Tohyama, R. W. Olsen, eds.). Plenum Press, New York, pp. 111-127 (1988).
46. Steranka, L. R., J. C. Manning, C. J. DeHaas, J. W. Ferkany, S. A. Borosky, J. R. Connor, R. J. Vavrek, J. M. Stewart, and S. H. Snyder. Bradykinin as a pain mediator: Receptors are localized to sensory neurons, and antagonists have analgesic actions. *Proc. Natl. Acad. Sci. USA* **85**:3245-3249 (1988).
47. Farmer, S. G., R. M. Burch, C. J. DeHaas, J. Togo, and L. R. Steranka. [Arg^1-$DPhe^7$]-substituted analogs of bradykinin inhibit vasopressin- and bradykinin-induced contractions of uterine smooth muscle. *J. Pharmacol. Exp. Ther.* **248**:677-681 (1989).
48. Antonio, A. The relaxing effect of bradykinin on intestinal smooth muscle. *Br. J. Pharmacol.* **32**:78-86 (1968).
49. Boschov, P., A. C. M. Paiva, T. B. Paiva, and I. S. Shimuta. Further evidence for the existence of two receptor sites for bradykinin responsible for the diphasic effect in the rat isolated duodenum. *Br. J. Pharmacol.* **83**:591-600 (1984).
50. Paiva, A. C. M., T. B. Paiva, C. C. Pereira, and S. J. Shimuta. Selectivity of bradykinin analogs for receptors mediating contraction and relaxation of the rat duodenum. *Br. J. Pharmacol.* **98**:206-210 (1989).
51. Calixto, J. B., M. Nicolau, M. G. Pizzolatti, and R. A. Yunes. A selective antagonist of bradykinin action from a crude extract of *Mandevilla velutina* Part II. Effect on non-uterine smooth muscles. *Brazilian J. Med. Biol. Res.* **18**:729A (1985).
52. Calixto, J. B., G. H. Strobel, A. B. Cruz, and R. A. Yunes. Blockade of bradykinin-evoked dyphasic responses of isolated rat duodenum by the crude extract of compounds obtained from *Mandevilla velutina*. *Brazilian J. Med. Biol. Res.* **21**:1015-1018 (1988).
53. Liebmann, C., S. Riessmann, P. Robberecht, and H. Arold. Bradykinin action in the rat duodenum: Receptor binding and influence on the cyclic AMP system. *Biomed. Biochim. Acta* **46**:469-478 (1987).
54. Farmer, S. G., R. M. Burch, S. A. Meeker, and D. E. Wilkins. Evidence for a pulmonary B_3 bradykinin receptor. *Mol. Pharmacol.* **36**:1-8 (1989).

55. Calixto, J. B., and R. A. Yunes. Effect of a crude extract of *Mandevilla velutina* on contractions induced by bradykinin and [desArg^9]-bradykinin in isolated vessels of the rabbit. *Br. J. Pharmacol.* **88**:937-941 (1986).
56. Palmer, R. M. J., A. G. Ferrige, and S. Moncada. Nitric oxide release accounts for the biological activity of endothelium-derived relaxing factor. *Nature* **327**:524-526 (1987).
57. Yanagisawa, M., H. Kurihara, S. Kimura, Y. Tomobe, M. Kobayashi, Y. Mitsui, Y. Yasaki, K. Goto, and T. Masaki. A novel potent vasoconstrictor peptide produced by vascular endothelial cells. *Nature* **332**:411-415 (1988).
58. Furchgott, R. F. The role of endothelium in the responses of vascular smooth muscle to drugs. *Ann. Rev. Pharmacol. Toxicol.* **24**:175-197 (1984).
59. Sung, C., A. J. Arleth, K. Shikano, and B. Berkowitz. Characterization and function of bradykinin receptors in vascular endothelial cells. *J. Pharmacol. Exp. Ther.* **247**:8-13 (1988).
60. D'Orleans-Juste, G., DeNucci, N., and J. R. Vane. Kinins act on B_1 or B_2 receptors to release conjointly endothelium-derived relaxing factor and prostacyclin from bovine aortic endothelial cells. *Br. J. Pharmacol.* **96**:920-926 (1989).
61. Lewis, G. P. Kinins in inflammation and tissue injury, in: *Handbook of Experimental Pharmacology*, vol. XXV (E. G. Erdos, ed.). Springer-Verlag, Berlin, pp. 516-530 (1970).
62. Marceau, F., A. Lussier, D. Regoli, and J. P. Giroud. Pharmacology of kinins: Their relevance to tissue injury and inflammation. *Gen. Pharmacol.* **14**:209-229 (1983).
63. Lerner, V. H., I. L. Jones, and G. T. Gustafson. Bradykinin, a new potential mediator of inflammation-induced bone resorption. *Arth. Rheum.* **30**: 530-540 (1987).
64. Hargreaves, K. M., E. S. Troullos, R. A. Dionne, E. A. Schmidt, S. C. Schaffer, and J. L. Joris. Bradykinin is increased during acute and chronic inflammation: Therapeutic implications. *Clin. Pharmacol. Ther.* **44**:613-621 (1988).
65. Trebien, H. A., and J. B. Calixto. Pharmacological evaluation of rat paw edema induced by *Bothrops jararaca* venom. *Agents Actions* **26**:292-300 (1989).
66. Henriques, M. G. M. O., V. B. Weg, M. A. Martins, P. M. R. Silva, P. D. Fernandes, R. S. B. Cordeiro, and B. B. Vargaftig. Differential inhibition by two hetrazepine PAF-antagonists of acute inflammation in the mouse. *Br. J. Pharmacol.* **99**:164-168 (1990).
67. Calixto, J. B., M. Nicolau, H. Trebien, M. G. M. O. Henriques, V. B. Weg, R. S. B. Cordeiro, and R. A. Yunes. Antiedematogenic actions of a hydroalcoholic crude water-alcohol extract of *Mandevilla velutina*. *Brazilian J. Med. Biol. Res.* **19**:575A (1986).
68. Neves, M. C. A., M. G. M. O. Henriques, R. S. B. Cordeiro, P. C. A. Neves, A. B. Cruz, R. A. Yunes, Y. S. Medeiros, and J. B. Calixto. Compounds from *Mandevilla velutina* inhibit bradykinin-induced paw oedema in rats and mice but do not affect enhanced vascular permeability, in: *Brazilian-Sino*

Symposium on Chemistry and Pharmacology of Natural Products, Rio de Janeiro, 253P (1989).
69. Rothschild, A. M. Some pharmacodynamic properties of cellulose sulphate, a kininogen-depleting agent in the rat. *Br. J. Pharmacol.* **33**:501-512 (1968).
70. Coelho, L., Y. S. Medeiros, R. A. Yunes, A. B. Cruz, and J. B. Calixto. Effect of compounds obtained from *Mandevilla velutina* on platelet aggregation in humans, rabbits and guinea pigs, in: *Brazilian-Sino Symposium on Chemistry and Pharmacology of Natural Products*, Rio de Janeiro, 263P (1989).
71. Inoue, H., T. Mori, and Y. Koshihara. Sulfidopeptide-leukotrienes are major mediators of arachidonic acid-induced mouse ear edema. *Prostaglandins* **36**: 731-739 (1988).
72. Griswold, D. E., E. Webb, L. Schwartz, and N. Hanna. Arachidonic acid-induced inflammation: Inhibition by dual inhibitor of arachidonic acid metaboblism, SK&F 86002. *Inflammation* **11**:189-199 (1987).
73. Crummey, A., G. P. Harper, E. A. Boyle, and F. R. Mangan. Inhibition of arachidonic acid-induced ear oedema as a model for assessing topical anti-inflammatory compounds. *Agents Actions* **20**:69-76 (1987).
74. Inoue, H. T., M. S. Shibata, and Y. Koshikara. Modulation by glycerrhetinic acid derivatives of TPA-induced ear oedema. *Br. J. Pharmacol.* **96**:204-210 (1989).
75. Marks, F., G. Furstenberger, and E. Kownatzki. Prostaglandin E-mediated mitogenic stimulation of mouse epidermis *in vivo* by divalent cation ionophore A23187 and by tumor promoter 12-0-tetradecanoyl-phorbol-13-acetate. *Cancer Res.* **41**:696-701 (1981).
76. Calixto, J. B., J. C. Zanini Jr., A. B. Cruz, R. A. Yunes, and Y. S. Medeiros. Inhibition of arachidonic acid-induced ear oedema by the crude extract and compounds obtained from *Mandevilla velutina*. *Third Interscience World Conference on Inflammation, Antirheumatics, Analgesics, Immunomodulators,* Monte Carlo (1989).
77. Nicolau, M., J. B. Calixto, M. L. Bittencourt, M. N. Beins, R. S. B. Cordeiro, M. G. O. Henriques, V. B. Weg, and R. A. Yunes. Effect of *Mandevilla velutina* crude extracts in cutaneous rat vascular permeability and mouse carrageenan-induced pleurisy, in: *Proc. French Brazilian Symposium on Chemistry and Pharmacology of Natural Substances in Inflammation, Allergy and Thrombosis*, Rio de Janeiro, 18P (1986).
78. Whalley, E. T., I. A. Nwator, J. M. Stewart, and R. J. Vavrek. Analysis of the receptors mediating vascular actions of bradykinin. *Naunyn-Schmiedeberg's Arch. Pharmacol.* **336**:430-433 (1987).
79. Greisbacher, T., and F. Lembeck. Effect of bradykinin antagonists on bradykinin-induced plasma extravasation, venoconstriction, prostaglandin E_2 release, and nociceptor stimulation and contraction of the iris sphincter muscle in the rabbit. *Br. J. Pharmacol.* **92**:333-340 (1987).
80. Bauman, Y., J. C. Gomes, Y. S. Medeiros, A. B. Cruz, R. A. Yunes, and J. B. Calixto. Action of *Mandevilla velutina* compounds on histamine release from rat mast cell and antigen-induced bronchoconstriction and hypotension

in actively sensitized guinea pigs, in: *Brazilian-Sino Symposium on Chemistry and Pharmacology of Natural Products*, Rio de Janeiro, 264P (1989).
81. Barnes, P. J., K. F. Chung, and C. P. Page. Inflammatory mediators and asthma. *Pharmacol. Rev.* **40**:49-84 (1988).
82. Vavrek, R. J., and J. M. Stewart. Competitive antagonists of bradykinin. *Peptides* **6**:161-164 (1985).
83. Steranka, L. R., S. G. Farmer, and R. M. Burch. Antagonists of B_2 bradykinin receptors. *FASEB J.* **3**:2019-2025 (1989).
84. Calixto, J. B., A. L. Silva, M. S. Reis, R. M. B. F. L. Costa, J. A. Yunes, A. B. Cruz, and R. A. Yunes. Demonstration of anti-bradykinin compounds by callus culture of *Mandevilla velutina. Brazilian J. Med. Biol. Res.* **22**: 1275-1279 (1989).
85. Silva, A. L., G. Cord Neto, M. S. Reis, J. A. Yunes, A. B. Cruz, C. Alberton, R. A. Yunes, and J. B. Calixto. Comparison of the constituents of *Mandevilla velutina* callus culture with those of the intact rhizome, in: *Brazilian-Sino Symposium on Chemistry and Pharmacology of Natural Products*, Rio de Janeiro, 262P (1989).
86. Silva, A. L., M. S. Reis, J. A. Yunes, G. Cord Neto, K. Honda, and L. L. Dalvesco. *In vitro* culture of *Mandevilla velutina* for mass propagation, in: *Brazilian-Sino Symposium on Chemistry and Pharmacology of Natural Products*, Rio de Janeiro, 161P (1989).

5
Conformational Properties of Bradykinin and Bradykinin Antagonists

Donald J. Kyle
Nova Pharmaceutical Corporation
Baltimore, Maryland

Paul R. Blake
University of Maryland
Baltimore County
Baltimore, Maryland

Rickey P. Hicks
Mississippi State University
Mississippi State, Mississippi

Valentine J. Klimkowski*
Polygen Corporation
Waltham, Massachusetts

A fundamental concept in medicinal chemistry is the determination of a relationship between the three-dimensional structure of a molecule and its corresponding biological activity. Synthetic manipulation of a given structure which is consistent with an established structure-activity relationship (SAR) is normally expected to result in compounds able to elicit an improvement in some pharmacologic property. Historically this approach has been used primarily in the development of nonpeptide molecules (1), however, recent advances in the synthetic methodology used to prepare peptides containing unnatural amino acids (which impose specific conformational restraints) have led to widespread application in this area as

**Present affiliation*: Eli Lilly and Company, Indianapolis, Indiana.

well (2). Thus, for those receptors whose natural ligands are peptides, the geometric and electronic requirements may be explored via restricted peptides whose conformations in solution likely remain unchanged upon binding to the receptor (3).

Coincident with the preparation of synthetic peptides, SARs of peptide ligands are being founded more frequently upon their conformational properties in solution. These conformations have been analyzed primarily by nuclear magnetic resonance (NMR) spectroscopy through the utilization of torsional dependent ^3J coupling constants (4-7) as well as by nuclear Overhauser enhancement spectrometry (NOESY) experiments (8-12). Since the peptide hormone bradykinin (Arg^1-Pro^2-Pro^3-Gly^4-Phe^5-Ser^6-Pro^7-Phe^8-Arg^9) has been implicated in a multitude of pathophysiological processes, the therapeutic value of a bradykinin receptor antagonist may be quite significant (13-16). To this end, bradykinin has been examined by virtually every spectroscopic technique available, including NMR, circular dichroism (CD), and optical rotary dispersion (ORD). Furthermore, several conformationally restricted peptide analogs have been reported.

On the basis of bradykinin's primary amino acid sequence alone, it is possible to extract several structural moieties that might be significant in stabilizing the biologically active conformation. The three Pro residues (one-third of the entire molecule) suggest that some ordering might prevail in solution due to the inherent restrictions about the angle ϕ within each. Furthermore, there is a likelihood of amide bond *cis/trans* isomerism since three of the eight total in bradykinin are of the type X-pro. On the basis of Chou and Fasman factors (7), the sequences Pro^2-Pro^3-Gly^4-Phe^5 and Ser^6-Pro^7-Phe^8-Arg^9 have significant β-turn probabilities (3.79×10^{-4} and 1.99×10^{-4}, respectively). These theoretical arguments can also be used as precedence for an ordered bioactive conformation.

In early CD and ORD experiments run in aqueous solution, Silva et al. suggested that bradykinin maintains considerable conformational freedom in spite of the presence of three order-inducing proline residues (18). Similar findings were reported by both Craig (19) and Bodanszky (20), the latter of whom noted the absence of several key absorption bands in both the CD and ORD spectra. These bands, which include absorptions at 233 nm, 190 nm, and a shoulder at 220 nm in the ORD spectrum, as well as a trough at 222 nm in the CD spectrum, had been previously characterized as fingerprints for helical structures in proteins by Holzworth (21).

In apparent contrast to these early results Cann later suggested, on the basis of CD data collected in water at 25 °C, that bradykinin was a time-average of two interconverting conformations, one being random, the other partially ordered (22,23). The ordering in the latter was proposed to be primarily due to a 3-1 hydrogen bond bridging Pro^7. It was reported that the relative population of this partially ordered state increased with temperature as the ordered waters of solvation were "melted off" leaving the amide protons free to hydrogen bond in an intramolecular fashion. Examination of the CD spectrum for bradykinin in a dioxane-water mixture led Cann (22,23) to propose the probable formation of three, 1-3 hydrogen bonds in this media. As shown in Figure 1, one of these bridged Pro^3, one Pro^7, and the other Phe^8. In particular, the adjacent hydrogen bonds were implicated by Cann as a segment within either a 2_7 ribbon or a 2.2_7 helix. On the basis of these findings, it was suggested that the adoption of a more highly ordered conformation in a nonpolar environment might have implications for the interaction of bradykinin with cell memranes housing the bradykinin receptor. This hypothesis was subsequently supported by other workers who reported that a series of bradykinin analogs maintained activity like bradykinin, yet their conformations, as determined by CD spectroscopy, were similar in hydrophobic media like trifluoroethanol (TFE) or sodium dodecylsulfate and dissimilar in an aqueous environment (24,25). These results were interpreted as proof that the pharmacologic actions were being expressed in a hydrophobic environment. Drawing upon this information, and incorporating the results of empirical energy conformational searches in vacuo, Chipens and colleagues proposed that the biologically active conformation of bradykinin is "quasicyclic" (26). According to these authors, a cyclic form of the peptide could be stabilized ionically, either through interactions between the guanidino side chain of Arg^1 and C-terminal carboxyl group, or through interaction between the N-terminal amino and C-terminal carboxyl groups directly. Due to the dominating forces of solvation, however, these conformational

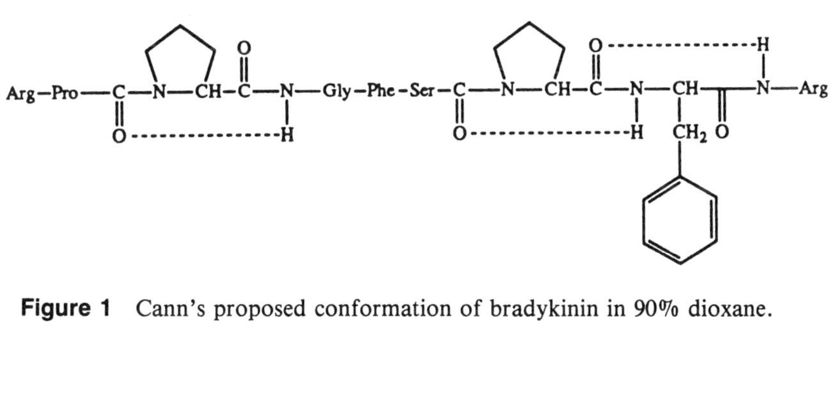

Figure 1 Cann's proposed conformation of bradykinin in 90% dioxane.

types would be unpopulated in polar aqueous solutions and, therefore, would be unobservable. In constrast, the solvated bradykinin molecule in vivo might first be dehydrated in the apolar biophase during hormone-receptor interaction, thereby negating the effect of solvation upon the conformation and making these "quasi-cyclic" forms more probable. This assumption is supported by the notion that dehydration of the contacting surfaces is the first step during enzyme-substrate interaction (27). The application of this information led to the preparation of a variety of cyclic peptides (28) including cyclo-[(N^{ξ}-Lys^{1},Gly^{6})bradykinin], which was reported to have potent depressor activity (of comparable magnitude but longer duration than bradykinin) and no myotropic activity.

Other than the cyclic analogs prepared by Chipens, there have been several other conformationally constrained but linear bradykinin analogs reported over the past several years. For example, Turk synthesized three analogs, each of which contained a C^{α}-methyl group at position 4, 5, or 8 in the primary sequence (29). The nature of the constraint imposed by the methyl group is best summarized by stating that the most probable values for the torsion angles ϕ and ψ, which describe a peptide's backbone conformation, fall primarily into two small areas centered around $\phi = -57°$, $\psi = -47°$, or $\phi = +57°$, $\psi = +47°$. None of the three analogs were bradykinin antagonists, and the [Ala^{4}] bradykinin molecule was completely inactive. [C^{α}-methyl, Phe^{8}]bradykinin was reported to exhibit tissue specificity and diminished pulmonary activation in the rat. Other analogs were prepared by Mazur, wherein single substitutions by N-methyl amino acids in the 1, 4, 5, 8, and 9 positions were made (30). [N-$MeArg^{1}$]bradykinin retained 60% of the muscle contracting activity of bradykinin in the guinea pig ileum assay. The other compounds were exceptionally weak agonists (<2%). Stewart has reported the preparation of analogs in which a hydroxyproline residue replaces one of the naturally occurring prolines in position 2, 3, or 7 of bradykinin (31). A progressive loss in potency was noted in all assays as the hydroxyproline residue was moved toward the C-terminus. This observation is consistent with the idea that the initial combination of bradykinin with its receptor is at the C-terminus, followed by a "zipping up" of the remainder of the peptide with the receptor. Still another series of analogs was reported by Fisher et al. (32). A set of three molecules was derived from bradykinin and contained a dehydrophenylalanine residue (Δ^{Z}Phe) in place of the naturally occurring phenylalanine at positions 5 and/or 8. It was reported that [$\Delta^{Z}Phe^{5}$]bradykinin showed high biological activity, particularly in terms of its systemic blood pressure lowering effect in rats, being more than 23 times as potent as bradykinin. [$\Delta^{Z}Phe^{8}$]bradykinin was less potent than bradykinin itself, and [$\Delta^{Z}Phe^{5,8}$]bradykinin was equipotent with bradykinin.

Although bradykinin has been the subject of intensive investigations over the past 20 years, surprisingly little is known about its mechanism of action at the molecular level. Additional insight could be obtained from an X-ray crystallographic study of bradykinin bound to its receptor, however, neither bradykinin nor the bradykinin receptor has been obtained in crystalline form. Furthermore, although several conformationally constrained analogs of bradykinin have been prepared and tested, most are either weak or inactive agonists, and none were tested in receptor binding assays. The overall result is that these analogs provide little in terms of establishing an SAR for peptide bradykinin antagonists.

Following established precedents for founding SARs of peptide ligands on their conformational preferences in solution, our approach was to complete a detailed examination of bradykinin using modern two-dimensional NMR methods in combination with empirical energy calculations. Incorporation of interproton distances obtained from NOESY spectra into molecular dynamics calculations in the form of restraints has been shown to be an effective method for establishing solution structures for both peptides and proteins (33,34). A typical problem encountered in this type of NMR work, however, is the quantification of the major conformational species present. This problem is potentially even more complex for bradykinin, where solvation is known to dominate the conformational preferences. The NMR analysis of bradykinin (35), bradykinin fragments (38,39), and bradykinin analogs (40) has been historically carried out in aqueous media capable of tremendous hydrogen bonding and, in each case, a random structure has been reported. Drawing on previously published spectral data, biological results from conformationally restricted analogs, as well as the relationship between ordering in bradykinin and the dielectric environment of the solvent as proposed by Cann and Chipens, the following hypothesis was established: Although in aqueous solution bradykinin exists randomly throughout multiple conformations, the biologically active form of the peptide is likely ordered and stabilized within the lipid bilayer of the cell membrane prior to binding with its receptor (41). Assuming that a solvent environment should be able to simulate, at least in terms of hydrophobicity and dielectric constant, the nature of a cell membrane, a 90% d_8-dioxane-H_2O mixture was selected for NMR experiments. It was anticipated that under these nonsolvating conditions the conformational diversity of bradykinin might be severely restricted. In this way, the aforementioned difficulties frequently encountered during analysis of the NMR spectral data could be minimized and the hypothesis could be tested without undertaking the experimentally difficult alternative of preparing micelles or a bilayer in the NMR tube (42,43).

Preliminary analysis of the two-dimensional NMR data collected at 500 MHz supports a single major conformational species in part due to the five HN-C^{α}H connectivities, one for each amide. This was confirmed in the ^{13}C NMR spectrum where only nine carbonyl resonances, one for each amino acid, were present. In order to provide a starting point for the molecular dynamics simulations the assumption was made, based on multiple observed long-range and amide to amide NOEs, that it was indeed a single major conformational species. Despite the fact that bradykinin contains three proline residues, the absence of any strong $C^{\alpha}H_i$-$C^{\alpha}H_{i+1}$ cross peaks in the NOESY spectrum was taken as proof that all peptide bonds were *trans*. In total, 35 interproton distances were extracted from the NOESY spectrum shown in Figure 2. Whenever possible, stereospecific assignments for pro-R and pro-S hydrogens were made explicitly. The specific values are listed in Table 1. A temperature-dependent study of the chemical shifts of the amide protons resulted in a near-linear dependence suggesting no major conformational changes were coinciding with the temperature change and therby allowing a comparison of slopes ($\Delta\delta/\Delta t$) (44). The lowest values obtained for these slopes corresponded to Phe^8 and Arg^9 suggesting solvent sequestering for these amides.

Given the high Chou and Fasman (17) probability of β-turns in the sequences Pro^2-Pro^3-Gly^4-Phe^5 and Ser^6-Pro^7-Phe^8-Arg^9 (3.79×10^{-4} and 1.99×10^{-4}, respectively), the computational strategy employed was to begin from two initial structures, (a) an extended β-strand, and (b) a structure containing these two predicted β-turns. These two starting structures are shon in Figure 3. Using the program CHARMM (45,46), version 21, the interproton distances were incorporated into the potential energy expression in the form of an additional potential energy term (33) given by:

$$E_{NOE} = \begin{cases} K_1 (R - R_0)^2 & \text{for } R < R_0 \\ K_2 (R - R_0)^2 & \text{for } R > R_0 \end{cases}$$

where R and R_0 are the calculated and target interproton distances, respectively, and K_1 and K_2 are force constants given by:

$$K_1 = \frac{S\,(k_B\,T/2)}{(D\,R_{LOW})^2}$$

$$K_2 = \frac{S\,(k_B\,T/2)}{(D\,R_{HIGH})^2}$$

where k_B is the Boltzmann constant, T is the absolute temperature, and S is a scale factor. ΔR_{LOW} and ΔR_{HIGH} are deviations above and below the target distance R_0, respectively. During the 3 ps heating step of the molecular dynamics, the temperature was raised from 0K to 300K in steps of 20K

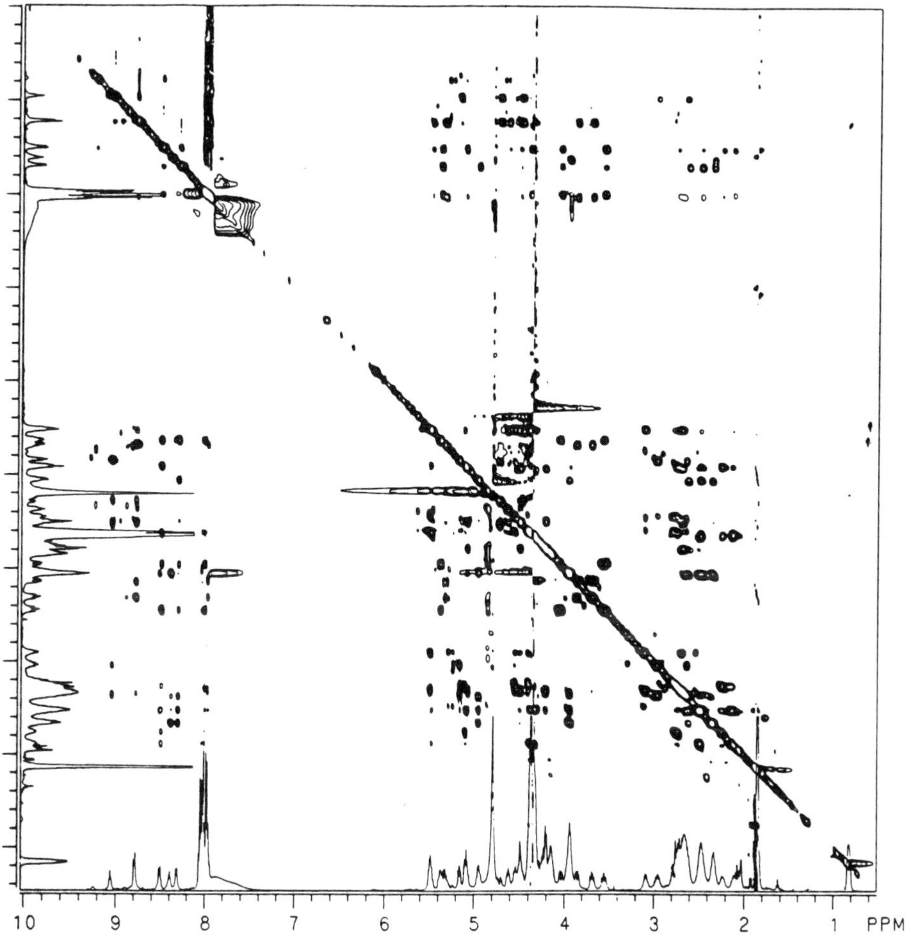

Figure 2 500 MHz NOESY spectrum of bradykinin collected at 25 °C in 90% d_8-dioxane-D_2O.

every 0.2 ps. Since the target distances were poorly satisifed in the starting structures, E_{NOE} was applied gradually by increasing the scale factor in a nonlinear fashion such that it was 0.0 after 0.2 ps, 0.1 after 1.2 ps, and 1.0 after the full 3.0 ps. Following 15 ps of equilibration, 7 ps of incremental production dynamics was completed. During this stage the NOE scale factor was raised from 1.0 to 4.5. By slowly raising the force constants for the NOE restraints as the target distances became better satis-

Table 1 Selected Interproton Distances Taken from the NOESY Spectrum Obtained at 500 MHz in 90% d_6-Dioxane/10% H_2O

A. Intraresidue	NH-C$^{\alpha}$H	NH-C$^{\beta}$H	C$^{\alpha}$H-C$^{\beta}$H
Pro^2			(H_R) 2.5(−0.3, +0.2) (H_S) 2.5(−0.3, +0.2)
Gly^4	(H_R) 2.7(−0.3, +0.5) (H_S) 2.5(−0.3, +0.2)		
Phe^5	2.5(−0.3, +0.2)	(H_R) 2.7(−0.3, +0.5) (H_S) 2.7(−0.3, +0.5)	(H_S) 2.7(−0.3, +0.5)
Ser^6	2.7(−0.3, +0.5)	(H_R) 4.0(−0.7, +0.5)	(H_S) 2.5(−0.3, +0.2)
Pro^7			(H_R) 2.7(−0.3, +0.5) (H_S) 2.7(−0.3, +0.5)
Phe^8	2.5(−0.3, +0.2)	(H_R) 2.7(+0.3, +0.5) (H_S) 4.0(−0.7, +0.5)	(H_R) 2.7(−0.3, +0.5)
Arg^9	2.7(−0.3, +0.5)	(H_S) 2.7(−0.3, +0.5)	
B. Interresidue	**NH$_i$-NH$_{i+1}$**	**C$^{\alpha}$H$_i$-NH$_{i+1}$**	**OTHER**
Arg^1-Pro^2			C$^{\alpha}$H$_i$-C$^{\delta}$H$_{i+1}$ (H_R) 2.7(−0.3, +0.5) (H_S) 2.5(−0.3, +0.2)
Pro^3-Gly^4		2.5(−0.3, +0.2)	C$^{\beta}$H$_i$-NH$_{i+1}$ (H_S) 4.0(−0.7, +0.5)
Gly^4-Phe^5	2.7(−0.3, +0.5)	(H_S) 2.5(−0.3, +0.2)	
Pro^7-Phe^8		2.5(−0.3, +0.2)	C$^{\beta}$H$_i$-NH$_{i+1}$ (H_R) 4.0(−0.7, +0.5)
Phe^8-Arg^9	2.7(−0.3, +0.5)	2.5(−0.3, +0.2)	
C. Long range	**C$^{\alpha}$H$_i$-NH$_{i+1}$**	**C$^{\beta}$H$_i$-NH$_{i+1}$**	**C$^{\beta}$H$_i$-NH$_{i+3}$**
Pro^2-Gly^4	4.0(−0.7, +0.5)		
Pro^3-Phe^5	4.0(−0.7, +0.5)		
Ser^6-Phe^8	4.0(−0.7, +0.5)	(H_R) 2.7(−0.3, +0.5)	
Ser^6-Arg^9			(H_R) 4.0(−0.7, +0.5)
Pro^7-Arg^9	4.0(−0.7, +0.5)		

fied, no dramatic increase in temperature was observed. This is in contrast to the results of other workers using this technique who raised scale factors in a single step from 1.0 to 5.0 which resulted in a dramatic increase in kinetic energy and, subsequently, temperature (33). Finally the NOE scale factor was set to 5.0, 10 ps of production dynamics were completed, and an average structure was extracted from the last 5 ps of the coordinate trajectory.

Analysis of the two average structures obtained from the two unique starting points demonstrated convergence to a similar conformational

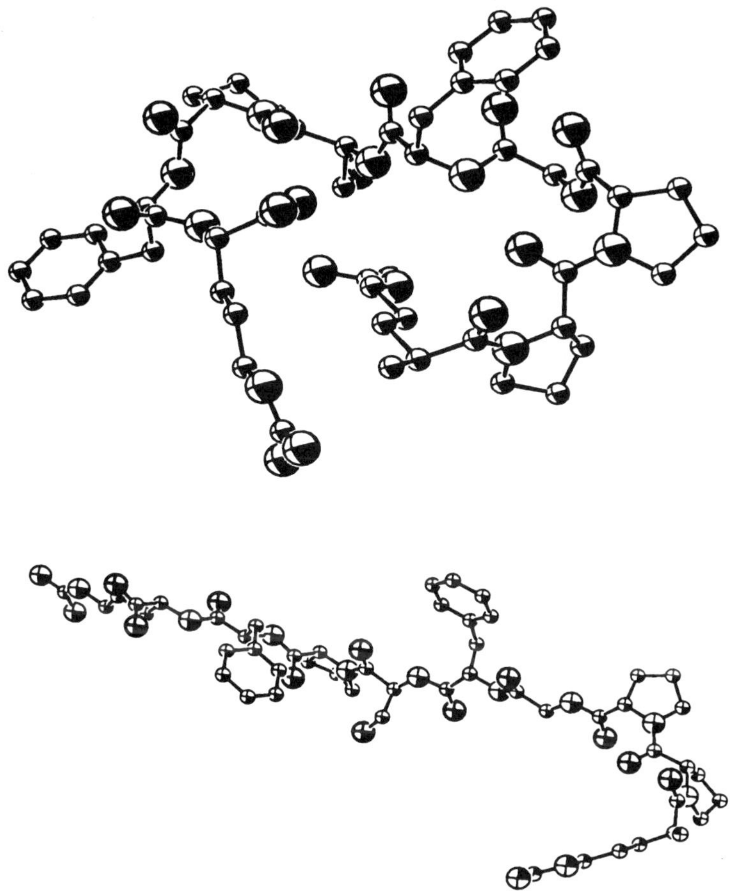

Figure 3 Initial bradykinin conformations used in molecular dynamics simulations. Two β-turn-containing models (above); fully extended β-strand (below).

species, which is shown in Figure 4. In each case the sum of the NOE restraint energy was less than 4.7 kcal/mol, and the RMS deviation from the target distances below 0.25 Å. Virtually identical results were obtained for each simulation when they were repeated without the electrostatic term included in the total potential energy function. This important data attests to the final structures as being derived from the NOE restraints and not by poorly represented electrostatic interactions. Table 2 lists the backbone dihedral angle values obtained at the end of the simulation starting from the fully extended form.

The average dynamic structures are characterized as having all *trans* peptide bonds, and the hydrophobic side chain groups are oriented outward into solution, perhaps ready to interact with the receptor. There ap-

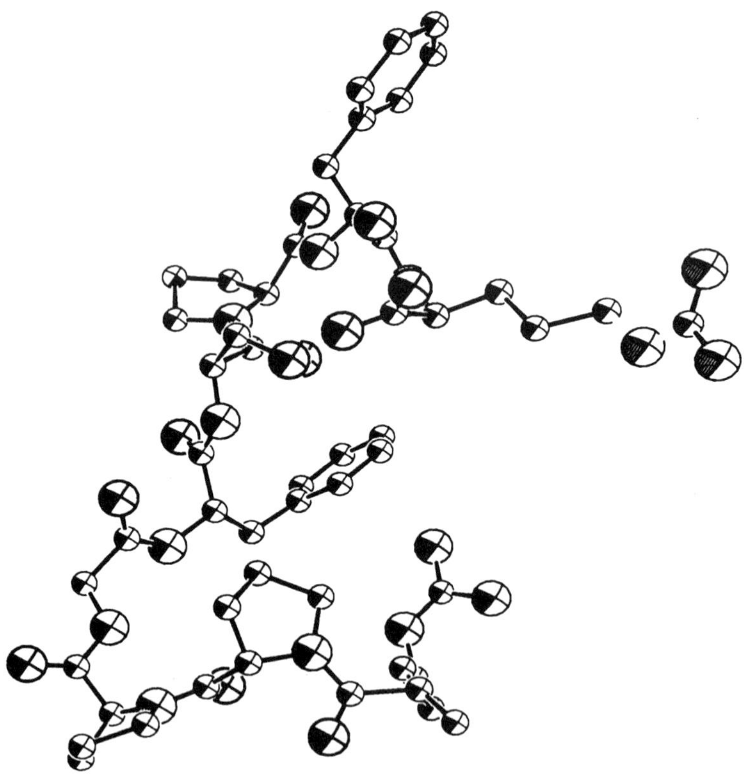

Figure 4 Converged dynamic structure of bradykinin obtained from β-strand start.

Table 2 Main Chain Dihedral Angle Values Corresponding to the Converged Average Structure

Residue	ϕ	ψ	χ
Arg		141.39	178.86
Pro	−86.89	170.27	168.54
Pro	−84.44	51.80	173.17
Gly	169.15	66.61	−176.76
Phe	−55.22	106.04	177.15
Ser	−68.63	141.72	167.21
Pro	−88.23	43.11	177.57
Phe	−177.73	60.81	−179.26
Arg	−74.34		

pear to be γ-turns (47) bridging Pro^3 as well as Phe^5, although the latter does not appear to be explicitly defined by the NOE data set. If present, then the preferred overall geometry is "U-shaped" and, if absent, an "S-shaped" geometry is also possible based on initial modeling results. According to ϕ, ψ dihedral angle values for Pro^7 and Phe^8, a type II β-turn (48) extending from Ser^6 to Arg^9 also exists.

Although at the time of this writing certain key NMR experiments are yet to be performed, results are supported by many of the previously reported data for bradykinin analogs. Recall first that Cann's proposed ordered conformation in both TFE and dioxane-water contained turns around both Pro^3 and Pro^7, as does our proposed conformation. Furthermore, all peptide bonds are *trans*, and the hydrophobic side chains are oriented outward into solution. This orientation of side chains is consistent with a conformation one would expect to find in a nonsolvating, hydrophobic environment like a cell membrane. Bach has shown that a Δ^ZPhe residue in the $i+1$ position of a γ-turn might stabilize a stronger conformational preference for the turn than its saturated counterpart (49). Interestingly, replacement of Phe^5 in bradykinin with Δ^ZPhe results in an agonist with 23 times the potency of bradykinin. Similarly, C^α-methyl Phe^5 bradykinin has been reported to be 100-fold less potent an agonist than the natural ligand. In this case the C^α-methyl group completely eliminates the possibility of the tight γ-turn bridging Phe^5 which our "U-shaped" conformer suggests to be present, thereby making the loss of potency quite reasonable. The adjacent γ-turns centered around Gly^4 offer possible insight into the diminished activity of all analogs, even [Ala^4]bradykinin, with substitutions at this position. It is conceivable that only glycine, the most flexible amino acid, could accommodate adjacent turns of this type. There have been no reported analogs containing restraints which might support the proposed β-turn, however, it is in agreement with the calculated Chou and Fasman probability factors, is supported by the temperature-dependent chemical shift studies done on the amide protons, and was included as a possibility during NMR studies on bradykinin in dimethylsulfoxide solution (37).

On the basis of the known analog data, it is clear that the simplest modification one can make to bradykinin in order to transform it from agonist to antagonist is to replace L-Pro^7 with D-Phe residue. Optimization of the D-Phe^7-bradykinin series led Stewart to prepare NPC 567 (D-Arg-Arg^1-Pro^2-Hyp^3-Gly^4-Phe^5-Ser^6-D-Phe^7-Phe^8-Arg^9) (50), which at the time of this writing is one of the most potent bradykinin antagonists known. As one approach toward understanding the conformational differences between NPC 567 and bradykinin, we are pursuing an examination of this antagonist in a fashion similar to that described previously for bradykinin. Hence NOE data was collected in a 90% d_8-dioxane-H_2O media, and the values were used subsequently in a series of molecular dynamics simulations. As was done for the bradykinin refinement, two different conformations were used to start the molecular dynamics simulations. These include an extended β-strand and a double β-turn containing conformation. For the latter, the turns were about Pro-Hyp-Gly-Phe, and Ser-D-Phe-Phe-Arg, again derived from high β-turn probabilities. At this time, the NMR results are preliminary, however, convergence of each starting structure to a β-turn at the C-terminal four residues was observed following the calculations. A complete lack of convergence was observed at the N-terminal portion of the peptide and has been attributed to lack of NOEs derived from a random N-terminal conformation, even in this nonpolar environment.

It is interesting that C-terminal β-turns were observed both in NPC 567 and bradykinin. Due to the inversion of allowed dihedral angles defining ϕ/ψ space for a D-amino acid residue, as well as the restricted angle ϕ inherent in proline, the two β-turns are of differing types. Since the $i+1$ position of the β-turn in bradykinin is the key site for causing antagonism of the receptor, it leads one to speculate that perhaps the difference between an agonist and an antagonist is the type of β-turn adopted at the C-terminus and the requisite orientation of the side chains afforded with it.

Although a comprehensive, systematic study has not yet, to our knowledge, been reported for bradykinin analogs, the work presented here could form the basis for such an approach. Conformationally restricted peptide analogs which inherently stabilize the turn structures proposed in this model are anticipated to have increased affinities for the bradykinin receptor. Current investigations in our laboratories are being focused in this direction.

REFERENCES

1. Jurs, P. C., T. R. Stouch, M. Czerwinski, and J. N. Narvaez. Computer-assisted studies of molecular structure biological activity relationships. *J. Chem. Inf. Comput. Sci.* **25**:296-308 (1985).
2. Spatola, A. F. Peptide backbone modifications: A structure-activity analyssis of peptides containing amide bond surrogates. Conformational constraints and relationships, in: *Peptides*, Proceedings of the Seventh American Peptide Symposium (D. H. Rich and E. Gross, eds.). Pierce Chemical Co., Rockford, IL, p. 613.
3. Hruby, V. J. Conformational restrictions of biologically active peptides via amino acid side chain groups. *Life Sciences* **31**:189-198 (1982).
4. Karplus, M. Contact electron-spin coupling of nuclear magnetic moments. *J. Chem. Phys.* **30**:11-20 (1959).
5. Garbish, E. W., Jr. Conformations VI. Vinyl-allelic proton spin couplings. *J. Am. Chem. Soc.* **86**:5561-5564 (1964).
6. Sternhell, S. Correlation of interproton spin-spin coupling constants with structure. *Quarterly Rev.* **23**:236-270 (1969).
7. Masamune, S., P. Ma, R. E. Moore, T. Fujiyoshi, C. Jaime, and E. J. Osawa. Computation of vicinal coupling constants in tetra- and hexaalditol peracetates using molecular mechanics. A rational approach to conformational analysis in solution. *J. Chem. Soc. Chem. Commun.* **3**:261-263 (1986).
8. Anet, F. A. L., and A. J. R. Bourn. Nuclear magnetic resonance spectral assignments from nuclear Overhauser effects. *J. Am. Chem. Soc.* **87**:5250-5253 (1965).
9. Bell, R. A., and J. K. Saunders. Correlation of the intramolecular nuclear Overhauser effect with internuclear distance. *Can. J. Chem.* **48**:1114-1122 (1970).
10. Hall, L. D., and J. K. Saunders. Complete analysis of 'H NMR spectra of complex natural products using a combination of one- and two-dimensional techniques, 1-dehydrotestosterone. *J. Am. Chem. Soc.* **102**:5703-5710 (1980).
11. Scheek, R. M., N. Russo, R. Boelens, R. Kaptein, and J. H. van Boom. Sequential resonance assignments in DNA proton NMR spectra by two-dimensional NOE spectroscopy. *J. Am. Chem. Soc.* **105**:2914-2916 (1983).
12. Neuhaus, D., R. N. Sheppard, and I. R. C. Bick. Structural and conformational study of repanduline using long-range nuclear Overhauser effect difference spectroscopy. *J. Am. Chem. Soc.* **105**:5996-6002 (1983).
13. Hilton, S. M., and G. P. Lewis. The mechanism of the functional hyperaemia in the submandibular salivary gland. *J. Physiol.* **129**:253-268 (1955).
14. Regoli, D., and J. C. Barabe. Pharmacology of bradykinin and related kinins. *J. Pharmacol. Rev.* **32**:1-46 (1980).

15. Naclerio, R. M., D. Proud, L. M. Lichtenstein, A. Kagey-Sobotka, J. O. Hendley, J. Sorrentino, and J. M. Gwaltney. Kinins are generated during experimental rhinovirus colds. *J. Infect. Dis.* **157**:133-142 (1988).
16. Proud, D., C. J. Reynolds, S. Lacapra, A. Kagey-Sobotka, L. M. Lichtenstein, and R. M. Naclerio. Nasal provocation with bradykinin induces symptoms of rhinitis and a sore throat. *Am. Rev. Respir. Dis.* **137**:613-616 (1988).
17. Chou, P. Y., and G. D. Fasman. Prediction of β-turns. *Biophys. J.* **26**:367-383 (1979).
18. Silva, A. S. Conformational analysis of bradykinin in aqueous solution. *Cien. Cult.* **1**:32-42 (1949).
19. Craig, L. C., A. C. Harfenist, and A. C. Paladini. The behavior of angiotensin, oxytocin, vasopressin, and some of their analogs. *Biochem.* **3**:764-770 (1964).
20. Bodanszky, A., M. A. Ondetti, V. Mutt, and M. Bodanszky. Synthesis of secretin. IV. Secondary structure in a miniature protein. *J. Am. Chem. Soc.* **91**:944-949 (1969).
21. Holzworth, A. The ultraviolet circular dichroism of polypeptides. *J. Am. Chem. Soc.* **87**:218-220 (1965).
22. Cann, J. P., R. E. London, J. M. Stewart, and N. A. Matwiyoff. Effect of temperature upon the circular dichroism of bradykinin. *Int. J. Pep. Prot. Res.* **14**:388-392 (1979).
23. Cann, J. P., J. M. Stewart, and G. P. Matsueda. Circular dichroism study of the secondary structure of bradykinin. *Biochem.* **12**:3780-3788 (1973).
24. Marlborough, D. I., J. W. Ryan, and A. M. Felix. Conformation of bradykinin in relation to solvent environment. *Adv. Exp. Meth. Biol.* **70**:43-51 (1976).
25. Felix, A. M., M. H. Jimenez, R. Vergona, and M. R. Cohen. Synthesis and biological studies of novel bradykinin analogs. *Int. J. Pep. Prot. Res.* **5**:201-206 (1973).
26. Chipens, G. I., F. K., Mutulis, B. S. Katayev, V. E. Klusha, I. P. Misina, and N. V. Myshlyiakova. Cyclic analogue of bradykinin possessing selective and prolonged biological activity. *Int. J. Pep. Prot. Res.* **18**:302-307 (1981).
27. Huber, R., and W. Bode. Structural basis of the activation and action of trypsin. *Acc. Chem. Res.* **11**:114-122 (1978).
28. Chipens, G. I., F. Mutulis, and N. Mishlyakova. Cyclic analogs of bradykinin and kallidin, in: *N. Chem. Rep. Prot.* Walter deGruyter & Co., Berlin, New York, p. 1 (1982).
29. Turk, J., P. Needleman, and G. R. Marshall. Analogs of bradykinin with restricted conformational freedom. *J. Med. Chem.* **18**:1139-1144 (1975).
30. Mazur, R. H., P. A. Jamer, D. A. Tyner, E. A. Halliman, J. H. Sanner, and R. Schulze. Bradykinin analogs containing N^{α}-methyl amino acids. *J. Med. Chem.* **23**:758-764 (1980).
31. Stewart, J. M., and D. W. Woolley. Importance of the carboxyl end of bradykinin and other peptides. *Nature* (London) 207:1160-1161 (1965).
32. Fisher, G. H., P. Berryer, J. W. Ryan, V. Chauhan, and C. H. Stammer. Dehydrophenylalanyl analogs of bradykinin: Synthesis and biological activities. *Arch. Biochem. Biophys.* **211**:269-275 (1981).

33. Clore, G. M., A. T. Brunger, M. Karplus, and A. M. Groneborn. Solution conformation of a heptadecapeptide comprising the DNA binding helix F of the cyclic AMP receptor protein of *Escherichia coli*. Combined use of proton nuclear magnetic resonance and restrained molecular dynamics. *J. Mol. Biol.* **191**:435-455 (1985).
34. Clore, G. M., A. M. Gronenborn, A. T. Brunger, and M. Karplus. Application of molecular dynamics with interproton distance restraints to three-dimensional protein structure determination. A model study of crambin. *J. Mol. Biol.* **186**:523-551 (1986).
35. London, R. E., J. M. Stewart, R. Williams, J. R. Cann, and N. A. Matwiyoff. Carbon-13 NMR spectroscopy of [20%-1,2-13C2-Gly6]-bradykinin. Role of serine in reducing structural heterogeneity. *J. Am. Chem. Soc.* **101**:2455-2462 (1979).
36. Litner, K., and S. Fermandjian. Proton NMR study of the conformation of bradykinin: pH titration. *Bioch. Bioph. Res. Comm.* **91**:803-811 (1979).
37. Saulitis, Y. B., E. E. Liepin'sh, F. K. Sekatsis, I. E. Mutulis, and G. I. Chipens. Two-dimensional proton NMR spectroscopy study of the bradykinin conformational state in dimethyl sulfoxide solution. *Biorg. Chem.* **12**:437-447 (1986).
38. Otter, A. P. G. Scott, J. R. Cann, R. J. Vavrek, J. M. Stewart, and G. Kotovych. High-field NMR and circular dichroism solvent-dependent conformational studies of the bradykinin C-terminal tetrapeptide Ser-Pro-Phe-Arg. *J. Biomol. Struct. Dyna.* **6**:609-625 (1988).
39. London, R. E., J. M. Stewart, J. R. Cann, and N. A. Matwiyoff. Carbon-13 and proton nuclear magnetic resonance studies of bradykinin and selected peptide fragments. *Biochem.* **17**:2270-2277 (1978).
40. Saulitis, Y. B., E. E. Liepin'sh, I. P. Sekatsis, M. D. Shenderovich, F. K. Mutulis, I. E. Mutule, and G. I. Chipens. Conformation of a cyclic analog of bradykinin in solution studied by two-dimensional proton NMR. *Biorg. Chem.* **11**:1013-1025 (1985).
41. Kyle, D. J., R. P. Hicks, P. R. Blake, W. J. Rzeszotarski, and V. J. Klimkowski. Manuscript in preparation.
42. Seelig, J., and P. M. MacDonald. Phospholipids and proteins in biological membrane. ^{3}H NMR as a method to study structure, dynamics, and interactions. *Acc. Chem. Res.* **20**:221-226 (1987).
43. Gierasch, L. M., J. E. Lacy, K. F. Thompson, A. L. Rockwell, and P. I. Watnick. Conformations of model peptides in membrane-mimetic environments. *Biophys. J.* **37**:275-284 (1982).
44. Kessler, H. Conformation and biological activity of cyclic peptides. *Angew. Chem. Int. Ed. Engl.* **21**:512-520 (1982).
45. Brooks, B. R., R. E. Bruccoleri, B. D. Olafson, D. J. States, S. Swaminathon, and M. J. Karplus. CHARMM: A program for macromolecular energy, minimization, and dynamics calculations. *J. Comp. Chem.* **4**:187-217 (1983).
46. Polygen Corporation, 200 Fifth Avenue, Waltham, MA 12254.
47. Nemethy, G., and M. P. Printz. The gamma turn, a possible folded conformation of the polypeptide chain. Comparison with the beta turn. *Macromolecules* **5**:755-758 (1972).

48. Venkatachalam, C. M. Stereochemical criteria for polypeptides and proteins. V. Conformation of a system of three linked peptide units. *Biopolymers* **6**: 1425-1436 (1968).
49. Bach, A. C., and L. M. Gierasch. Dehydrophenylalanine can occur in various reverse-turn sites: conformational analysis of Dehydro Phe-containing model peptides. *Biopolymers* **25**:175-191 (1986).
50. Steranka, L. R., S. G. Farmer, and R. M. Burch. Antagonists of B_2 bradykinin receptors. *FASEB J* **3**:2019-2025 (1989).

6
Metabolism of Bradykinin and Bradykinin Analogs

Patrick E. Ward
The Ohio State University
Columbus, Ohio

I. INTRODUCTION

Bradykinin and kallidin (Lys-bradykinin), collectively referred to as kinins, are produced by the action of plasma and glandular kallikreins on both high and low molecular weight kininogens (1). Acting primarily through B_2 kinin receptors, kinins display a range of biologic activities (1,2) including the ability to lower systemic blood pressure (3), increase capillary permeability, produce natriuresis and diuresis, stimulate pain and sensitize pain fibers to noxious stimuli (4,5), and mimic coryza elicited by rhinoviruses (6-8). Despite their considerable intrinsic potency, kinins are degraded rapidly in vivo, and endogenous levels of circulating plasma kinins are difficult to determine accurately (9). The half-life of bradykinin in plasma is less than one minute (10,11). In vivo, where even more rapid degradation occurs at the cell surface of vascular endothelium, the half-life is considerably less (12,13).

Due to their nearly complete degradation across the pulmonary vascular bed (14-17), kinins are considered local hormones normally exerting their actions at or near their sites of production. The two principal enzymes involved in the degradation of circulating kinins are angiotensin I converting enzyme (ACE, EC 3.4.15.1) and carboxypeptidase N (CPN: EC 3.4.17.3). ACE hydrolyzes the C-terminal Pro^7-Phe^8 bond of bradykinin to produce desPhe^{8}Arg^9-bradykinin, and CPN hydrolyzes the C-terminal Phe^8-Arg^9 bond to produce desArg^9-bradykinin (Fig. 1).

Although bradykinin has been suggested to play a role in many physiological and pathophysiological conditions, definitive cause-effect relationships have seldom been established due to the lack of kinin antagonists. In 1985, Vavrek and Stewart (18) reported that D-Phe^7-kinin analogs are specific kinin antagonists. However, in view of the rapid degradation of bradykinin in vivo, the development of potent kinin analogs based on modifications of the parent molecule (Fig. 2) must include factors relevant not only to receptor interactions, but also stability from enzymatic degradation (19,20). Since peptide structure relative to receptor interactions are considered elsewhere, this review will focus on the metabolism of kallidin and bradykinin, how modifications in the basic kinin molecule alter metabolism, and, in certain instances, how such metabolism affects analog specificity for B2 and B1 kinin receptors. In view of their role in the degradation of kallidin and bradykinin, there can be little doubt that resistance to hydrolysis by ACE and CPN are important factors in the development of potent and long-acting kinin agonists and antagonists. However, as will be seen in subsequent sections, such resistance in itself may be insufficient since numerous circulating and cell-surface peptidases have been implicated in the degradation of kinins in vivo.

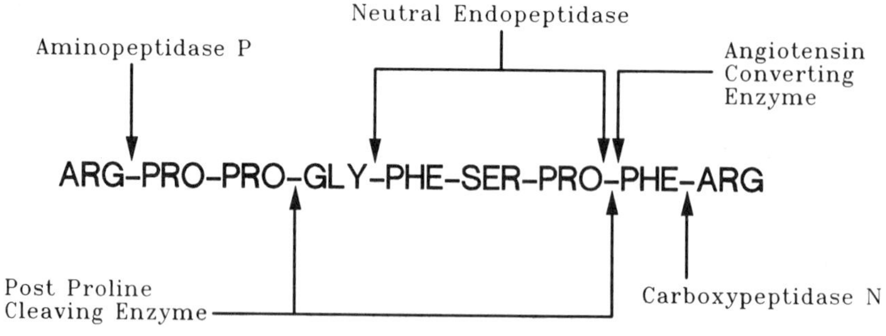

Figure 1 Sites of hydrolysis of bradykinin by amino-, endo-, and carboxypeptidases.

B_2 KININ AGONISTS	
$ARG^1-PRO^2-PRO^3-GLY^4-PHE^5-SER^6-PRO^7-PHE^8-ARG^9$	Bradykinin
LYS -ARG -PRO -PRO -GLY -PHE -SER -PRO -PHE -ARG	Kallidin
LYS -LYS -ARG -PRO -PRO -GLY -PHE -SER -PRO -PHE -ARG	Lys-Kallidin
B_1 KININ AGONISTS	
ARG -PRO -PRO -GLY -PHE -SER -PRO -PHE	desArg^9-Bradykinin
LYS -ARG -PRO -PRO -GLY -PHE -SER -PRO -PHE	desArg^{10}-Kallidin
B_2 KININ ANTAGONIST	
D-ARG -ARG -PRO -HYP -GLY -THI -SER -DPHE -THI -ARG	D-Arg^0[Hyp^3,Thi^{5,8},D-Phe^7]Bradykinin
B_1 KININ ANTAGONIST	
ARG -PRO -PRO -GLY -PHE -SER -PRO -LEU	desArg^9[Leu^8]-Bradykinin

Figure 2 Structures of kallidin and bradykinin and related kinin analogs.

II. ANGIOTENSIN CONVERTING ENZYME (EC 3.4.15.1)

Several detailed reviews are available regarding the distribution and characterization of ACE (12,21). ACE, also known as peptidyldipeptide hydrolase and kininase II, converts angiotensin I to angiotensin II and degrades kinins. In addition to circulating plasma ACE (22), ACE is concentrated on the cell surface of endothelial cells (13,23) in a variety of vascular beds including pulmonary, mesenteric, renal, adrenal, cerebral, and retinal vessels and microvessels (24-27). In particular, ACE on pulmonary endothelium prevents kinins in the venous circulation from reaching arterial resistance vessels. Comparisons of the depressor effects of bradykinin given i.v. and i.a. have demonstrated that 80-95% of i.v. infused bradykinin is degraded in one pass across the pulmonary vascular bed (19). Further, even under experimental conditions designed to inhibit pulmonary ACE, bradykinin continues to be subject to rapid degradation by ACE throughout systemic vasculature (28). Perhaps the clearest demonstration of the importance of ACE in the degradation of circulating kinins comes from numerous studies demonstrating that the depressor effects of infused kinins are potentiated 10-fold or more by ACE inhibitors.

In addition to the degradation of kallidin and bradykinin (B2 kinins), ACE may also degrade kinin agonists specific for the B1 kinin receptor, namely desArg^9-bradykinin and desArg^{10}-kallidin (4,29-32). ACE has a relatively broad substrate specificity and can hydrolyze both di- and tripeptides from many low molecular weight peptides with varying C-terminal sequences (33). In vitro, purified ACE can rapidly degrade desArg^9-bradykinin (34,35). However, in contrast to the high affinity of bradykinin for ACE ($K_m = 1\ \mu M$) (36), the affinity of desArg^9-bradykinin for ACE is considerably lower (K_m = 130-240 μM) (34,35). This lower affinity may account, at least in part, for the data of Regoli and coworkers (29), which we have confirmed in unpublished studies, that desArg^9-bradykinin is not significantly degraded in vivo across the pulmonary circulation of the rabbit. These conflicting data may also relate to species variations and differences in peptide/enzyme interactions in vitro and in vivo.

A. Analogs Resistant to Angiotensin Converting Enzyme

Based on the above, a primary consideration in the development of kinin analogs is resistance to degradation by ACE. As noted earlier, ACE inactivates bradykinin by hydrolysis of the Pro^7-Phe^8 bond to produce the inactive metabolites Phe-Arg and desPhe^{8}Arg^9-bradykinin. Previous studies have demonstrated that angiotensin I analogs containing D-residues in positions 8, 9, and 10 and [D-Pro^7]bradykinin are not hydrolyzed by ACE

(19,37). Thus, it might be anticipated that B2 kinin antagonists, nearly all of which contain D-Phe in position 7, would also be resistant to degradation by ACE. Recently, Togo et al. (38) have shown that three D-Phe^7-substituted bradykinin analogs, [D-Phe^7]bradykinin, D-Arg^0[Hyp^3,D-Phe^7] bradykinin, and D-Arg^0[Hyp^3,Thi^{5,8},D-Phe^7]bradykinin, are resistant to hydrolysis by purified rabbit lung ACE. Similarly, we have found that all [D-Phe^7]bradykinin antagonists tested to date are resistant to purified porcine and rat plasma ACE (39). As will be detailed in subsequent sections, additional N- and C-terminal modifications of bradykinin have also been used to develop potent B2 kinin agonists resistant to degradation by ACE.

Substitution of a D-amino acid residue at the C-terminus of desArg^9-bradykinin (B1 agonist) also confers resistance to degradation by ACE (39). Consistent with such resistance, desArg^9[D-Phe^8]bradykinin is reported to be a more potent B1 agonist than is desArg^9-bradykinin (5). However, it remains to be determined whether this increased potency is directly related to resistance to degradation by ACE.

Despite the resistance of D-Phe^7-containing B2 kinin antagonists to hydrolysis by ACE, these analogs are not resistant to CPN. Incubation of D-Arg^0[Hyp^3,D-Phe^7]bradykinin with diluted rat serum resulted in complete degradation in less than 2 minutes (38). Hydrolysis was due to serum CPN since a single product was produced with HPLC characteristics consistent with identification as the desArg^9 metabolite. Further, all three of the [D-Phe^7]bradykinin analogs examined by Togo et al. (38) were short-lived when injected in vivo, being degraded into small unidentified metabolites. These data indicate that despite resistance to metabolism by ACE, [D-Phe^7]bradykinin antagonists are rapidly hydrolyzed by CPN and other as yet unidentified peptidases in vivo.

III. CARBOXYPEPTIDASE N (EC 3.4.17.3)

Plasma CPN, also known as kininase I, hydrolyzes C-terminal basic amino acids from a variety of biologically active peptides including kinins, anaphylatoxins, fibrinopeptides, and enkephalins (40-44). Unlike ACE, CPN is primarily a circulating plasma enzyme (12). However, a CPN or CPN-like enzyme is also present in vasculature and microvasculature. Vascular homogenates hydrolyze synthetic carboxypeptidase substrates, and an enzyme immunologically related to plasma CPN has been identified on pulmonary endothelium (17). These reports are consistent with observations that a plasma membrane fraction purified from porcine aorta contains a carboxypeptidase which hydrolyzes the C-terminal Phe[8]-Arg[9] bond of bradykinin. Activity was higher on cultured endothelium than on smooth muscle (44), was present in isolated cerebral microvessels (42), and displayed characteristics similar to those of plasma CPN. Kinin hydrolysis was optimal at physiologic pH, was activated by $CoCl_2$, and was inhibited by the carboxypeptidase inhibitor MERGETPA (DL-mercapto-methyl-3-guanidinoethylthiopropanoic acid) (42,44). Also, like plasma CPN, the affinity of bradykinin for the endothelial plasma membrane carboxypeptidase (K_m = 20-50 μM) (42) was considerably lower than that of bradykinin for ACE (36). Similarly, Skidgel et al. (45) have identified a membrane-bound CPN-like activity, referred to as carboxypeptidase M, in numerous tissue sites including human placenta. These data demonstrate an extensive distribution of CPN and CPN-like activity capable of hydrolyzing the C-terminal Phe[8]-Arg[9] bond of bradykinin. Since the resultant desArg[9]-bradykinin metabolite is inactive on B2 kinin receptors (4,19), CPN and the comparable vascular and tissue enzymes could represent an important pathway for the degradation for B2 kinins in vivo.

Despite the above, the importance of carboxypeptidase-mediated metabolism of kallidin and bradykinin (relative to that of ACE) is controversial. Ryan et al. (46) have reported that the carboxypeptidase inhibitor MERGETPA, unlike ACE inhibitors, does not potentiate the systemic depressor effect of exogenously administered bradykinin. Similarly, Salgado et al. (47) have found only slight bradykinin potentiation with MERGETPA, and such potentiation could not clearly be ascribed to CPN inhibition since nonspecific potentiation of other vasoactive agents was also observed. These data stand in marked contrast to the 10-fold or greater potentiation of the depressor effect of kinins produced by ACE inhibitors in vivo, and the results of Huey et al. (40) demonstrating that MERGETPA can produce significant potentiation of anaphylatoxins in vivo through inhibition of carboxypeptidase-mediated degradation of anaphylatoxin C3a and C4a. Collectively, these studies suggest that ACE is far more important than CPN and CPN-like activity in the metabolism of circulating kallidin and bradykinin.

In contrast, other studies support a role for carboxypeptidase(s) in kinin metabolism in vivo. Carboxypeptidase-mediated kinin hydrolysis in human serum is reported to be more rapid than that due to ACE (41,43). Significant circulating levels of the desArg[9]-bradykinin metabolite have been found in vivo (48), and Streeten et al. (49) have observed that patients with low levels of circulating CPN have elevated plasma kinin levels and physiologic symptoms consistent with the biologic action of kinins. Further, although the affinity of kinins for CPN is lower than that for ACE, carboxypeptidase-mediated metabolism may be significant at tissue and vascular sites of kinin synthesis and release (50), where local levels may be considerably higher than in plasma.

In contrast to their possible importance in the metabolism of the B2 agonists kallidin and bradykinin, plasma CPN and vascular CPN-like activity cannot play any significant role in the degradation of kinins specific for B1 receptors. Due to their inability to hydrolyze amino acids bound to proline, neither CPN nor CPN-like vascular activities hydrolyze C-terminal Pro-Phe or Pro-Leu bonds (44). Thus, the B1 receptor specific kinin agonists desArg^9-bradykinin and desArg^{10}-kallidin (Pro-Phe C-terminus), and antagonists [Leu^8]desArg^9-bradykinin and [Leu^9]desArg^{10}-kallidin (Pro-Leu C-terminus), are resistant to CPN-mediated degradation. As noted earlier, however, these B1 agonists and antagonists are susceptible to degradation by ACE, at least in vitro.

Regarding the metabolism of bradykinin and bradykinin analogs active on B2 receptors, debate about the importance of carboxypeptidase-mediated metabolism relative to ACE is not purely an academic matter. If metabolism by ACE predominates, the resultant metabolite (desPhe^{8}Arg^9-bradykinin) represents a completely inactive product. In contrast, if carboxypeptidase-mediated metabolism predominates under some conditions (e.g., kinin analogs resistant to ACE), such metabolism can result in the formation of desArg^9-bradykinin analogs active on B1 kinin receptors. As detailed below, CPN-mediated kinin metabolism has been shown to have substantial effects on the ability of kinins and kinin antagonists to act on B1 kinin receptors (51).

A. CPN-Mediated Conversion of B2 Kinin Agonists and Antagonists

CPN-mediated hydrolysis of the C-terminal Phe^8-Arg^9 bond of bradykinin results in the formation of the desArg^9-bradykinin metabolite, which does not stimulate the B2 kinin receptor. Thus, CPN (kininase I) kinin metabolism has traditionally been viewed as a degradative pathway. Although this remains true for B2 agonist activity, the demonstration by Regoli and coworkers (4) that kallidin and bradykinin metabolites lacking their C-terminal arginine are potent agonists for B1 receptors has led to the recognition that CPN-mediated kinin metabolism also represents a kinin conversion pathway. Such CPN conversion of kinins (B2 agonists) to desArg-kinins (B1 agonists) could alter the relative balance between B1- and B2-mediated effects, particularly in inflammatory states (5,52) or in patients receiving ACE inhibitors (where kinin metabolism may be shunted toward conversion of kinins to desArg-kinins). Indeed, whereas both kallidin and bradykinin were originally thought to be effective though less potent B1 agonists (4,52), it has now been demonstrated that their apparent ability to stimulate vascular B1 receptors is indirect, dependent on local conversion to desArg^{10}-kallidin and desArg^{9}-bradykinin by vascular carboxypeptidase (i.e., MERGETPA inhibits the B1 agonist activity of kallidin and bradykinin) (51). These data demonstrate that desArg^{10}-kallidin and desArg^{9}-bradykinin are the specific agonists for B1 receptors, and that local conversion by cell surface carboxypeptidase activity can have direct effects on the type of kinin receptor stimulated (44,51). Such conversion to B1 agonists could be particularly important not only in the presence of ACE inhibitors, but also at localized sites containing high levels of carboxypeptidase activity relative to ACE (42,53).

Such carboxypeptidase-mediated metabolism may be even more important in the case of [D-Phe^{7}]kinin antagonists resistant to degradation by ACE (38). As noted earlier, the ACE-resistant kinin antagonist D-Arg^{0}[Hyp^{3},D-Phe^{7}]bradykinin was rapidly metabolized by rat serum CPN (38). In recent studies we have found that the presence of D-Phe^{7} in a number of kinin analogs has little or no effect on C-terminal hydrolysis by rat serum CPN (39). Even the presence of a number of additional modifications of the C-terminal sequence had little effect on C-terminal Arg hydrolysis by CPN. For instance, in addition to analogs with the C-terminal sequence: D-Phe^{7}-Phe^{8}-Arg^{9}, analogs containing D-Phe^{7}-Thi^{8}-Arg^{9} and Pro^{7}-Tyr-(OMe)^{8}-Arg^{9} were also hydrolyzed. In general, neither the V_{max} nor the K_m values were significantly different from those obtained for kallidin or bradykinin (39). Thus, since C-terminal desArg-antagonists do not block B2 kinin receptors (18,52), the activities of CPN and vascular CPN-like enzymes are likely to be important in the degradation of many B2 antagonist analogs.

Carboxypeptidase-mediated removal of the C-terminal Arg from B2 kinin antagonists may also explain the ability of several [D-Phe^{7}]kinin antagonists to block both B2 and B1 kinin receptors (30). Although desArg^{9}-[Leu^{8}]-bradykinin is the prototype B1 kinin antagonist (4), other desArg^{9}-kinin analogs may also be able to block B1 kinin receptors. In order to investigate this possibility, Regoli and coworkers (51) examined the ability of [Thi^{5,8},D-Phe^{7}]bradykinin and [Thi^{6,9},D-Phe^{8}]kallidin to block both B2 and B1 vascular receptors in the presence of the carboxypeptidase inhibitor MERGETPA. MERGETPA did not alter the ability of either analog to block B2 receptors, but significantly attenuated their B1 antagonist activity. These data suggest that B2 kinin receptor antagonists are converted by vascular carboxypeptidase into active B1 antagonists, and that such local metabolism may account for the mixed B2/B1 antagonism seen for some [D-Phe^7]kinin analogs (30,51).

B. Analogs Resistant to Both ACE and CPN

Based on the above, the development of kinin analogs resistant to both ACE and CPN could result in agonists and antagonists which are both more potent and specific for B2 receptors. With this in mind, Drapeau et al. (54) have synthesized a kinin agonist [Phe$^8\psi$(CH_2-NH)Arg^9]bradykinin, in which the Phe^8-Arg^9 peptide bond was replaced by the isosteric CH_2-NH bond. This agonist, which is resistant to hydrolysis by both ACE and CPN (39,54), was found to be selective for vascular B2 receptors (due to resistance to CPN), and to be nearly fivefold more potent than bradykinin in lowering systemic blood pressure in the rat (primarily due to resistance to ACE). Similarly, D-Arg^0[Hyp^3,D-Phe^7-Phe$^8\psi$(CH_2-NH)Arg^9]bradykinin, due to its resistance to hydrolysis by vascular CPN-like activity, has been found to be a specific B2 kinin antagonist (5).

C. Kinin Metabolism by Serum and Circulating Blood Cells

Erythrocytes, lymphocytes, neutrophils, and macrophages have been reported to contain amino-, endo-, and carboxypeptidases (55-59). However, due to the relatively small amount of information available, it is too early to speculate regarding their possible role in kinin metabolism.

Sheikh and Kaplan (41,43) have recently reported that although kinin hydrolysis by plasma is due to ACE and CPN, the rate of hydrolysis of C-terminal Arg by serum was five times faster than could be accounted for by the level of CPN. Although not ruling out a serum cofactor which augments CPN activity, they suggest that serum may contain a carboxypeptidase B-like enzyme, perhaps released as a result of blood clotting, that rapidly converts bradykinin to desArg^9-bradykinin. Similarly, Hendriks et al. (60) have reported that fresh human serum contains a labile carboxypeptidase activity which hydrolyzes the CPN synthetic substrate hippuryl-L-arginine three times more rapidly than plasma CPN. Although preliminary, these observations suggest the possibility that changes in blood chemistry in vivo can alter both the degradation of B2 kinins and the formation of B1 kinins.

IV. KININ METABOLISM BY OTHER PEPTIDASES

As noted earlier, the effects of three D-Phe^7-containing kinin antagonists infused into the rat were short-lived despite their resistance to ACE (38).

Similarly, the depressor effect produced by infusion of a kinin agonist resistant to both ACE and CPN ([Phe$^8\psi$(CH_2-NH)Arg^9]bradykinin), although sustained over that produced by bradykinin, was also relatively short-lived (54). The duration of action of these peptides in vivo, together with the detection of numerous small antagonist metabolites (38), strongly suggest that peptidases other than ACE, CPN, and vascular carboxypeptidases are involved in the degradation of kinin analogs in vivo.

Although relatively little direct information is available regarding the identities of the responsible enzymes, a number of candidates should be considered. In general, tissues and vasculature contain substantial levels of numerous peptidases capable of kinin degradation. However, the majority of such activity is cytosolic and is probably irrelevant to kinin metabolism under normal conditions. Thus subsequent sections will focus on peptidases present in the circulation and/or localized to cell surface membranes.

A. Neutral Endopeptidase (EC 3.4.24.11)

Neutral endopeptidase (NEP), which specifically cleaves peptide substrates on the amino side of hydrophobic amino acids, can degrade numerous biologically active peptides including kinins, angiotensins, neurokinins, opioids, and atrial natriuretic peptides (59,61). NEP is a cell surface peptidase that, although most abundant on renal brush border (62,63), has also been identified in lymph nodes, chondrocytes from articular cartilage, neutrophils, and pulmonary and CNS tissues (59,64).

The initial site of hydrolysis of bradykinin by NEP occurs at the Pro^7-Phe^8 bond (i.e., the same site bond hydrolyzed by ACE) (59,65). Thus, [D-Phe^7]kinin analogs resistant to ACE may also be resistant to NEP. However, this remains to be determined. Further, since NEP also hydrolyzes bradykinin at a secondary site (Gly^4-Phe^5), additional modifications at or near the Gly^4-Phe^5 bond would be required to produce analogs completely resistant to NEP.

Consistent with the high levels of NEP within the kidney, and despite the colocalization of numerous brush border peptidases including ACE, renal NEP has been shown to participate in the degradation of intrarenal kinins (66). However, its role in the degradation of circulating kinins is less clear. Unlike the endothelial localization of ACE, pulmonary NEP activity is primarily associated with the alveolar septa (67). Although serum NEP levels are reported to increase in patients with adult respiratory distress syndrome (68) and sarcoidosis (69), normal levels in vasculature and serum are low (64,68). Further, in contrast to studies demonstrating that

NEP is involved in the metabolism of circulating atrial natriuretic peptides in vivo (70-72), Seymour et al. (73) have reported that infusion of the NEP inhibitor SQ 29,072 only slightly potentiates the depressor action of infused bradykinin in the conscious SHR.

Collectively, these data suggest that NEP is not an important factor in the metabolism of circulating kinins. However, in view of the normally rapid degradation of kinins by ACE, it is possible that NEP-mediated kinin degradation may be significant only in the presence of ACE inhibitors or in the case of kinin analogs resistant to both ACE and CPN. Nevertheless, this interpretation is not supported by the data of Ishida et al. (74). These investigators found that although potentiation of plasma kinin levels is seen after ACE inhibition, no further potentiation is seen after addition of a cocktail of peptidase inhibitors including the NEP inhibitor phosphoramidon.

B. Aminopeptidase M (EC 3.4.11.2)

Aminopeptidase M (AmM), also known as aminopeptidase N, is routinely assayed with the synthetic substrates alanyl- and leucyl-naphthylamide. AmM hydrolyzes neutral and basic amino acids from the N-terminus of low molecular weight peptides (62,63). Although the neutral/basic amino acid naphthylamidase activity in plasma has often been attributed to a number of enzymes including leucine aminopeptidase (EC 3.4.11.1) and aminopeptidase B (EC 3.4.11.6) (63,75), recent studies have established that the majority of alanyl-naphthylamidase activity in human, rat, and rabbit plasma is AmM (76,77). AmM is also present within the vascular compartment as an intrinsic cell surface peptidase (78) on both endothelium and smooth muscle (79). In addition to aorta and mesenteric arteries, AmM has also been identified in isolated porcine, rabbit (80), and rat (81,82) cerebral microvessels. AmM can degrade low molecular weight opioid peptides (80,83) and has been shown to play a physiologically significant role in the degradation of circulating desAsp^{1}-angiotensins (77). However, its role in the metabolism of kinins is less clear.

Due to an inability to hydrolyze N-terminal amino acids bound to proline, AmM does not degrade bradykinin (Arg^{1}-Pro^{2} N-terminus) (84). Further, although AmM can convert kallidin to bradykinin by N-terminal hydrolysis of the Lys^{1}-Arg^{2} bond, it is unlikely that such metabolism is physiologically significant, since kallidin and bradykinin display similar potencies on B2 receptors. However, such AmM-mediated metabolism may be important in the N-terminal conversion of desArg^{10}-kallidin to desArg^{9}-bradykinin. Since desArg^{10}-kallidin is an order of magnitude more potent than desArg^9-bradykinin in stimulating B1 receptors (4,31), AmM-mediated conversion would result in a significant decrease in B1 kinin receptor stimulation.

Regarding N-terminally extended kinin analogs, Stewart and coworkers (19,85) have found that the addition of an N-terminal lysine to kallidin resulted in a kinin agonist, Lys-kallidin, which is relatively resistant to degradation to ACE both in vivo (19,85,86) and in vitro (87). Consistent with such resistance, Lys-kallidin is significantly more potent than kallidin or bradykinin in lowering blood pressure in the rat (19,85). Thus, since AmM can convert Lys-kallidin to kallidin (84), AmM could convert a potent ACE-resistant kinin agonist into a significantly less potent ACE-susceptible agonist. In view of this, the use of D-amino acids for N-terminal extensions of kinin agonists (19) would seem useful since such analogs are resistant to hydrolysis by AmM and most other aminopeptidases. Nevertheless, if the major reason for the increased potency of Lys-kallidin is resistance to degradation by ACE, such N-terminal extensions will have little value in extending the duration of action of D-Phe^7-containing B2 kinin antagonists, which, as noted earlier, are already resistant to ACE (38).

Based on the observation that Lys-kallidin is partially resistant to degradation by ACE, there has been a tendency to believe that N-terminal extensions may also confer resistance to degradation by other peptidases. Although analogs extended at their N-termini with D-amino acids are undoubtedly resistant to metabolism by aminopeptidases, a generalized resistance to endo- and carboxypeptidase-mediated degradation can be ruled out. In contrast to the resistance of Lys-kallidin to metabolism by ACE, we have found that Lys-kallidin and a number of other N-terminally extended kinin analogs are susceptible to C-terminal hydrolysis by rat plasma CPN. Both the K_m and V_{max} values obtained with these analogs were not significantly different from those for kallidin and braydkinin (39). Thus, N-terminal extensions of bradykinin do not prevent CPN and vascular CPN-like metabolism.

C. Aminopeptidase A (EC 3.4.11.7)

In addition to its presence on renal and intestinal brush border membranes, aminopeptidase A (AmA) (62,63) has been identified in plasma, endothelium, glomeruli (88), and adrenal (25) and cerebral microvessels (89). AmA, routinely assayed with the synthetic substrates glutamyl- and aspartyl-naphthylamide, hydrolyzes acidic amino acids from the N-terminus of low molecular weight peptides. Vascular and plasma AmA plays a major role in the conversion of angiotensin II to angiotensin III by hydrolysis of the N-terminal Asp^1-Arg^2 bond of angiotensin II (77). However, due to its specificity for N-terminal acidic amino acids, it is unlikely that AmA plays any significant role in in vivo conversion of kallidin to bradykinin. Similarly, due to the inability of AmA to hydrolyze N-terminal amino acids bound to proline, AmA can be ruled out as an enzyme involved in the N-terminal degradation of bradykinin (Arg^1-Pro^2 N-terminus).

D. Aminopeptidase P (EC 3.4.11.9)

Despite the well-established role of ACE in the degradation of kinins across the pulmonary circulation, significant evidence indicates that other less well-characterized pulmonary enzymes may also be involved. Perfusion of radiolabeled bradykinin through the isolated rat lung has been reported to result in peptide bond cleavages which could not be accounted for by the known specificity of ACE (90). Further, a bradykinin analog resistant to ACE was rapidly degraded when perfused through both isolated guinea pig and rat lungs (91). Despite the fact that most aminopeptidases are unable to hydrolyze bonds involving amino acids bound to proline, significant hydrolysis of the N-terminal Arg^1-Pro^2 bond of bradykinin was detected.

Aminopeptidase P (AmP), also known as aminoacylproline aminopeptidase, can remove a variety of N-terminal amino acids provided they are bound to proline (62,63). In addition to its presence in kidney brush border, Simmons and coworkers (92,93) have detected apparent AmP-mediated hydrolysis of Arg^1-Pro^2 bond of bradykinin in pulmonary microsomes and in the isolated perfused rat lung. N-terminal metabolism has also been found in a preparation enriched in cerebral microvasculature (42). These data suggest that AmP may play a role in the degradation of circulating bradykinin and, if so, provide a specific rationale for the use of D-amino acids at the N-terminus of bradykinin analogs. Nevertheless, since tissue damage during perfusion of isolated lungs can expose enzyme(s) not normally in contact with the circulation, a definitive conclusion regarding the role of AmP must await clear histologic localization and the identification and use of specific and selective AmP inhibitors (92,93).

E. Dipeptidyl(amino)peptidase IV (EC 3.4.14.5)

Dipeptidyl(amino)peptidase IV (DAP IV) has been identified in plasma (78) and on the cell surface membrane of isolated vessels and cultured endothelium and smooth muscle (94,95). DAP IV, which hydrolyzes X-Pro dipeptides from the N-terminus of low molecular weight peptides, sequentially removes the N-terminal Arg-Pro and Lys-Pro dipeptides from substance P to produce the biologically active metabolite hepta[5-11]-substance P (94,96). However, it is unlikely that DAP IV plays any role in the degradation of bradykinin. Although bradykinin contains the same N-terminal dipeptide as substance P (Arg-Pro), bradykinin is resistant to hydrolysis by DAP IV due to the presence of a second proline residue in position 3 (Arg-Pro-Pro) (94,96).

F. Post Proline Cleaving Enzyme (EC 3.4.21.26)

Post proline cleaving enzyme (PPCE) is a cytosolic endopeptidase which hydrolyzes internal peptide bonds on the carboxyl side of proline residues (65,97). PPCE can degrade a variety of vasoactive peptides including angiotensins, neurokinins, vasopressin, oxytocin, and kinins (65,98). As with ACE and NEP, bradykinin is initially hydrolyzed by purified PPCE at the Pro^7-Phe^8 bond to produce Phe-Arg and des$Phe^8$$Arg^9$-bradykinin (98). Similarly, both the B1 agonist desArg^9-bradykinin and antagonist desArg^9[Leu^8]bradykinin are inactivated by hydrolysis of their Pro^7-Phe^8 and Pro^7-Leu^8 bonds, respectively.

Kinin degradation by PPCE is optimal at a neutral pH, and maximal velocities of degradation are similar for both agonists and antagonists. The K_m of bradykinin for PPCE (7.5 μM) (98) is comparable to that of bradykinin for ACE. Further, in contrast to the relatively low affinity of desArg^9-bradykinin for ACE (K_m = 130-240 μM) (34,35), the affinity of desArg^9-bradykinin for PPCE is considerably higher (K_m = 10μM) (98).

Despite the above, the majority of vascular and tissue PPCE activity is cytosolic and probably not relevant to normal extracellular kinin metabolism. However, PPCE is present in the circulation, and a PPCE (or like) activity has been reported associated with membrane-enriched fractions. Thus, it remains to be determined whether specific inhibition of PPCE in vivo potentiates the action of kinins or kinin analogs. Although the majority of aminopeptidase inhibitors, including o-phenanthroline, amastatin, bestatin, and puromycin, have no effect on PPCE (65), kinin degradation can be inhibited in vitro by the specific PPCE inhibitor Z-Pro-prolinal (98), which has also been shown to be an effective inhibitor of PPCE in vivo.

As previously noted for NEP, [D-Phe^7]kinin analogs resistant to ACE may also be partially resistant to PPCE since the initial site of bradykinin hydrolysis by PPCE is the same Pro^7-Phe^8 bond. Such resistance would not necessarily be due to the presence of a D-amino acid, but rather to the absence of proline in position 7. Nevertheless, PPCE also hydrolyzes bradykinin at the Pro^3-Gly^4 bond, and it remains to be determined whether the substitution of hydroxyproline in position 3 (18,19) alters such metabolism.

G. Carboxypeptidase P (EC 3.4.12.__)

As noted earlier, the C-termini of desArg-kinin agonists (Pro^7-Phe^8) and antagonist (Pro^7-Leu^8) are not hydrolyzed by CPN due to the presence of Pro in the penultimate position. However, incubations of $desArg^9$-bradykinin with plasma can result in hydrolysis of the C-terminal Pro^7-Phe^8 bond (99). Although such metabolism may be due to the previously detailed plasma PPCE activity (98), an alternate candidate is carboxypeptidase P (CPP).

CPP is found on renal and intestinal brush border and hydrolyzes C-terminal amino acids from peptides containing Pro at the penultimate position (62,63). Since many peptidases found on renal brush border are also found in plasma and on the cell surface of vasculature (e.g., ACE, AmM, DAP IV) (78,100,101), it is tempting to speculate that the observed C-terminal metabolism of $desArg^9$-bradykinin is due to vascular CPP. Identifying and characterizing this enzyme could be particularly important due to its potential to inactivate both $desArg^9$-bradykinin analogs and angiotensin II (Pro-Phe C-terminus) (79).

An enzyme with a substrate specificity similar to CPP is prolylcarboxypeptidase (EC 3.4.12.4) (102). However, due to its lysosomal localization and acidic pH optimum, it is probably not significant to $desArg^9$-bradykinin or angiotensin II metabolism under normal circumstances. However, the release of this lysosomal enzyme at sites of inflammation and/or other pathologic situations could result in increased rates of $desArg^9$-bradykinin inactivation.

V. KININ METABOLISM BY UNIDENTIFIED PLASMA PEPTIDASES

Ishida et al. (74) have reported that the degradation of bradykinin by rat plasma is only decreased 50% in the presence of inhibitors of ACE (enalapril), CPN (MERGETPA), NEP (phosphoramidon), and AmM (bestatin). These data suggest that a significant fraction of kinin degradation in plasma is due to enzymes resistant to the above inhibitors. As detailed earlier, although plasma AmA or DAP IV are not inhibited by these agents, their substrate specificities preclude significant roles in kinin metabolism. However, based on their abilities to degrade bradykinin and their relative resistance to inhibition by the above agents, PPCE, CPP, and AmP could be considered reasonable candidates for such metabolism.

VI. RENAL METABOLISM OF KININS

The kidney clearly plays a significant role in the metabolism of circulating kinins. As noted throughout this review, brush border membranes of renal proximal tubules contain high levels of a number of peptidases including ACE, AmM, AmA, NEP, AmP, and CPP (62,101,103). These peptidases are thought to play a role in the degradation of circulating peptides filtered into the renal proximal tubule (101,103-105). Based on the substantial levels and variety of enzymes, it is unlikely that any kinin analog would survive filtration and subsequent passage through the proximal tubule.

Nasjletti et al. (106) have reported that kallidin and bradykinin are also rapidly degraded in the renal circulation. Although both ACE and vascular carboxypeptidase activities would seem the likely agents of such metabolism, Ishida et al. (74) have obtained data indicating that other enzymes must be involved. In rats infused with bradykinin, plasma kinin levels increased 20-fold during infusion of a cocktail of inhibitors for ACE, CPN, and NEP. However, after nephrectomy, plasma kinin levels increased another twofold. This subsequent increase was not due to decreased degradation of filtered kinin since no secondary increase was seen after ureteral ligation.

VII. KININ METABOLISM AT SPECIALIZED SITES

The majority of this review has focused on the metabolism of circulating kinins and kinin analogs. However, although ACE may be primarily responsible for the degradation of circulating kinins, some of the other peptidases detailed in this review may predominate in the metabolism of kinins acting at local sites. For instance, although ACE is present in cerebral microvessels and ACE inhibitors block the local formation of angiotensin II, they do not potentiate the local action of bradykinin (53). Rather, kinins are rapidly hydrolyzed by a microvascular carboxypeptidase (42). A similar predominance of CPN-like activity has been noted for kinin metabolism in nasal secretions during experimentally induced allergic rhinitis (6). Although few studies have examined local kinin metabolism by NEP, NEP inhibitors have been shown to potentiate the actions of substance P in gut smooth muscle (107) and the guinea pig airway (108). In view of the potential for rapid kinin analog degradation in particular sites (103,104), and the demonstrated ability of local metabolism to alter both agonist and antagonist activities (30,51), these data underscore the importance of local kinin metabolism to kinin agonist and antagonist studies.

VIII. ENZYME INHIBITION BY KININ ANALOGS

Numerous studies infusing high levels of bradykinin antagonists (e.g., 500 μg/kg/min) have been conducted to determine if endogenous kinins affect blood pressure and flow in normotensive and hypertensive animal models (20). Although this matter has yet to be decided, caution should be exercised in the interpretation of data obtained with such high doses of antagonist. D-Phe[7]-substituted kinin antagonists have been shown to be weak, noncompetitive inhibitors of ACE (38), and inhibition of ACE and other kinin-metabolizing peptidases might be expected to potentiate endogenous kinin levels. Conversely, these analogs also have the potential to decrease endogenous kinin formation via inhibition of plasma and glandular kallikreins.

ACKNOWLEDGMENTS

I would like to thank Dr. Guy Drapeau for his thoughtful advice and criticisms and Ms. Ana Chow for her help in the preparation of this manuscript.

REFERENCES

1. Bradykinin, kallidin and kallikrein, in: *Handbook of Experimental Pharmacology*, Vol 25, Suppl. I (E. G. Erdos, ed.). Springer-Verlag, Heidelberg, 1979.
2. Braas, K. M., D. C. Manning, D. C. Perry, and S. H. Snyder. Bradykinin analogues: Differential agonist and antagonist activities suggesting multiple receptors. *Br. J. Pharmacol.* **94**:3-5 (1988).
3. Aubert, J. F., B. Waeber, J. Nussberger, R. Vavrek, J. M. Stewart, and H. Brunner. Influence of endogenous bradykinin on acute blood pressure response to vasopressors in normotensive rats assessed with a bradykinin antagonist. *J. Cardiovasc. Pharmacol.* **11**:51-55 (1988).
4. Regoli, D., and J. Barabe. Pharmacology of bradykinin and related kinins. *Pharmacol. Rev.* **32**:1-46 (1980).
5. Regoli, D., N-E. Rhaleb, G. Drapeau, and S. Dion. The kinin system: Current concepts and perspectives. *Biochem. Inflam.* (in press).

6. Proud, D., C. R. Baumgarten, R. M. Naclerio, and P. E. Ward. Kinin metabolism in human nasal secretions during experimentally-induced allergic rhinitis. *J. Immunol.* **138**:428-434 (1987).
7. Proud, D., and A. P. Kaplan. Kinin formation: Mechanisms and role in inflammatory disorders. *Ann. Rev. Immunol.* **6**:49-83 (1988).
8. Proud, D., C. J. Reynolds, S. Lacapra, A. Kagey-Sobotka, L. M. Lichtenstein, and R. M. Naclerio. Nasal provocation with bradykinin induces symptoms of rhinitis and a sore throat. *Am. Rev. Respir. Dis.* **137**:613-616 (1988).
9. Carretero, O. A., A. G. Scicli, S. F. Rabito, and A. Nasjletti. Kinins. in: *The Heart and Cardiovascular System* (H. A. Fozzard et al., eds.). Raven Press, New York, pp. 1663-1677 (1986).
10. McCarthy, D. A., D. E. Potter, and E. D. Nicolaides. An in vivo estimation of the potencies and half-lives of synthetic bradykinin and kallidin. *J. Pharmacol. Exp. Ther.* **148**:117-122 (1965).
11. Ferreira, S. H., and J. R. Vane. Half-lives of peptides and amines in the circulation. *Nature* **215**:1237-1240 (1967).
12. Erdos, E. G. Kininases, in: *Bradykinin, Kallidin and Kallikrein. Handbook of Experimental Pharmacology*, Vol 25, Suppl. I (E. G. Erdos, ed.). Springer-Verlag, Heidelberg, pp. 427-487 (1979).
13. Ryan, J. W. Processing of endogenous polypeptides by the lungs. *Ann. Rev. Physiol.* **44**:241-255 (1982).
14. Ryan, J. W., J. Roblero, and J. M. Stewart. Inactivation of bradykinin in the pulmonary circulation. *Biochem. J.* **110**:795-797 (1968).
15. Aiken, J. W., and J. R. Vane. The renin angiotensin system. Inhibition of converting enzyme in isolated tissues. *Nature* **228**:30-34 (1970).
16. Ryan, J. W., J. M. Stewart, W. P. Leary, and J. G. Ledingham. Metabolism of angiotensin I in the pulmonary circulation. *Biochem. J.* **120**:221-223 (1970).
17. Ryan, U. S., and J. W. Ryan. Endothelial cells and inflammation. *Clin. Lab. Med.* **3**:577-599 (1983).
18. Vavrek, R. J., and J. M. Stewart. Competitive antagonists of bradykinin. *Peptides* **6**:161-164 (1985).
19. Stewart, J. M. Chemistry and biologic activity of peptides related to bradykinin, in: *Bradykinin, Kallidin and Kallikrein. Handbook of Experimental Pharmacology*, Vol 25, Suppl. I (E. G. Erdos, ed.). Springer-Verlag, Heidelberg, pp. 227-272 (1979).
20. Steranka, L. R., S. G. Farmer, and R. M. Burch. Antagonists of B_2 bradykinin receptors. *FASEB J.* **3**:2019-2025 (1989).
21. Soffer, R. L. Angiotensin converting enzyme and the regulation of vasoactive peptides. *Ann. Rev. Biochem.* **45**:73-94 (1976).
22. Das, M., J. L. Hartley, and R. L. Soffer. Serum angiotensin converting enzyme. Isolation and relationship to the pulmonary enzyme. *J. Biol. Chem.* 252:1316-1319 (1977).
23. Das, M., and R. L. Soffer. Pulmonary angiotensin converting enzyme. Structural and catalytic properties. *J. Biol. Chem.* **250**:6762-6768 (1975).

24. Ward, P. E., T. A. Stewart, K. J. Hammon, R. C. Reynolds, and R. P. Igic. Angiotensin I converting enzyme (kininase II) in isolated retinal microvessels. *Life Sci.* **24**:1419-1424 (1979).
25. Del Vecchio, P. J., J. W. Ryan, A. Chung, and U. S. Ryan. Capillaries of the adrenal cortex possess aminopeptidase A and angiotensin converting enzyme activities. *Biochem. J.* **186**:605-608 (1980).
26. Brecher, P., V. Hingorani, K. Reininga, and A. V. Chobanian. Distribution and properties of angiotensin converting enzyme in cerebral microvessels of the rabbit and rat. *Clin. Sci.* **61**:249s-251s (1981).
27. Ryan, J. W., U. S. Ryan, A. Chung, and G. H. Fisher. Metabolism of bradykinin by endothelial cells in culture. *Adv. Exp. Med. Biol.* **156B**:775-781 (1983).
28. Oparil, S., T. Koerner, and J. K. O'Donoghue. Mechanism of angiotensin I converting enzyme inhibition by SQ 20881. Further evidence for extrapulmonary conversion. *Hypertension* **I**:13-22 (1979).
29. Regoli, D., F. Marceau, and J. Lavigne. Induction of B_1-receptors for kinins in the rabbit by a bacterial lipopolysaccharide. *Eur. J. Pharmacol.* **71**:105-115 (1981).
30. Regoli, D., G. Drapeau, P. Rovero, S. Dion, P. D'Orleans-Juste, and J. Barabe. The action of kinin antagonists in B_1 and B_2 receptor systems. *Eur. J. Pharmacol.* **123**:61-65 (1986).
31. Churchill, L., and P. E. Ward. Conversion of B_1 kinin receptor-mediated vascular relaxation to contraction. *Hypertension* **9**[Suppl III]:III-1-III-5 (1987).
32. Guimaraes, J. A., M. A. R. Vieira, M. J. F. Camargo, and T. Maack. Renal vasoconstrictive effect of kinins mediated by B_1-kinin receptors. *Eur. J. Pharmacol.* **130**:177-185 (1986).
33. Cascieri, M. A., H. G. Bull, R. A. Mumford, A. A. Patchett, N. A. Thornberry, and T. Liang. Carboxyl-terminal tripeptidyl hydrolysis of substance P by purified rabbit lung angiotensin converting enzyme and the potentiation of substance P activity in vivo by captopril and MK-422. *Mol. Pharmacol.* 25:287-293 (1984).
34. Inokuchi, J-I., and A. Nagamatsu. Tripeptidyl carboxypeptidase activity of kininase II (angiotensin converting enzyme). *Biochim. Biophys. Acta* **662**: 300-307 (1981).
35. Oshima, G., Y. Hiraga, K. Shirono, S. Oh-ishi, S. Sakakibara, and T. Kinoshita. Cleavage of des-Arg^9-bradykinin by angiotensin I converting enzyme from pig kidney cortex. *Experientia* **41**:325-328 (1985).
36. Dorer, F. E., J. R. Kahn, K. E. Lentz, M. Levine, and L. T. Skeggs. Hydrolysis of bradykinin by angiotensin converting enzyme. *Circ. Res.* **34**:824-827 (1974).
37. Oparil, S., T. Koerner, G. W. Tregear, B. A. Barnes, and E. Haber. Substrate requirements for angiotensin I conversion in vivo and in vitro. *Circ. Res.* **32**:415-423 (1973).

38. Togo, J., R. M. Burch, C. J. DeHaas, J. R. Connor, and L. R. Steranka. D-Phe[7]-substituted peptide bradykinin antagonists are not substrates for kininase II. *Peptides* **10**:109-112 (1989).
39. Drapeau, G., and P. E. Ward. Metabolism of bradykinin and bradykinin analogs. *Fed. Proc.* **4**:A990 (1990).
40. Huey, R., C. M. Bloor, M. S. Kawahara, and T. E. Hugli. Potentiation of the anaphylatoxins in vivo using an inhibitor of serum carboxypeptidase N (SCPN). I. Lethality and pathologic effects on pulmonary tissue. *Am. J. Pathol.* **112**:48-60 (1983).
41. Sheikh, I. A., and A. P. Kaplan. Studies of the digestion of bradykinin, lysyl-bradykinin, and kinin-degradation products by carboxypeptidases A, B, and N. *Biochem. Pharmacol.* **35**:1957-1963 (1986).
42. Bausback, H. H., and P. E. Ward. Kallidin and bradykinin metabolism by isolated cerebral microvessels. *Biochem. Pharmacol.* **37**:2973-2978 (1988).
43. Sheikh, I. A., and A. P. Kaplan. Mechanism of digestion of bradykinin and lysyl-bradykinin (kallidin) in human serum. *Biochem. Pharmacol.* **38**:993-1000 (1989).
44. Palmieri, F. E., H. H. Bausback, L. Churchill, and P. E. Ward. Kinin and enkephalin conversion by an endothelial plasma membrane carboxypeptidase. *Biochem. Pharmacol.* **35**:2749-2756 (1986).
45. Skidgel, R. A., R. M. Davis, and F. Tan. Human carboxypeptidase M. Purification and characterization of a membrane-bound carboxypeptidase that cleaves peptide hormones. *J. Biol. Chem.* **264**:2236-2239 (1989).
46. Ryan, J. W., A. Chung, and U. S. Ryan. A radioassay for carboxypeptidase N. *Adv. Exp. Med. Biol.* **156B**:867-874 (1983).
47. Salgado, H. C. O. A. Carretero, A. G. Scicli, and R. D. Murray. Effect of DL-2-mercaptomethyl-3-guanidinoethylthiopropanoic acid on the blood pressure response to vasoactive substances. *J. Pharmacol. Exp. Therp.* **237**:204-208 (1986).
48. Odya, C. E., F. P. Wilgis, J. F. Walker, and S. Oparil. Immunoreactive bradykinin and [des-Arg[9]]-bradykinin in low renin essential hypertension—before and after treatment with enalapril (MK421). *J. Lab. Clin. Med.* **102**:714-721 (1983).
49. Streeten, D. H., L. P. Kerr, C. B. Kerr, J. C. Prior, and T. G. Dalakos. Hyperbradykininism: A new orthostatic syndrome. *Lancet* **2**:1048-1053 (1972).
50. Nolly, H., A. G. Scicli, G. Scicli, and O. A. Carretero. Characterization of a kininogenase from rat vascular tissue resembling tissue kallikrein. *Circ. Res.* **56**:816-821 (1985).
51. Regoli, D., G. Drapeau, P. Rovero, S. Dion, N-E. Rhaleb, J. Barabe, P. D'Orleans-Juste, and P. E. Ward. Conversion of kinins and their antagonists into B_1 receptor activators and blockers in isolated vessels. *Eur. J. Pharmacol.* **127**:219-224 (1986).
52. Marceau, F., A. Lussier, D. Regoli, and J. P. Giroud. Pharmacology of kinins: Their relevance to tissue injury and inflammation. *Gen. Pharmacol.* **14**:209-229 (1983).

53. Whalley, E. T., H. Fritz, and R. Greiger. Kinin receptors and angiotensin converting enzyme in rabbit basilar arteries. *Naunyn-Schmiedeberg's Arch. Pharmacol.* **324**:296-301 (1983).
54. Drapeau, G., N-E. Rhaleb, S. Dion, D. Jukic, and D. Regoli. [Phe^8(CH_2-NH)Arg^9]bradykinin, a B_2 receptor selective agonist which is not broken down by either kininase I or kininase II. *Europ. J. Pharmacol.* **155**:193-195 (1988).
55. Wachsmuth, E. D., and F. G. Staber. Changes in membrane-bound aminopeptidase on bone marrow-derived macrophages during their maturation in vitro. *Exp. Cell Res.* **109**:269-276 (1977).
56. Behal, F. J., W. Sidorowicz, and P. C. Canizaro. Kinin cleavage by intact human erythrocytes. *Fed. Proc.* **43**:652 (Abst.) (1984).
57. Nagaoka, I., and T. Yamashita. Possible involvement of aminopeptidase, an ecto-enzyme, in the inactivation of bradykinin by intact neutrophils. *Biochim. Biophys. Acta* **847**:67-76 (1985).
58. Amoscato, A. A., J. W. Alexander, and G. F. Babcock. Surface aminopeptidase activity of human lymphocytes. I. Biochemical and biologic properties of intact cells. *J. Immunol.* **142**:1245-1252 (1989).
59. Erdos, E. G., and R. A. Skidgel. Neutral endopeptidase 24.11 (enkephalinase) and related regulators of peptide hormones. *FASEB J.* **3**:145-151 (1989).
60. Hendriks, D., S. Scharpe, M. Van Sande, and M. P. Lommaert. A labile enzyme in fresh human serum interferes with the assay of carboxypeptidase N. *Clin. Chem.* **35**:177 (1989).
61. Gafford, J. T., R. A. Skidgel, E. G. Erdos, and L. B. Hersh. Human kidney "enkephalinase," a neutral metalloendopeptidase that cleaves active peptides. *Biochemistry* **22**:3265-3271 (1983).
62. Kenny, A. J. Proteinases associated with cell membranes, in: *Proteinases in Mammalian Cells and Tissues* (A. J. Barrett, ed.). Biomedical Press, Elsevier/North Holland, pp. 393-444 (1977).
63. McDonald, J. K., and A. J. Barrett. *Mammalian Proteases, a Glossary and Bibliography*, Vol. 2: *Exopeptidases*. Academic Press, New York, 1986.
64. Gee, N. S., M. A. Bowes, P. Buck, and A. J. Kenny. An immunoradiometric assay for endopeptidase-24.11 shows it to be a widely distributed enzyme in pig tissues. *Biochem. J.* **228**:119-126 (1985).
65. Orlowski, M. Pituitary endopeptidases. *Mol. Cell. Biochem.* **52**:49-74 (1983).
66. Ura, N., O. A. Carretero, and E. G. Erdos. Role of renal endopeptidase 24.11 in kinin metabolism in vitro and in vivo. *Kidney Int.* **32**:;507-513 (1987).
67. Johnson, A. R., J. Ashton, W. W. Schulz, and E. G. Erdos. Neutral metalloendopeptidase in human lung tissue and cultured cells. *Am. Rev. Respir. Dis.* **132**:564-568 (1985).
68. Johnson, A. R., J. J. Coalson, J. Ashton, M. Larumbide, and E. G. Erdos. Neutral endopeptidase in serum samples from patients with adult respiratory distress syndrome. Comparison with angiotensin converting enzyme. *Am. Rev. Respir. Dis.* **132**:1262-1267 (1985).

69. Almenoff, J., A. S. Teirstein, J. C. Thornton, and M. Orlowski. Identification of a thermolysin-like metalloendopeptidase in serum: Activity in normal subjects and in patients with sarcoidosis. *J. Lab. Clin. Med.* **103**:420-431 (1984).
70. Gros, C., A. Souque, J-C. Schwartz, J. Duchier, A. Cournot, P. Baumer, and J-M. Lecomte. Protection of atrial natriuretic factor against degradation: Diuretic and natriuretic responses after in vivo inhibition of enkephalinase (EC 3.4.24.11) by acetorphan. *Proc. Natl. Acad. Sci.* **86**:7580-7584 (1989).
71. Olins, G. M., P. A. Krieter, A. J. Trapani, K. L. Spear, and P. R. Bovy. Specific inhibitors of endopeptidase 24.11 inhibit the metabolism of atrial natriuretic peptides in vitro and in vivo. *Mol. Cell. Endocrinol.* **61**:201-208 (1989).
72. Webb, R. L., G. D. Yasay, Jr., C. McMartin, R. B. McNeal, Jr., and M. B. Zimmerman. Degradation of atrial natriuretic peptide: Pharmacologic effects of protease EC 24.11 inhibition. *J. Cardiovasc. Pharmacol.* **14**:285-293 (1989).
73. Seymour, A. A., J. N. Swerdel, S. A. Fennell, S. P. Druckman, R. Neubeck, and N. G. Delaney. Potentiation of the depressor responses to atrial natriuretic peptides in conscious SHR by an inhibitor of neutral endopeptidase. *J. Cardiovasc. Pharmacol.* **14**:194-204 (1989).
74. Ishida, H., A. G. Scicli, and O. A. Carretero. Role of angiotensin converting enzyme and other peptidases in in vivo metabolism of kinins. *Hypertension* **14**:322-327 (1989).
75. Sanderink, G-J., Y. Artur, and G. Siest. Human aminopeptidases: A review of the literature. *J. Clin. Chem. Clin. Biochem.* **26**:795-807 (1988).
76. Tokioka-Terao, M., K. Hiwada, and T. Kokubu. A radioimmunoassay for the measurement of aminopeptidase (microsomal) in human serum. *Enzyme* 33:181-187 (1985).
77. Ahmad, S. A., and P. E. Ward. Role of aminopeptidase activity in the regulation of the pressor activity of circulating angiotensins. *J. Pharmacol. Exp. Therap.* **252**:643-650 (1990).
78. Ward, P. E. Immunoelectrophoretic analysis of vascular, membrane-bound angiotensin I converting enzyme, aminopeptidase M and dipeptidyl(amino)peptidase IV. *Biochem. Pharmacol.* **33**:3183-3193 (1984).
79. Palmieri, F. E., H. H. Bausback, and P. E. Ward. Metabolism of vasoactive peptides by vascular endothelium and smooth muscle aminopeptidase M. *Biochem. Pharmacol.* **38**:173-180 (1989).
80. Churchill, L., H. H. Bausback, M. E. Gerritsen, and P. E. Ward. Metabolism of opioid peptides by cerebral microvascular aminopeptidase M. *Biochim. Biophys. Acta* **923**:35-41 (1987).
81. Hersh, L. B., N. Aboukhair, and S. Watson. Immunohistochemical localization of aminopeptidase M in rat brain and periphery: Relationship of enzyme localization and enkephalin metabolism. *Peptides* **8**:523-532 (1987).
82. Solhonne, B., C. Gros, H. Pollard, and J. C. Schwartz. Major localization of aminopeptidase M in rat brain microvessels. *Neuroscience* **22**:225-232 (1987).

83. Bausback, H. H., and P. E. Ward. Degradation of low molecular weight opioid peptides by vascular plasma membrane aminopeptidase M. *Biochim. Biophys. Acta* **882**:437-444 (1986).
84. Palmieri, F. E., J. J. Petrelli, and P. E. Ward. Vascular, plasma membrane aminopeptidase M: Metabolism of vasoactive peptides. *Biochem. Pharmacol.* **34**:2309-2317 (1985).
85. Roblero, J., J. W. Ryan, and J. M. Stewart. Assay of kinins by their effects on blood pressure. *Res. Commun. Chem. Pathol. Pharmacol.* **6**:207-212 (1973).
86. Ahmad, S. A., G. Drapeau, and P. E. Ward. Depressor effect of bradykinin agonists resistant to degradation by angiotensin converting enzyme and/or carboxypeptidase N. *Fed. Proc.* **4**:A990 (1990).
87. Dorer, F. E., J. W. Ryan, and J. M. Stewart. Hydrolysis of bradykinin and its higher homologues by angiotensin converting enzyme. *Biochem. J.* **141**: 915-917 (1974).
88. Kugler, P. Aminopeptidase A is angiotensinase A. I. Quantitative histochemical studies in the kidney glomerulus. *Histochemistry* **74**:229-245 (1982).
89. Bausback, H. H., L. Churchill, and P. E. Ward. Angiotensin metabolism by cerebral microvascular aminopeptidase A. *Biochem. Pharmacol.* **37**:155-160 (1988).
90. Ryan, J. W., J. Roblero, and J. M. Stewart. Inactivation of bradykinin in rat lung. *Adv. Exp. Med. Biol.* **8**:263-281 (1970).
91. Bakhle, Y. S. Pulmonary metabolism of bradykinin analogues and the contribution of angiotensin converting enzyme to bradykinin inactivation in isolated lungs. *Brit. J. Pharmacol.* **59**:123-128 (1977).
92. Orawski, A. T., J. P. Susz, and W. H. Simmons. Aminopeptidase P from bovine lung: Solubilization, properties, and potential role in bradykinin degradation. *Mol. Cell. Biochem.* **75**:123-132 (1987).
93. Orawski, A. T., J. P. Susz, and W. H. Simmons. Metabolism of bradykinin by multiple coexisting membrane-bound peptidases in lung: Techniques for investigating the role of each peptidase using specific inhibitors. *Adv. Exp. Med. Biol.* (in press).
94. Palmieri, F. E., and P. E. Ward. Mesentery vascular metabolism of substance P. *Biochim. Biophys. Acta* **755**:522-525 (1983).
95. Palmieri, F. E., and P. E. Ward. Dipeptidyl(amino)peptidase IV and post proline cleaving enzyme in cultured endothelial and smooth muscle cells. *Adv. Exp. Med. Biol.* **247A**:305-311 (1989).
96. Heymann, E., and R. Mentlein. Liver dipeptidylaminopeptidase IV hydrolyzes substance P. *FEBS Lett.* **91**:360-364 (1978).
97. Bausback, H. H., and P. E. Ward. Vascular post proline cleaving enzyme: Metabolism of vasoactive peptides. *Adv. Exp. Med. Biol.* **198A**:397-404 (1986).
98. Ward, P. E., H. H. Bausback, and C. E. Odya. Kinin and angiotensin metabolism by purified renal post-proline cleaving enzyme. *Biochem. Pharmacol.* **36**:3187-3193 (1987).

99. Marceau, F., M. Gendreau, J. Barabe, S. St-Pierre, and D. Regoli. The degradation of bradykinin (BK) and des-Arg^9-BK in plasma. *Can. J. Physiol. Pharmacol.* **59**:131-138 (1981).
100. Ward, P. E., W. Schultz, R. C. Reynolds, and E. G. Erdos. Metabolism of kinins and angiotensins in the isolated glomerulus and brush border of rat kidney. *Lab. Invest.* **36**:599-606 (1977).
101. Ward, P. E., and M. A. Sheridan. Immunoelectrophoretic analysis of renal and intestinal brush border converting enzyme. *Biochem. Pharmacol.* **32**: 265-274 (1983).
102. Odya, C. E., D. V. Marinkovic, K. J. Hammon, T. A. Stewart, and E. G. Erdos. Purification and properties of prolylcarboxypeptidase (angiotensinase C) from human kidney. *J. Biol. Chem.* **253**:5927-5931 (1978).
103. Ward, P. E., M. A. Sheridan, K. J. Hammon, and E. G. Erdos. Angiotensin I converting enzyme (kininase II) of the brush border of human and swine intestine. *Biochem. Pharmacol.* **29**:1525-1529 (1980).
104. Oparil, S., F. A. Carone, T. N. Pullman, and S. Nakamura. Inhibition of proximal tubular hydrolysis and reabsorption of bradykinin by peptides. *Am. J. Physiol.* **231**:743-748 (1976).
105. Martin, L. C., J. W. Ryan, G. H. Fisher, A. Chung, M. Epstein, and J. M. Stewart. Fate of bradykinin-potentiating peptide 9a after intravenous injection. *Biochem. J.* **184**:713-716 (1979).
106. Nasjletti, A., J. Colina-Chourio, and J. C. McGiff. Disappearance of bradykinin in the renal circulation of dogs. *Circ. Res.* **37**:59-65 (1975).
107. Djokic, T. D., K. Sekizawa, D. B. Borson, and J. A. Nadel. Neutral endopeptidase inhibitors potentiate substance P-induced contraction in gut smooth muscle. *Am. J. Physiol.* **256**:G39-G43 (1989).
108. Frossard, N., K. J. Rhoden, and P. J. Barnes. Influence of epithelium on guinea pig airway responses to tachykinins: Role of endopeptidase and cyclooxygenase. *J. Pharmacol. Exp. Ther.* **248**:292-298 (1989).

7

Effects of Bradykinin Antagonists on the Cardiovascular System

Haralambos Gavras and Irene Gavras
Boston University School of Medicine
Boston, Massachusetts

I. INTRODUCTION

One of the most important aspects in the development of bradykinin antagonists is their use as pharmacological probes in studying the cardiovascular effects of bradykinin. The possible role of bradykinin in cardiovascular regulation has intrigued scientists for many years. A member of the kinin system discovered in the late 1920s, bradykinin is a nonapeptide whose existence was first recognized by Rocha e Silva et al. (1) from its effects on intestinal smooth muscle. Since then, several other actions of bradykinin have been described, including vascular contraction and relaxation, participation in the process of inflammatory reactions, interaction with central and peripheral neural structures, stimulation of synthesis and release of various vasoactive substances, and so on.

Several factors have hindered the investigation of bradykinin's effects over the years. Most important among them are the ubiquitous nature of the substance, which is found in almost every organ tissue, and the fact that it appears to be primarily a "tissue hormone" acting mostly at its site of release because of its quick degradation in the systemic circulation. Despite the recent development of assays for its evaluation, the results produced to date, although helpful, have not been entirely consistent. The fact that some effects might be direct, whereas others appear to be mediated and/or modulated by a variety of locally released humoral agents and can differ in different organ systems, has further complicated the issue.

Interest in the cardiovascular effects of bradykinin has accelerated rapidly in recent years due to the work of many investigators, which produced a lot of new information with potential clinical relevance: for example, the discoveries that the kininase II which degrades bradykinin is identical to the angiotensin-converting enzyme (ACE) (2), that the bradykinin-potentiating factors isolated from a snake venom are ACE inhibitors that could act as antihypertensives in experimental hypertension (3), that renal and vascular wall prostaglandins synthesized locally were both stimulated by and found to mediate the action of locally generated kinins (4-7), that various types of hypertension were associated with, and probably affected by the changes in the renal kallikrein-kinin system (8-11), that cyclooxygenase inhibitors, which interrupt prostaglandin synthesis, could induce renal failure through their effects on kinins as well as on the renin-angiotensin system (12), and that part of the blood pressure-lowering effect of ACE inhibitors must be accounted for by potentiation of bradykinin since antibodies to bradykinin could partly reverse this effect (13). But the synthesis of a variety of polypeptide bradykinin analogs with various combinations of agonistic and antagonistic properties for different bradykinin receptors was the most recent major advance in the field (14,15).

II. BRADYKININ RECEPTORS AND ANTAGONISTS

At least two types of bradykinin receptors have been characterized in vascular and other tissues. Their classification is based both on their ability to respond to specific pharmacological agonists and antagonists and on the type of functional or biochemical response elicited by these compounds (16-25).

In summary, the evidence suggests that B1 receptors (characterized by their particular sensitivity to the selective agonist desArg^9-BK and the selective antagonist desArg^9[Leu^8]-BK) are of low affinity; they are coupled to adenylate cyclase and use cAMP as intracellular second messenger; their stimulation can induce vasoconstriction directly (i.e., not mediated by other locally released vasoactive substances) and vasorelaxation (i.e., via release of the vasodilatory prostaglandins PGI_2 and PGE_2 as well as release of endothelium-derived relaxing factor [EDRF]); their function is independent from the arachidonic acid cascade; and B1 receptors can form de novo under the influence of injury and various agents, including endotoxins and ACE inhibitors, in vivo and in vitro.

The classical B2 receptors are of high affinity; their excitation generates inositol phosphates, with $I_{1,4,5}P_3$ being the most likely intracellular second messenger coupling bradykinin receptor stimulation to CA^{2+} release in the cytosol; B2 receptors may also directly cause contraction of vascular smooth muscle, but their most prominent effect in vessels with intact endothelium is indirect vascular relaxation, mediated via release of EDRF and PGE_2 and PGI_2; and their action is dependent on activation of the arachidonic acid cascade and therefore subject to blockade by cyclooxygenase inhibitors. Accumulated evidence indicates that most of the clinically relevant vascular effects of bradykinin, including vasodilation, vascular permeability, pain from stimulation of sensory neurons, release of histamine by mast cells, and release of catecholamines from sympathetic nerve terminals, are functions of the B2 receptors.

Stewart and Vavrek discovered that the key modification of the nonapeptide bradykinin that confers B2 antagonistic properties to an analog is replacement of the Pro residue at position 7 with a D-Phe residue (14,15, 26,27) (see Chapter 3). Antagonist potency was further increased by extension of the N-terminus with a basic residue, such as D-Arg, replacement of the Phe residues at positions 5 and 8 with β-(2-thienyl)-L-alanine (Thi), and replacement of Pro by 4-hydroxy-Pro at positions 2 and/or 3. The resulting decapeptide, NPC 349, is the most potent vascular B2 antagonist synthesized by these investigators. It is the one that most effectively inhibits production of intracellular second messengers (28), and when infused at a rate of 10 μg/min in dog hind limbs it was found to produce a full log shift in the dose-response curve to exogenous bradykinin (29). Unlike other similar bradykinin analogs which appear to act as partial agonists on sympathoadrenal tissue bradykinin receptors, causing an outpouring of epinephrine, this compound at the usually employed doses has no evidence of agonistic activity (30). For this reason it is now the most widely used bradykinin antagonist in recent experiments designed to assess the cardiovascular effects of bradykinin.

It should be kept in mind that, unlike the B1 binding analogs, B2 receptor agonists or antagonists are not selective (25). They may, however, be tissue-specific, so that a given compound may act on some tissues as a pure antagonist, on others as a partial agonist, and in some cases as a "superagonist" eliciting a specific response more powerfully than bradykinin itself (25). It is also noteworthy that bradykinin antagonists, although more resistant than bradykinin itself to enzymatic degradation, are still rapidly inactivated in the circulation by enzymes degrading bradykinin; ACE inhibition can partly block the degradation of both bradykinin and its analogs (31). Finally, it must be acknowledged that surgery and instrumentation of experimental animals might activate plasma kallikrein and lead to artifactually enhanced generation of kinin; blockade of bradykinin under these conditions may not accurately reflect the physiological role of bradykinin in the normal resting state (32).

III. SYSTEMIC AND REGIONAL VASCULAR EFFECTS OF BRADYKININ ANTAGONISTS

Since ACE inhibitors have become increasingly popular as drugs of first choice in the treatment of hypertension and congestive heart failure, a question that has drawn the interest of many investigators is how much of the vasorelaxant effect of ACE inhibition is due to diminished formation of angiotensin II and how much to diminished degradation of bradykinin. In this respect, it is important to note that, although initially the circulating plasma levels of angiotensin II are markedly suppressed, at a later stage they return toward the baseline despite continuing effective inhibition of ACE and continuing maintenance of antihypertensive effect (33). On the other hand, accumulation of bradykinin could not be convincingly demonstrated, as some authors found it with teprotide but not with captopril (34-37); others suggested on the contrary that captopril might be unique among ACE inhibitors in augmenting the synthesis of vasodilatory prostaglandins by reducing inactivation of bradykinin (38); however, most support the view that potentiation of bradykinin and interaction with prostaglandins is a function of ACE inhibition per se regardless of which ACE-inhibiting compound is used. The lack of measurable change in plasma bradykinin concentration during ACE inhibition is probably due to the rapid degradation of the circulating peptide by alternative enzymatic pathways, whereas the potentiation of its effect is probably due to increased concentration within the vascular wall tissue (39).The doses of bradykinin antagonist necessary to inhibit the vasodepressor effect of exogenously infused bradykinin are much lower than those required to demonstrate the effect of endogenous bradykinin (40). The most likely explanation for this is that much higher concentrations of bradykinin antagonist are needed to displace tissue-bound bradykinin that was locally generated and accumulated than the concentrations sufficient to inhibit circulating hormone (32,39,40).

In our earlier studies, we used as pharmacological probes two bradykinin antagonists, NPC 394 and NPC 392. The specificity of these compounds as bradykinin antagonists in vitro has been well established (14, 15). In pilot experiments they were tested in vivo to ascertain their capacity to block the vasodilatory effect of bradykinin infused intraarterially (41,42) or intravenously (43). We found that NPC 394 infused i.a. at a rate of 40 μg/kg/min in unanesthetized rats could inhibit the vasodepressor effect of a 200 ng bolus of bradykinin by 55%, and infusion at twice that rate did not change the magnitude of bradykinin inhibition or produce any effect of its own on blood pressure (41). Other investigators found that NPC 341 could block exogenous bradykinin by 69% (43). NPC 392 infused at a rate of 500 μg/kg/min could inhibit by 60% the hypotensive effect of a bradykinin bolus.

Our first series of experiments was designed to assess the contribution of bradykinin to the blood pressure lowering obtained by ACE inhibition in a high-renin model, the renovascular hypertensive rat with one renal artery clipped and the other left intact (41). After their blood pressure was lowered with the ACE inhibitor enalapril, i.a. infusion of the bradykinin antagonist NPC 394 raised blood pressure an average of 30% of the original fall, suggesting that this much was the contribution of bradykinin to the blood pressure lowering achieved by ACE inhibition. In other renovascular hypertensive rats whose blood pressure had been lowered by the angiotensin II antagonist saralasin or the nonspecific vasodilator sodium nitroprusside, infusion of the bradykinin antagonist produced no further changes in blood pressure; this suggested that bradykinin did not contribute to the antihypertensive effect of these agents, nor did the analog produce a nonspecific pressor effect related to the lowered blood pressure per se or the magnitude of blood pressure lowering. Comparable results were obtained by other investigators, using a similar high-renin hypertensive rat model (aortic ligation between the renal arteries) treated with enalaprilat and the bradykinin antagonist NPC 349 (40).

The next question to be answered was whether endogenous bradykinin participates in the maintenance of normal blood pressure in intact conscious untreated rats (39). In our experiment, doses of 40-80 μg/kg/min of NPC 394 had failed to produce any blood pressure change in such animals, but a large bolus of 1 mg produced acute blood pressure rises on the order of 12-15 mmHg. As mentioned earlier, we interpreted these findings as evidence suggesting that bradykinin does contribute to the maintenance of normal blood pressure, but that high doses of the inhibitors are necessary to demonstrate this effect, possibly because high concentration of the compound may be needed to displace tissue-bound bradykinin that is probably generated locally, as opposed to the lower concentration required to inhibit the circulating hormone (39). Other investigators, however, have recently reported that i.v. injection of this same compound at doses of 25, 50, and 100 μg could increase blood pressure in normal anesthetized rats in a dose-dependent manner (43). These conflicting results are difficult to reconcile, but they all point to a variable contributory role of bradykinin in the maintenance of normotension, its extent differing with various concurrent factors, such as the conditions of each experiment (e.g., presence or absence of anesthesia). The finding that a bradykinin antagonist, in this case NPC 394, could make previously subpressor doses of vasopressor hormones increase significantly the blood pressure of normotensive rats is compatible with this view (44). This finding suggests that, even though circulating endogenous bradykinin may not be directly involved in normal blood pressure regulation, it still contributes to blood pressure control by attenuating the pressor reaction to other vasoconstrictors, i.e., to angiotensin II, vasopressin, and α-adrenoceptor stimulation (44). When normotensive animals had been pretreated with an ACE inhibitor (ramipril or captopril), the bradykinin antagonist, just as with hypertensive models, could in part reverse the ACE inhibitor-induced blood pressure fall (39,43). Interestingly, in anesthetized or conscious spontaneously hypertensive rats, the bradykinin antagonist produced only minor elevation in blood pressure unless their renin-angiotensin system had been stimulated by salt depletion, suggesting that this strain may be deficient in bradykinin and that this deficiency could in part be responsible for the development and/or maintenance of hypertension in this model (45,46). Moreover, salt loading per se tends to suppress kinins regardless of blood pressure levels attained (47), suggesting that this mechanism may also contribute to salt-induced hypertension in general.

Studies of renal hemodynamics revealed that bradykinin antagonist analogs can affect autoregulation of renal perfusion and decrease renal blood flow and/or glomerular filtration rate (43,46,48). In a series of recent experiments in normal conscious rats using NPC 349, we found that not only the renal blood flow, but also the regional blood flow to the heart, liver, spleen, stomach, and testes was significantly diminished after bradykinin inhibition, whereas blood flow to brain, skin, and skeletal muscle remained mostly unchanged (49). Although total systemic vascular resistance did not change appreciably following bradykinin inhibition, the cardiac output did fall significantly, probably as a result of the marked decrease in coronary perfusion in these otherwise healthy hearts.

This pattern of blood flow changes is of particular interest because it is almost, but not quite, the reverse of the redistribution of regional blood flow obtained by ACE inhibition or by angiotensin II blockade with saralasin (50,51). The two notable exceptions are the regional flows to the brain and the adrenal glands, which were significantly augmented by angiotensin II receptor blockade or ACE inhibition, but totally unaffected by bradykinin antagonism. Blood flow to musculocutaneous tissues remained unaffected by either intervention. Taken together, these studies suggest that the redistribution of regional blood flow in favor of some vital organs, heart and kidney, induced by ACE inhibition, appears to be due in part to elimination of angiotensin II, but also to a large extent to potentiation of bradykinin. Indeed, the patterns of sensitivity of regional vascular trees to angiotensin II and bradykinin appear to be similar, with the exception of the cerebral and adrenal vasculature, which seem to be sensitive to vasoconstriction by angiotensin II but not to vasodilation by bradykinin.

These findings are of great clinical relevance because they explain how ACE inhibition, which is used to treat not only hypertension, but also congestive heart failure and coronary disease with normal or low baseline blood pressures, can still successfully maintain adequate perfusion of vital organs despite substantial reductions in systemic pressure. They also suggest that pharmacological interventions affecting the actions of bradykinin but not those of angiotensin II might be expected to interfere with coronary and renal blood flow, but not the cerebral blood flow of patients treated with ACE inhibitors. An example of such a pharmacological intervention is the use of nonsteroidal anti-inflammatory drugs (NSAIDs), which are inhibitors of cyclooxygenase and therefore block the synthesis of prostaglandins. The vascular B2 receptor-mediated effects of bradykinin on arterial walls with intact endothelium are known to be partly exerted via EDRF and partly via activation of the arachidonic acid cascade and synthesis of prostaglandins, as mentioned earlier, and therefore subject to attenuation by NSAIDs. Treatment with a NSAID in a patient receiving ACE inhibition might diminish the coronary and renal perfusion (and hence attenuate the protective effect of ACE inhibitors on these organs) but would not be expected to affect cerebral perfusion.

Most of the studies described up to this point have used single injections or short infusions of bradykinin antagonists. In one study, we attempted a continuous 5-minute infusion of NPC 392 in intact awake normotensive rats at the rate of 500 μg/min (42). We observed an immediate blood pressure rise of 15 mmHg within the first minute, increasing gradually by another 10 mmHg over the next 4 minutes, and decreasing sharply within seconds after discontinuation of the infusion. In normotensive bilaterally nephrectomized rats, this procedure caused a similar time-course of blood pressure rise, but of half the magnitude. The problem with this particular antagonist, however, is that it has a pronounced agonistic bradykinin-like effect on the adrenal medulla, causing a marked stimulation of catecholamine release which can confound the interpretation of its results (30).

Other bradykinin antagonists, such as NPC 394 and NPC 349, have no agonistic properties at the commonly used doses. In intact rats pretreated with the cyclooxygenase inhibitor indomethacin, a 5-minute infusion of NPC 349 at 250 μg/min produced a progressive increase in blood pressure, whereas in intact untreated rats it failed to produce a blood pressure change (52). A large bolus of 4 mg/kg of this antagonist was found to produce a biphasic effect: first a pressor action that was unaffected by a variety of concurrent vasoactive treatments, then a depressor action apparently caused by a release of vasodilator renal prostaglandins because it was abolished by nephrectomy or treatment with indomethacin (53). In a recent study, Beierwaltes and Carretero (54) showed that this bradykinin antagonist could in part reverse the ACE inhibitor-stimulated synthesis of the vasodilatory PGI_2 by arterial wall tissue. Taken together, these studies indicate that the blood pressure rise produced by bradykinin antagonists—or their attenuation of the hypotensive effect of ACE inhibition—is counteracted by vasodilatory prostaglandins and confirm the notion that bradykinin's vascular action is to a large extent mediated via the local effect of prostaglandins generated by the activation of the cyclooxygenase pathway.

Another aspect of the role of bradykinin in blood pressure regulation, is its participation in endotoxic shock. Sepsis from *E. coli*, or treatment with lipopolysaccharides derived from *E. coli*, can induce septic shock associated with a sixfold increase in levels of circulating bradykinin (55). Various primarily B2 antagonists of bradykinin have been recently used to reverse the profound hypotension in response to endotoxin. NPC 413 and NPC 567 were found to attenuate the hypotension of endotoxic shock, diminish the increase in prostaglandin metabolites associated with this condition, and reduce the overall mortality rates of rats submitted to this procedure from 100% to 50% (55-57). However, as mentioned earlier, during endotoxic shock there may be de novo generation of B1 receptors; earlier studies (58) had suggested that this may be, at least in part, a B1-mediated effect, since it was accentuated by desArg-kinins and blocked by desArg^{10}[Leu^{9}]kallidin, all of which are specific B1-binding analogs. It should be kept in mind, on the other hand, that B2 antagonists are nonselective, as mentioned earlier, and can be transformed in vivo into B1 antagonists, thus binding to both types of receptors (25). Therefore, it is unclear at this point whether B1 or B2 receptors are responsible for the hypotensive reaction, and which type of bradykinin antagonists might have a potential clinical value in the treatment of septic shock. Likewise, in diabetics with orthostatic hypotension, it was found that bradykinin increments correlated significantly with the fall in systemic blood pressure (59). It would be interesting to assess the potential corrective action of a bradykinin antagonist in such patients.

In contrast to the peripheral vascular action of systemically injected bradykinin, which is more depressor than pressor, its central action when introduced into the CNS is clearly pressor (60,61). Intracerebroventricular injection of bradykinin causes a dose-dependent increase in blood pressure, which can be antagonized by i.c.v. phentolamine, suggesting an α-adrenergic-mediated mechanism. I.c.v. administration of desArg^{9}-BK, a specific B1 agonist, produced no pressor effect, and i.c.v. desArg^{9}[Leu^{8}]-BK, a specific B1 antagonist, could not prevent the pressor response to i.c.v. bradykinin, which the B2 antagonist NPC 349 could prevent (62-64). Furthermore, this last B2 antagonist, given i.c.v. by itself, produced no blood pressure changes, whereas the B2 antagonist NPC 392 produced on its own a blood pressure rise similar to that elicited by bradykinin (64, 65). Both the latter bradykinin analog and bradykinin itself were found to increase substantially the local release of norepinephrine (61) and the circulating levels of epinephrine (65). Taken together, the data suggest that the centrally mediated pressure action of bradykinin (and of those of its analogs with partial agonistic properties) is a B2 receptor function effected via stimulation mostly of the sympathoadrenal system, although an interaction with vasopressin (66) and possibly with serotonin (67) may also contribute to this response. Other actions of centrally administered bradykinin may be mediated by other neurotransmitters, e.g., the hyperthermic effect of i.c.v. bradykinin and possibly its nociceptive effect appear to be dependent on stimulation of brain tissue concentrations of serotonin and PGE_2 (68-69). The possible influence of bradykinin analogs on these functions has not yet been studied.

IV. CARDIAC EFFECTS OF BRADYKININ ANTAGONISTS

Bradykinin, in addition to its systemic vascular effects which would indirectly affect the cardiac function, appears to also act directly on the coronary vasculature and the myocardium. The long-known coronary dilation induced by bradykinin appears to be mediated in part by prostaglandins and in part by other endothelial humoral factors (70,71), most likely EDRF (72). Experimental myocadial ischemia in animals is followed by an immediate sharp increase in bradykinin concentration in the coronary sinus blood (73), a finding subsequently confirmed also in patients with acute myocardial infarction (74). The possible implications of this finding are multiple, since bradykinin may exert both beneficial and deleterious actions on the heart.

On the one hand bradykinin may improve ischemia by local EDRF-mediated vasodilation, although this action may already be significantly attenuated in the atherosclerotic coronary arteries (75). It can also reduce the workload of the injured heart as a result of the systemic vasodilation. Furthermore, bradykinin-stimulated EDRF may reduce the platelet adhesiveness and enhance the nonadhesive properties of vascular endothelium (76). The early finding that survivors of acute myocardial infarct had lower kininase activity than nonsurvivors (74,77) is consistent with the subsequent reports that ACE inhibitors may attenuate the reperfusion injury soon after release of coronary obstruction (78-81), as well as the later progression of ischemic cardiomyopathy in survivors of myocardial infarction (82,83). Over the years, these cardioprotective effects of ACE inhibition had mostly been attributed to partial elimination of angiotensin II (84), which is known to have a positive inotropic effect on the myocardium (85), a strong vasoconstrictor influence on the coronary arteries (86), and a facilitatory action on sympathetic neurotransmission (87), all of which are detrimental to the ischemic heart. However, the fact that part of the benefits of ACE inhibitors can be abolished by a bradykinin antagonist suggests that bradykinin also plays a major role in this process. Indeed, it was recently reported that infusion of the B2 antagonist NPC 349 in isolated hearts submitted to ischemia and reperfusion could abolish the beneficial effects of the ACE inhibitor ramipril (88). This corroborated the earlier finding by the same team that perfusion with bradykinin in this model had reduced the postischemic reperfusion arrythmias (89).

On the other hand, bradykinin may also exert a detrimental effect on the ischemic heart, either directly or via stimulation of sympathoadrenal neurons. Direct application of bradykinin in the epicardium has a direct vasopressor effect, although this effect is attenuated during ischemia (90). Bradykinin is known to stimulate sympathetic nerve terminals, resulting in rise of blood pressure and acceleration of heart rate (91,92), both of which are reversible by α- and β-adrenergic blockade. However, they could also be prevented by prior application of the local anesthetic lidocaine, suggesting that they may be partially reflex in nature in response to local pain elicited by stimulation by bradykinin of cardiac sensory nerve fibers. Therefore, the well-known nociceptive action of bradykinin may contribute significantly to the pain of myocardial ischemia; consequently, via this action as well as via its action on sympathetic neurons, bradykinin may indirectly cause a vasopressor and arrythmogenic effect, even though its direct local effects are mostly vasodepressor and antiarrythmic. It has repeatedly been demonstrated that B2 but not B1 antagonists have an antinociceptive effect (93-96). Accordingly, it would be difficult to speculate at this point what might be the overall cardiac effect of a B2 bradykinin antagonist in vivo. Unlike the isolated perfused heart model used in the studies mentioned above (88,89), in the live animal, the bradykinin antagonist would also affect the modulatory action of bradykinin on sympathetic neurons and on the synthesis of other vasoactive local hormones (97). The final result would be the sum of these interactions, where either the beneficial or the detrimental effects might prevail.

One aspect of bradykinin function that has not yet been investigated with the use of antagonists, but may be especially relevant to the preservation of ischemic myocardium, is the influence of bradykinin on glucose metabolism. Bradykinin not only increases the supply of substrate to the affected tissues through vasodilation and augmented blood perfusion, but it also improves utilization of the nutrient because it stimulates glucose uptake and metabolism via its potentiation of insulin action (98,99). Indeed, the reported beneficial effects of ACE inhibition on the insulin resistance of non-insulin-dependent diabetes mellitus and even on the insulin resistance of essential hypertension without overt diabetes (100-103) is probably attributable to the potentiation of all of bradykinin's effects, including the metabolic ones. The effect of bradykinin antagonists on this function would greatly help clarify the implications of bradykinin stimulation under ischemic conditions in cardiovascular tissues.

In summary, the use of bradykinin analogs with different patterns of antagonistic and partial agonistic activities for different tissues has already helped elucidate some of bradykinin's effects on the heart and the regulation of systemic or regional organ circulation under various conditions of health and disease. It has demonstrated the participation of bradykinin in normal blood pressure maintenance; its interaction with local vasoactive hormones and neurotransmitters, including endothelium-derived relaxing factor, prostaglandins, catecholamines, serotonin, and others; its contribution to the antihypertensive and cardioprotective effects of ACE inhibition; and its possible role in the development and maintenance of certain types of experimental hypertension, especially those induced or aggravated by salt excess. Much remains to be done to further define the vasoregulatory, neural, and metabolic effects of bradykinin and its inhibition under various conditions. Development of new, more potent bradykinin analogs with selective effects on specific vascular, neural, humoral, or metabolic actions of bradykinin promises to yield not only invaluable pharmacological tools for research but potentially useful therapeutic agents as well.

ACKNOWLEDGMENTS

This work was supported in part by NIH grant HL-18318 and by a grant from the Thomas A. Pappas Foundation.

REFERENCES

1. Rocha e Silva, M., W. T. Beraldo, and G. Rosenfeld. Bradykinin: A hypotensive and smooth muscle stimulating factor released from plasma globulin by snake venom and by trypsin. *Am. J. Physiol.* **156**:261 (1949).
2. Yang, H. Y. T., E. G. Erdos, and Y. Levin. A dipeptidyl carboxypeptidase that converts angiotensin I and inactivates bradykinin. *Biochem. Biophys. Acta* **214**:374-376 (1970).
3. Krieger, E. M., H. C. Salgado, C. J. Assan, L. L. J. Greene, and S. H. Ferreira. Potential screening test for detection of overactivity of renin-angiotensin system. *Lancet* **1**:269-271 (1971).
4. McGiff, J. C., and A. Nasjletti. Kenins, renal function, and blood pressure regulation. Introduction. *Fed. Proc.* **35**:172-174 (1976).
5. McGiff, J. C., H. D. Itskovitz, A. Terragno, and P. Y. K. Wong. Modulation and mediation of the action of the renal kallikrein-kinin system by prostaglandins. *Fed. Proc.* **35**:175-180 (1976).
6. Nasjletti, A., and J. Colina-Chourio. Interaction of mineralocorticoids, renal prostaglandins, and the renal kallikrein-kinin system. *Fed. Proc.* **35**:189-193 (1976).
7. Nasjletti, A., and K. U. Malik. Minireview: Relationships between the kallikrein-kinin and prostaglandin systems. *Life Sci.* **25**:99-110 (1979).
8. Carretero, O. A., N. B. Oza, A. G. Scicli, and A. Schork. Renal tissue kallikrein plasma renin, and plasma aldosterone in renal hypertension. *Acta Physiol. Lat. Am.* **24**:448-452 (1974).
9. Ward, P. E., and H. S. Margolius. Renal and urinary kallikreins, in: *Bradykinin, Kallidin, and Kallikrein* (E. G. Erdos, ed.). Springer-Verlag, New York, pp. 525-548 (1979).

10. Roman, R. J., M. L. Kaldunski, D. L. Mattson, M. Mistry, and A. Nasjletti. Influence of eicosanoids on renal function of DOCA-Salt hypertensive rats. *Hypertension* **12**:287-294 (1988).
11. Mills, I. H. Renal kallikrein and regulation of blood pressure in man, in: *Bradykinin, Kallidin, and Kallikrein* (E. G. Erdos, ed.). Springer-Verlag, New York, pp. 549-567 (1979).
12. Romero, J. C., C. L. Dunlop, and C. G. Strong. The effect of indomethacin and other anti-inflammatory drugs on the renin-angiotensin system. *J. Clin. Invest.* **58**:282-288 (1976).
13. Carretero, O. A., S. Miyazaki, and A. G. Scicli. Role of kinins in the acute antihypertensive effect of the converting enzyme inhibitor captopril. *Hypertension* **3**:18-22 (1981).
14. Vavrek, R. J., and J. M. Stewart. Competitive antagonists of bradykinin. *Peptides* **6**:161-164 (1985).
15. Stewart, J. M., and R. J. Vavrek. Bradykinin competitive antagonists for classical kinin systems, in: *Kinins IV* (L. M. Greenbaum and J. S. Margolius, eds.). Plenum Press, New York, pp. 537-547 (1986).
16. Regoli, D. Kinins, receptors, antagonists. *Adv. Exp. Med. Biol.* **198**:549-558 (1986).
17. Palmer, R. M., A. G. Ferrige, and S. Moncada. Nitric oxide release accounts for the biological activity of endothelium-derived relaxing factor. *Nature* **327**: 524-526 (1987).
18. Toda, N., K. Bian, T. Akiba, and T. Okamura. Heterogeneity in mechanisms of bradykinin action in canine isolated blood vessels. *Eur. J. Pharmacol.* **135**:321-329 (1987).
19. Jackson, T. R., T. J. Hallam, C. P. Downes, and M. R. Hanley. Receptor coupled events in bradykinin action: Rapid production of inositol phosphates and regulation of cytosolic free Ca^{2+} in a neural cell line. *EMBO J.* **6**:49-54 (1987).
20. Gadd, A. L., and K. Bhoola. Activation by bradykinin and vasoactive intestinal peptide of adenylate cyclase from immunologically sensitized lung membranes. *Adv. Exp. Med. Biol.* **198**:577-583 (1986).
21. Cooper, C. L., and K. U. Malik. Evidence that bradykinin stimulates renal prostaglandin synthesis by a mechanism distinct from that of other vasoactive substances. *Circ. Res.* **60**:914-922 (1987).
22. Sung, C. P., A. J. Arleth, K. Shikano, and B. A. Berkowitz. Characterization and function of bradykinin receptors in vascular endothelial cells. *J. Pharmacol. Exp. Ther.* **247**:8-13 (1988).
23. Loeb, A. L., N. J. Izzo, Jr., R. M. Johnson, J. C. Garrison, and M. J. Peach. Endothelium-derived relaxing factor release associated with increased endothelial cell inositol trisphosphate and intracellular calcium. *Am. J. Cardiol.* **62**:36G-40G (1988).
24. Conklin, B. R., R. M. Burch, L. R. Steranka, and J. Axelrod. Distinct bradykinin receptors mediate stimulation of prostaglandin synthesis by endothelial cells and fibroblasts. *J. Pharmacol. Exp. Ther.* **244**:646-649 (1988).

25. Regoli, D., N. E. Rhaleb, G. Drapeau, S. Dion, C. Tousignant, P. D'Orleans-Juste, and P. Devillier. Basic pharmacology of kinins: Pharmacologic receptors and other mechanisms. in: *Kinins V* (K. Abe, H. Moriya, and S. Fuji, eds.). Plenum Press, New York, pp. 398-407 (1989).
26. Stewart, J. M., and R. J. Vavrek. Bradykinin competitive antagonists for classical kinin systems. *Adv. Exp. Med. Biol.* **198** pt A:537-542 (1986).
27. Vavrek, R. J., and J. M. Stewart. Smooth muscle selectivity in bradykinin analogs with multiple D-amino acid substitutions. *Adv. Exp. Med. Biol.* **198** Pt A:543-547 (1986).
28. Francel, P. C., J. F. Keefer, and G. Dawson. Bradykinin analogs antagonize bradykinin-induced second messenger production in a sensory neuron cell line. *Mol. Pharmacol.* **35**:34-38 (1989).
29. Beierwaltes, W. H., O. A. Carretero, A. G. Scicli, R. J. Vavrek, and J. M. Stewart. Competitive analog antagonists of bradykinin in the canine hindlimb. *Proc. Soc. Exp. Biol. Med.* **186**:79-83 (1987).
30. Mulinari, R., A. Benetos, I. Gavras, and H. Gavras. Vascular and sympathoadrenal responses to bradykinin and a bradykinin analogue. *Hypertension* **11**:754-757 (1988).
31. Griesbacher, T., F. Lembeck, and A. Saris. Effects of the bradykinin antagonist B4310 on smooth muscles and blood pressure in the rat, and its enzymatic degradation. *Br. J. Pharmacol.* **96**:531-538 (1989).
32. Carretero, O. A., and A. G. Scicli. Kinins as regulators of blood flow and blood pressure, in: *Hypertension: Pathophysiology, Diagnosis and Management* (J. H. Laragh and B. M. Brenner, eds.). Raven Press, New York, pp. 805-817 (1990).
33. Biollaz, J., H. R. Brunner, I. Gavras, B. Waeber, and H. Gavras. Antihypertensive therapy with MK-421: Angiotensin II-renin relationships to evaluate efficacy of converting enzyme blockade. *J. Cardiovasc. Pharmacol.* **4**:966-972 (1982).
34. Swartz, S. L., G. H. William, N. K. Hollenberg, T. J. Moore, and R. G. Dluhy. Converting enzyme inhibition in essential hypertension: The hypotensive response does not reflect only angiotensin II formation. *Hypertension* **1**:106-111 (1979).
35. Crantz, F. R., S. L. Swartz, N. K. Hollenberg, T. J. Moore, R. G. Dluhy, and G. H. Williams. Differences in response to peptidyldipeptide hydrolase inhibitors SR20881 and SQ14225 in normal-renin essential hypertension. *Hypertension* **2**:604-609 (1980).
36. Johnston, C. I., B. P. McGrath, J. A. Millar, and P. G. Matthews. Long term effect of captopril (SQ14225) on blood pressure and hormone levels in essential hypertension. *Lancet* **2**:493-495 (1979).
37. Rasmussen, S., A. Leth, H. Ibsen, M. Damkjaer Nielsen, F. Nielsen, and J. Giese. Converting enzyme inhibition in mild and moderate essential hypertension. II. *Acta Med. Scand.* **219**:29-36 (1986).
38. Zussman, R. M. Effects of converting-enzyme inhibitors on the renin-angiotensin-aldosterone, bradykinin, and arachidonic acid-prostaglandin systems:

Correlation of chemical structure and biologic activity. *Am. J. Kidney Dis.* **10**(1 Suppl 1):13-23 (1987).
39. Benetos, A., I. Gavras, and H. Gavras. Hypertensive effect of a bradykinin antagonist in normotensive rats. *Hypertension* **8**:1089-1092 (1986).
40. Carbonell, L. F., O. A. Carretero, J. M. Stewart, and A. G. Scicli. Effect of a kinin antagonist on the acute antihypertensive activity of enalaprilat in severe hypertension. *Hypertension* **11**:239-243 (1988).
41. Benetos, A., H. Gavras, J. M. Stewart, R. J. Vavrek, S. Hatinoglou, and I. Gavras. Vasodepressor role of endogenous bradykinin assessed by a bradykinin antagonist. *Hypertension* **8**:971-974 (1986).
42. Gavras, H., A. Benetos, and I. Gavras. Contribution of bradykinin to maintenance of normal blood pressure. *Hypertension* **9** (Suppl. III):III-147-III-149 (1987).
43. Seino, M., K. Abe, N. Nushiro, K. Omata, Y. Kasai, and K. Yoshinaga. Effects of a competitive antagonist of bradykinin on blood pressure and renal blood flow in anaesthetized rats. *J. Hypertension* **6**:867-871 (1988).
44. Aubert, J. F., B. Waeber, J. Nussberger, R. Vavrek, J. M. Stewart, and H. R. Brunner. Influence of endogenous bradykinin on acute blood pressure response to vasopressors in normotensive rats assessed with a bradykinin antagonist. *J. Cardiovasc. Pharmacol.* **11**:51-55 (1988).
45. Waeber, B., J. F. Aubert, J. Nussberger, R. Vavrek, J. M. Stewart, and H. R. Brunner. Influence of bradykinin on blood pressure regulation of spontaneously hypertensive rats maintained on different sodium intakes. *Clin. Exp. Pharmacol. Physiol.* **14**:659-664 (1987).
46. Seino, M., K. Abe, N. Nushiro, K. Omata, Y. Kasai, and K. Yoshinaga. Contribution of bradykinin to maintenance of blood pressure and renal blood flow in anaesthetized spontaneously hypertensive rats. *J. Hypertens. Suppl.* **6**:8401-8403 (1988).
47. Nakagawa, M., and A. Nasjletti. Plasma kinin concentration in deoxycorticosterone-salt hypertension. *Hypertension* **11**:411-415 (1988).
48. Beierwaltes, W. H., O. A. Carretero, and A. G. Scicli. Renal hemodynamics in response to a kinin analogue antagonist. *Am. J. Physiol.* **255**:F408-414 (1988).
49. Wang, Y-X., B. Lammek, M. Brasnahan, I. Gavras, and H. Gavras. Systemic and regional hemodynamic effects of a bradykinin antagonist in normal conscious rats. (Abstract) 13th Congress of the ISH, Montreal, 1990.
50. Liang, C., H. Gavras, and W. B. Hood, Jr. Renin-angiotensin system inhibition in conscious sodium-depleted dogs: Effects on systemic and coronary hemodynamics. *J. Clin. Invest.* **61**:874-883 (1978).
51. Gavras, H., C. Liang, and H. R. Brunner. Redistribution of regional blood flow after inhibition of the angiotensin converting enzyme. *Cir. Res.* **43** (Suppl 1):59-63, 1978.
52. Mulinari, R., I. Gavras, R. Franco, and H. Gavras. Bradykinin antagonism and prostaglandins in blood pressure regulation. *Hypertension* **13**:960-963 (1989).

53. Carbonell, L. F., O. A. Carretero, P. Madeddu, and A. G. Scicli. Effects of a kinin antagonist on mean blood pressure. *Hypertension* **11**:184-188 (1988).
54. Beierwaltes, W. H., and O. A. Carretero. Kinin antagonist reverses converting enzyme inhibitor-stimulated vascular prostaglandin I_2 synthesis. *Hypertension* **13**:754-758 (1989).
55. Wilson, D. D., L. de Garavilla, W. Kuhn, J. Togo, R. M. Burch, and L. R. Steranka. D-Arg-[Hyp3-D-Phe7]-bradykinin, a bradykinin antagonist, reduces mortality in a rat model of endotoxic shock. *Cir. Shock* **27**:93-101 (1989).
56. Weipert, J., H. Hoffman, M. Siebeck, and E. T. Whalley. Attenuation of arterial blood pressure fall in endotoxin shock in the rat using the competitive bradykinin antagonist Lys-Lys-[Hyp2, Thi5,8, DPhe7]-BK (B4148). *Br. J. Pharmacol.* **94**:282-284 (1988).
57. Weipert, J., H. Hoffman, M. Siebeck, and E. T. Whalley. Endotoxin shock in the rat: Reduction of arterial blood pressure fall by the bradykinin antagonist B4148. *Prog. Clin. Biol. Res.* **308**:983-387 (1989).
58. Regoli, D., F. Marceau, and J. Lavigne. Induction of B_1-receptors for kinins in the rabbit by a bacterial lipopolysaccharide. *Eur. J. Pharmacol.* **71**:105-115 (1981).
59. Miyamori, I., Y. Takeda, H. Koshida, M. Ikeda, S. Yasuhara, K. Nagai, T. Morise, H. Takimoto, and R. Takeda. Role of bradykinin for orthostatic hypotension in diabetes mellitus. *Exp. Clin. Endocrinol.* **87**:169-175 (1986).
60. Correa, F. M. A., and F. G. Graef. Central mechanism of the hypertensive action of intraventricular bradykinin in the unanesthetized rat. *Neuropharmacology* **13**:65-75 (1974).
61. Correa, F. M., J. Ueta, and I. R. Pel'a. Central adrenergic mediation of the cardiovascular effect of intraventricular bradykinin. *Naunyn Schmiedebergs Arch. Pharmacol.* **333**:139-142 (1986).
62. Lindsey, C. J., K. Fujita, and T. O. Martins. The central pressor effect of bradykinin in normotensive and hypertensive rats. *Hypertension* **11**:1126-1129 (1988).
63. Lindsey, C. J., C. R. Nakaie, and D. T. Martins. Central nervous system kinin receptors and the hypertensive response mediated by bradykinin. *Br. J. Pharmacol.* **97**:783-788 (1989).
64. Yang, X. P., O. A. Carretero, M. Akahoski, and A. G. Scicli. Effects on blood pressure on intracerebroventricular administration of a kinin antagonist, in: *Kinins V* (K. Abe, H. Moriya, and S. Fuji, eds.). Plenum Press, New York, pp. 439-445 (1989).
65. Franco, R., I. Gavras, Y-X. Wang, R. Mulinari, and H. Gavras. Comparative effects of intracerebroventricular microinjection of bradykinin and analogues in normal rats (submitted).
66. Brooks, D. P., L. Share, J. T. Crofton, and A. Nasjletti. Interrelationship between central bradykinin and vasopressin in conscious rats. *Brain Res.* **371**:42-48 (1986).

67. Pirola, C. J., A. Scheucher, M. S. Balda, S. M. Dabsys, S. Finkielman, and V. E. Nahmod. Serotonin mediates cardiovascular responses to acetylcholine, bradykinin, angiotensin II and norepinephrine in the lateral septal area of the rat brain. *Neuropharmacology* **26**:561-566 (1987).
68. Bhattacharya, S. K., P. J. Rao, S. J. Brumleve, and S. S. Parmar. Effects of intracerebroventricular administration of bradykinin on rat brain serotonin and prostaglandins. *Res. Commun. Chem. Pathol. Pharmacol.* **54**: 355-366 (1986).
69. Rao, P. J., and S. K. Bhattacharya. Hyperthermic effect of centrally administered bradykinin in the rat: Role of prostaglandins and serotonin. *Int. J. Hyperthermia* **4**:183-189 (1988).
70. Nakano, J. Effects of bradykinin, eledoisin, and physalaemin on cardiovascular dynamics. *Adv. in Exp. Med. Biol.* **8**:157-170 (1970).
71. Needleman, P. The synthesis and function of prostaglandins in the heart. *Fed. Proc.* **35**:2376-2381 (1976).
72. Toda, N., K. Bian, T. Akiba, and T. Okamura. Heterogeneity in mechanisms of bradykinin action in canine isolated blood vessels. *Eur. J. Pharmacol.* **135**:321-329 (1987).
73. Kimura, E., K. Hashimoto, S. Furukawa, and H. Hayakawa. Changes in bradykinin level in coronary sinus blood after the experimental occlusion of a coronary artery. *Am. Heart J.* **85**:635-647 (1973).
74. Hashimoto, K., H. Hamamoto, Y. Honda, M. Hirose, S. Furukawa, and E. Kimura. Changes in components of kinin system and hemodynamics in acute myocardial infarction. *Am. Heart J.* **95**:619-626 (1978).
75. Förstermann, U., A. Mügge, U. Alheid, A. Haverich, and J. C. Frölich. Selective attenuation of endothelium-mediated vasodilation in atherosclerotic human coronary arteries. *Cir. Res.* **62**:185-190 (1988).
76. Sneddon, J. M., and J. R. Vane. Endothelium-derived relaxing factor reduces platelet adhesion to bovine endothelial cells. *Proc. Natl. Acad. Sci. USA* **85**:2800-2804 (1988).
77. Hashimoto, K., J. Wanka, R. N. Kohn, H. J. Wilkens, R. Steger, and N. Back. The vasopeptide kinin system in acute clinical cardiac diseases. *Adv. Exp. Med. Biol.* **70**:245-259 (1976).
78. Van Gilst, W. H., P. A. De Graeff, J. H. Kingma, H. Wesseling, and C. D. J. DeLanges. Captopril reduces purine loss and reperfusion arrhythmias in the rat heart after coronary artery occlusion. *Eur. J. Pharmacol.* **100**:113-117 (1984).
79. Linz, W., B. A. Schoelkens, and Han Yi-Fan. Beneficial effects of the converting enzyme inhibitor ramipril in ischemic hearts. *J. Hypertension* **8**(Suppl 10):S91-S99 (1986).
80. Li, K., and X. Chen. Protective effects of captopril and enalapril on myocardial ischemia and reperfusion damage of rat. *J. Mol. Cell Cardiol.* **19**: 909-915 (1987).
81. Westlin, W., and K. Mullane. Does captopril attenuate reperfusion-induced myocardial dysfunction by scavenging free radicals? *Circulation* **77** (Suppl 1):30-39 (1988).

82. Pfeffer, M. A., J. M. Pfeffer, C. Steinburg, and P. Finn. Survival after an experimental myocardial infarction: beneficial effects of long-term therapy with captopril. *Circulation* **72**:406-412 (1985).
83. Pfeffer, M. A., G. A. Lamas, D. E. Vaughn, A. F. Parisi, and E. Braunwald. Effect of captopril on progressive ventricular dilatation after anterior myocardial infarction. *New Engl. J. Med.* **319**:80-86 (1988).
84. Gavras, H. The place of angiotensin-converting enzyme inhibition in the treatment of cardiovascular diseases. *New Engl. J. Med.* **319**:1541-1543 (1988).
85. Bonnardeaux, J. L., and D. Regoli. Action of angiotensin and analogues on the heart. *Can. J. Physiol. Pharmacol.* **52**:50-60 (1974).
86. Britton, S., and J. DiSalvo. Effects of angiotensin I and II on hindlimb and coronary vascular resistance. *Am. J. Physiol.* **225**:1226-1231 (1973).
87. Malik, K. U., and A. Nasjletti. Facilitation of adrenergic transmitter by locally generated AII in rat mesenteric arteries. *Cir. Res.* **38**:26-30 (1975).
88. Schölkens, B. A., W. Linz, and W. König. Effects of the angiotensin converting enzyme inhibitor, ramipril, in isolated ischaemic rat heart are abolished by a bradykinin antagonist. *J. Hypertension* 6(Suppl 4):S25-S28 (1988).
89. Linz, W., and B. A. Schölkens. Influence of local converting enzyme inhibition on angiotensin and bradykinin effects in ischemic rat hearts. *J. Cardiovasc. Pharmacol.* (10 Suppl) **7**:S75-82 (1987).
90. Inoue, H., B. T. Skale, and D. P. Zipes. Effects of ischemia on cardiac afferent sympathetic and vagal reflexes in dog. *Am. J. Physiol.* **255**:H26-35 (1988).
91. Staszewska-Barczak, J., and G. J. Dusting. Sympathetic cardiovascular reflex initiated by bradykinin-induced stimulation of cardiac pain receptors in the dog. *Clin. Exp. Pharmacol. Physiol.* **4**:443-452 (1977).
92. Rioux, F., H. Bachelard, S. St-Pierre, and J. Barabé. Epicardial application of bradykinin elicits pressor effects and tachycardia in guinea pigs. Possible mechanisms. *Peptides* **8**:863-868 (1987).
93. Whalley, E. T., S. Clegg, J. M. Stewart, and R. J. Vavrek. The effect of kinin agonists and antagonists on the pain response of the human blister base. *Naunyn Schmiedebergs Arch. Pharmacol.* **336**:652-655 (1987).
94. Laneuville, O., and R. Couture. Bradykinin analogue blocks bradykinin-induced inhibition of a spinal nociceptive reflex in the rat. *Eur. J. Pharmacol.* **137**:281-285 (1987).
95. Steranka, L. R., C. J. DeHaas, R. J. Vavrek, J. M. Stewart, S. J. Enna, and S. H. Snyder. Antinociceptive effects of bradykinin antagonists. *Eur. J. Pharmacol.* **136**:261-262 (1987).
96. Steranka, L. R., D. C. Manning, C. J. DeHaas, J. W. Ferkany, S. A. Borosky, J. R. Connor, R. J. Vavrek, J. M. Stewart, and S. H. Snyder. Bradykinin as a pain mediator: Receptors are localized to sensory neurons, and antagonists have analgesic actions. *Proc. Natl. Acad. Sci. USA* **85**:3245-3249 (1988).

97. Beierwaltes, W. H., and O. A. Carretero. Kinin antagonist reverses converting enzyme inhibitor-stimulated vascular prostaglandin I_2 synthesis. *Hypertension* **13**:754-758 (1989).
98. Jaffa, A. A., J. Pratt, A. Ashford, and G. S. Bailey. Studies of the effects of insulin, bradykinin, and captopril on blood glucose levels of alloxan-diabetic rats. *Adv. Exp. Med. Biol.* **198** Pt B:373-378 (1986).
99. Goldman, J., D. Pfister, and R. Vukmirovich. Potentiation of insulin stimulation of hexose transport by kallikrein and bradykinin in isolated rat adipocytes. *Mol. Cell Endocrinol.* **50**:183-191 (1987).
100. Rett, K., K. W. Jauch, M. Wicklmayr, G. Dietze, E. Fink, and H. Mehnert. Angiotensin converting enzyme inhibitors in diabetes: Experimental and human experience. *Postgrad. Med. J.* **62** (Suppl 1):59-64 (1986).
101. Ferrannini, E., G. Buzzioli, R. Bonadonna, M. A. Giordino, M. Oleggin, L. Graziadei, R. Pedrinelli, L. Brandi, and S. Bevilagna. Insulin resistance in essential hypertension. *New Engl. J. Med.* **317**:350-357 (1987).
102. Pollare, T., H. Lithell, and C. Berne. A Comparison of the effects of hydrochlorothiazide and captopril on glucose and lipid metabolism in patients with hypertension. *New Engl. J. Med.* **321**:868-873 (1989).
103. Rett, K., K. W. Jauch, M. Wicklmayr, E. Fink, G. J. Dietze, and H. Mehnert. Increased insulin-responsiveness by ACE-inhibition in non-insulin dependent diabetes mellitus, in: *Kinins V* (K. Abe, H. Moriya, and S. Fuji, eds.). Plenum Press, New York, pp. 207-213 (1989).

8

Bradykinin Antagonists in Pain and Inflammation

Larry R. Steranka and Ronald M. Burch
Nova Pharmaceutical Corporation
Baltimore, Maryland

I. INTRODUCTION

In the first century A.D., Cornelius Celsus noted the cardinal signs of inflammation: *rubor, tumor, calor, and dolor* (redness, swelling, heat, and pain) (1). To this list was added *sensio lato* (loss of function) by Virchow (1), and to these can be added accumulation of leukocytes. Bradykinin has, from the beginning of its study, been implicated in the pathogenesis of inflammation. To be considered as an inflammatory mediator, levels of the substance in question should be elevated during the inflammatory response, administration of the substance itself must produce inflammation, whereas antagonists should be anti-inflammatory. Bradykinin elicits all the cardinal signs of inflammation, and bradykinin has been identified in inflammatory exudates. The availability of bradykinin antagonists is making testing of the third criterion possible. This chapter considers the effects of peptide bradykinin antagonists and certain kallikrein inhibitors on models of inflammation. Chapter 4 considers nonpeptide agents in pain and inflammation.

II. PAIN AND INFLAMMATORY HYPERALGESIA

Considerable evidence supports a role for bradykinin as a physiological mediator of pain. Bradykinin is a potent algesic agent (2). In man, bradykinin causes a burning, stinging pain after application to a blister base, as well as after intradermal, intraarterial, or intraperitoneal injection (3). In addition, bradykinin is present in damaged tissues at concentrations sufficient to cause pain (4).

Nociceptive neurotransmission involves small-diameter, poorly myelinated fibers with small cell bodies in the dorsal root ganglion, which terminate in the superficial layers of the dorsal spinal cord. Bradykinin receptors are selectively localized to sites involved in nociception: superficial layers of the spinal cord, thin unmyelinated fibers, and small neuronal cells in sensory ganglia (5). Bradykinin produces its algesic effects by stimulating these nociceptive afferent fibers (6-8).

There is also good evidence that bradykinin plays an important role in hyperalgesia. Hyperalgesia is the perceptual companion of inflammation, whether it is from infection, abrasion, or burn injury. Hyperalgesia is characterized by a decrease in pain threshold, an enhanced response to suprathreshold stimulation, and sometimes spontaneous pain. Using standard teased-fiber techniques to record from the radial nerves in anesthetized monkeys, Kahn et al. (6) reported a bradykinin-induced decrease in the heat threshold of and an increase in response to suprathreshold stimulation of A- and C-fiber nociceptive afferents sensitive to mechanical and heat stimulation. This sensitization parallels the changes in the responsiveness of nociceptors that follows burn injury (9), supporting a role for bradykinin in hyperalgesia.

A. Pain

1. Bradykinin-Induced Pain

When bradykinin is injected into the right common carotid artery of a conscious, freely moving rat, a stereotypic flexion of the right forelimb and dextrorotation of the head is produced. Both of these effects are blocked by opiate and nonopiate analgesic compounds (10), suggesting that the behavior is an algesic response. Further supporting this conjecture is the observation that intraarterial injection of bradykinin in human subjects elicits pain (11). In one study using the rat model (5), animals that exhibited stereotypic response after injection of bradykinin at 2 nmol/kg were injected 5 minutes later with the same dose of bradykinin, and a bradykinin antagonist at 1-100 times that dose. At the lowest dose, NPC 414,

NPC 566, and NPC 722 blocked the effects of bradykinin in all or most animals, whereas NPC 349 and NPC 567 were less effective, and NPC 573 was without effect. At a dose 10-fold higher than bradykinin, all antagonists except NPC 573 blocked the effect of bradykinin. Curiously, at the highest dose tested, NPC 414 became less effective, consistent with a weak bradykinin agonist-like effect.

In more quantitative studies using the same model, K_b values were determined for inhibition of the bradykinin-induced response (12). Using a protocol similar to that described above, but with dose-percent responding curves being generated to bradykinin at each dose of antagonist, K_b values of 6.7 and 7.2 were determined for NPC 567 and NPC 414, respectively. In neither these experiments nor those described above did the response to bradykinin change with subsequent challenges. In a series of animals in which dose-response curves were obtained, when saline substituted for the antagonist on the subsequent trial, the second EC_{50}/first EC_{50} ratio was 1.1:1.

Another algesic model consists of a rabbit ear prepared such that it remains in contact with the head only by the intact auricular nerve. Injection of bradykinin or acetylcholine into the circulation of the ear elicits a reflex fall in systemic blood pressure, which is used as a quantitative index of the intensity of nociceptor stimulation in the ear. Using this model, Griesbacher and Lembeck (13) measured the reflex fall in blood pressure before, during, and after infusion of NPC 415. NPC 415 caused rightward, parallel shifts in the bradykinin dose-response curve of 8.7-fold and 26.4-fold when 50 nmol and 500 nmol of NPC 415 were infused, respectively. If bradykinin was injected 15 minutes after termination of infusion of NPC 415, the dose-response curves were shifted back to the left. Injection of acetylcholine also caused dose-dependent decreases in blood pressure, but this was unaffected by NPC 415.

Intraperitoneal injection of bradykinin (0.5 mg/kg) does not induce writhing in mice (14). However, if mice are pretreated with PGE_2 (1 mg/kg i.p.), which by itself is without effect, then bradykinin induces writhing. Morphine completely blocked bradykinin-induced writhing, consistent with writhing being a response to pain. At concentrations up to 25 mg/kg, the B1 agonist, desArg^9-BK, did not induce writhing. Consistent with the lack of activity of a B1 agonist, the B1 antagonist desArg^9[Leu^8]-BK did not inhibit bradykinin-induced writhing. However, several DPhe^7-BK antagonists inhibited bradykinin-induced writhing; IC_{50}s were 0.10, 0.45, 0.60, 6, and >10 mg/kg for NPC 567, NPC 568, NPC 349, NPC 361, and NPC 394. None of the D-Phe^7 antagonists displayed agonist activity.

2. Chemical and Mechanical Nociception

In another writhing assay, kaolin was used (15). Kaolin activates factor XII, leading to bradykinin formation. Each mouse was injected intraperitoneally with kaolin, then writhes were counted for 10 minutes. Soybean trypsin inhibitor (SBTI) was used to inhibit kallikrein and block kinin formation. At a concentration of 25 mg/kg i.p., SBTI completely blocked kaolin induced writhing. Conversely, captopril, which blocks kinin degradation by kininase II, increased the number of writhes in response to kaolin.

Acetic acid-induced writhing is a standard test for pain perception in which opiates as well as nonopiate analgesics exert antinociceptive effects. When injected intraperitoneally with acetic acid, NPC 567 and NPC 349 were found to inhibit writhing (16).

In another study, recordings were made from single neurons in the dorsal horn of the spinal cord at L1-L3. When formalin was injected into the hind toe or foot, a two-phase response was apparent (17). No treatment affected the first phase. However, NPC 349 blocked the second phase. Further, repeated injection of bradykinin desensitized the ability of formalin to induce the second phase. The receptor mediating nociception was of the B2 subtype since desArg^9[Leu^8]bradykinin was unable to antagonize formalin.

B. Hyperalgesia

1. Bradykinin-Induced Hyperalgesia

Bradykinin antagonists also inhibit bradykinin-induced hyperalgesia in the rat paw. Hyperalgesia was measured using a Randal-Sellito apparatus to measure mechanical pain threshold (5,16). Intradermal injection of 2 nmol bradykinin into the dorsum of the paw caused about a 50% decrease in pressure threshold, which was maximal between 5 and 15 minutes after injection, and gradually dissipated over the course of an hour. In independent experiments, animals were injected with 2 nmol bradykinin, 2 or 20 nmol of a bradykinin antagonist, or both bradykinin and an antagonist. Pain threshold was measured 5 minutes after injection. Both NPC 567 and NPC 349 blocked the hyperalgesic effect of bradykinin.

2. Inflammatory Hyperalgesia

To evaluate the potential role of bradykinin in the pain elicited by an inflammatory stimulus, hyperalgesia was elicited with the injection of urate crystals into the hind paws of rats (5,16). Urate crystals activate the kallikrein-kinin system in vitro (18), and in vivo induce an inflammatory process in which kinins are found in the exudate (19). Injection of sodium urate crystals into the dorsum of a hindpaw caused a marked decrease in the mechanical pain threshold 4 hours after injection. In some animals bradykinin antagonists were injected with the urate crystals, and mechanical pain threshold determined 4 hours later. NPC 349 completely blocked urate-induced hyperalgesia at a dose of 2 nmol/paw. NPC 567 also completely blocked the hyperalgesic response, but was less potent. NPC 414 and NPC 722 significantly inhibited hyperalgesia, but both agents appeared to be partial agonists. In clinical gout, urate crystals are present for a substantial time before analgesic therapy can commence. Accordingly, experiments were performed in which NPC 567 was administered 2 hours after sodium urate crystals. In this protocol NPC 567 was completely effective in blocking urate-induced hyperalgesia.

Carrageenan injection into rat hind paws increases local bradykinin synthesis (20,21, and see below) and causes hyperalgesia as well as inflammation (see below). Soybean trypsin inhibitor, at a concentration that inhibited plasma kallikrein, as well as the bradykinin antagonist NPC 567 blocked hyperalgesia in response to carrageenan (20,22).

C. Human Studies

A human experimental model of pain involves the verbal report of the degree of pain produced by the application of bradykinin to the exposed base of a blister. Using an exposed blister base model in human volunteers, Whalley and colleagues (23) reported significance antagonism of bradykinin-induced pain by NPC 349 at a concentration which did not affect pain induced by serotonin or potassium chloride. NPC 349 by itself did not elicit pain, even though it and other D-Phe^7-bradykinin antagonists have been reported to degranulate skin mast cells (24,25-27).

The kallikrein-kinin system is activated following burn injury (28). Thus, studies have been undertaken in human patients following superficial burn injury. NPC 567 is administered topically, and subjective pain is scored by the patient at various times afterward. Results from these studies should be available late in 1990.

III. INFLAMMATION

Bradykinin, when injected into the skin of experimental animals and human volunteers, elicits responses that mimic all the cardinal signs of inflammation, as well as accumulation of leukocytes (29). Further, myriad metabolic imbalances and minor trauma dramatically activate the cascade of events leading to formation of bradykinin, and all components of the system have been reported from inflammatory exudates (29). Thus, trauma, which exposes negatively charged collagen surfaces (30) or articular cartilage (31), or deposition of immune complexes, may serve to activate the contact system of coagulation and activate kallikrein, and urate crystals may activate the system directly (18), resulting in the formation of kinins.

Released kinins cause contraction of vascular endothelial cells to increase permeability, resulting in edema formation; they relax resistance vessels to increase blood flow while restricting venous outflow, resulting in further edema, as well as erythema and warmth. Extravasation of vascular fluid further activates the contact system and complement cascade, recruiting leukocytes to the site. Leukocytes contain kallikrein-like enzymes (32,33) and may contribute further to kinin accumulation.

Bradykinin does not elicit leukocyte chemotaxis in vitro (29,34). However, application of bradykinin in vivo leads to accumulation of leukocytes (35), an effect caused by increased adherence of the cells to the vascular endothelium (36). Necrotaxis of rat polymorphonuclear leukocytes was found to be inhibited by bradykinin (37), leading Marceau and colleagues (29) to speculate that kinins may recruit inflammatory cells by causing fixation of leukocytes at sites where they come into contact with kinins. The receptor mediating the adherence of polymorphonuclear leukocytes in vitro appear to be of the B2 subtype, since B1 agonists had little activity and B1 antagonists did not inhibit bradykinin's actions (37). Bradykinin also causes murine macrophages to become fixed to their substrate (38,39). Certain leukocytes also have kinin receptors that mediate release of cytokines that further increase inflammation (40). Finally, kinins released in the inflammatory lesion directly stimulate sensory neurons, resulting in pain, as discussed above, as well as releasing other inflammatory substances from the sensory terminals, including substance P (41).

The role of bradykinin in chronic inflammation has also been considered. Bradykinin has been demonstrated to be elevated, or substrate depleted, in several chronic inflammatory diseases, including rheumatoid arthritis (12,20,29). At least two classes of hypotheses may be formulated to account for a role for kinins in chronic inflammation. First, biologic expression of B1 receptors has been demonstrated to be induced in a variety of inflammatory diseases, especially in rabbits. This hypothesis is discussed in detail elsewhere in this book (Chapter 2).

The second hypothesis is based on the ability of bradykinin to interact with several other mediators to amplify inflammatory reactions. In this scenario, bradykinin receptors are not increased in number, instead, upregulation of signal transduction systems allows even very low concentrations of kinins to elicit large biological effects. Interactions can occur with a variety of other mediators, including the cytokines interleukin 1 (42,43) and tumor necrosis factor (44). The mechanism for the interactions have been examined in detail in a model system, the 3T3 fibroblast.

In 3T3 fibroblasts, bradykinin elicits PGE_2 synthesis (45). Bradykinin is potent, its EC_{50} for stimulation of PGE_2 synthesis being about 300 pM, and PGE_2 synthesis is increased about fourfold, from 100 to 400 pg/well. In these cells the bradykinin receptor is of the B2 subtype (46) and is coupled by means of a GTP binding regulatory protein to phospholipase A_2, which frees arachidonate for PGE_2 synthesis by cyclooxygenase and PGE isomerase (45). Incubation of the cells with interleukin 1 (42) or tumor necrosis factor (44) causes a rise in PGE_2 synthesis. In these cytokine-primed cells bradykinin-stimulated PGE_2 synthesis is greatly amplified, up to 40-fold (42,44). The amplification is not due to any change in bradykinin receptor number or affinity (42), being instead associated with increases in the coupling GTP-binding regulatory protein(s) and phospholipase A_2 and cyclooxygenase metabolic enzymes.

Amplification may be an important mechanism in maintaining chronic inflammation. We have speculated that a positive feedback loop may exist among the cells in a chronic inflammatory lesion (47) (Fig. 1). Cytokines are present in high concentration in inflammatory lesions such as rheumatic joints (48), where kinin production has also been shown to be elevated (49). Kinins may well be involved in mitogenesis (pannus formation), eicosanoid formation, and hyperalgesia. In addition, as mentioned above and in Section F, below, kinins may cause increased cytokine release, at least from murine macrophages, and cytokines increase activation of leukocytes and inflammatory fibroblast-like cells, probably leading to enhanced enzymatic conversion of kininogens to kinins. Kinins have also been found to stimulate mitogenesis of at least certain T lymphocytes (50,51), cells which also play important roles in chronic inflammation.

A. Vascular Permeability

Intradermal injection of bradykinin into animals and man results in increased vascular permeability to plasma fluid and proteins. Bradykinin-induced increases in vascular permeability appear to be mediated by B2 receptors. B1 agonists do not elicit increases in vascular permeability, and B1 antagonists do not block bradykinin-induced increases (29).

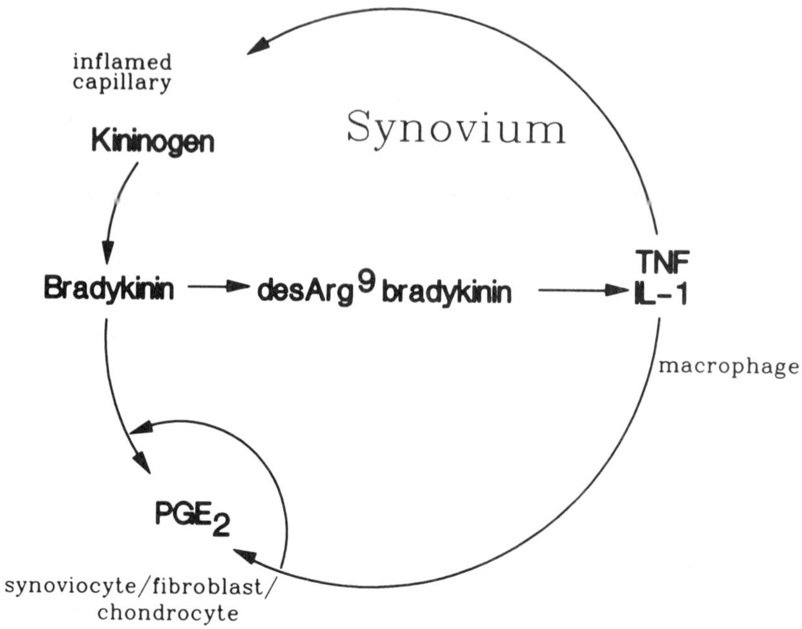

Figure 1 The role of kinins in chronic inflammation. Inflammation in the synovium, induced by acute mediators, increases vascular permeability, which activates kallikrein to release kinins. Kinins then bind to their receptors on macrophages, stimulating release of cytokines including interleukin 1 (IL-1) and tumor necrosis factor (TNF), which chronically inflame the tissue. In cytokine-primed tissues, bradykinin-induced prostaglandin synthesis is amplified, leading to enhanced chondrocyte and bone erosion. (Used with permission from Ref. 47, Birkhauser Verlag, Basel.)

In one study in rats, animals were pretreated with mepyramine and cimetidine (13). Bradykinin, a bradykinin antagonist, or a combination of the two, was injected intracutaneously, and dye leakage was measured 20 minutes later. All the bradykinin antagonists tested, NPC 431, NPC 394, NPC 413, NPC 349, NPC 414, and NPC 415, blocked bradykinin-induced plasma extravasation when 1.6 nmol bradykinin was administered with 20 or 60 nmol antagonist. NPC 415 was most potent, completely blocking bradykinin's effect when 20 nmol was coinjected. NPC 431 and NPC 394 were the weakest, achieving only modest blockade when coinjected at 60 nmol. NPC 413 and NPC 349 demonstrated weak agonist activity when injected by themselves at 60 nmol. However, both agents blocked bradykinin-induced extravasation.

In a study in untreated rabbits, similar results were reported (52). Thus, NPC 431, NPC 394, NPC 349, NPC 420, and NPC 419 all blocked bradykinin-induced plasma extravasation. However, when untreated rats received the same compounds, no blockade of bradykinin was observed, and NPC 349 augmented bradykinin-induced plasma extravasation. These findings were interpreted as evidence for species differences in cutaneous vascular bradykinin receptors (52).

Bradykinin and D-Phe[7]-substituted bradykinin analogs can release stored mast cell mediators by a non-receptor mediated mechanism (24-27). Since skin contains a high density of mast cells, and mast cell mediators can increase vascular permeability, it seemed likely that increased vascular permeability elicited by D-Phe[7]-substituted bradykinin analogs might well have been secondary to mast cell degranulation. To invstigate this possibility, NPC 567 was injected intradermally in untreated rats. NPC 567, in a dose-dependent fashion, increased vascular permeability (Fig. 2), similar to the effect previously reported (53). Similarly, NPC 567 increased vascular permeability in untreated mice (Fig. 3).

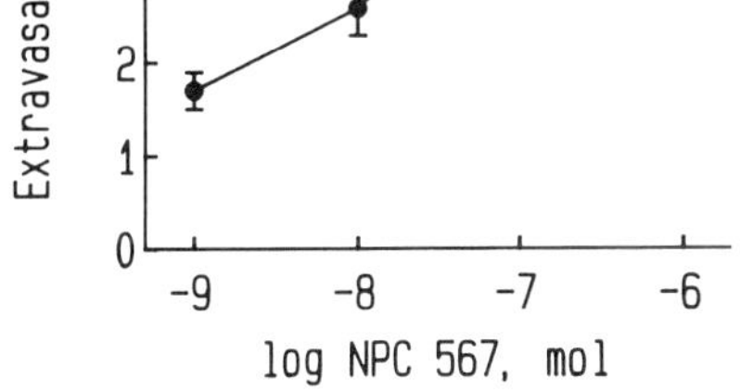

Figure 2 NPC 567 increases vascular permeability in rats. Evan's blue dye (10 mg/kg i.v.) was injected intradermally with 10 μl saline or NPC 567. After 20 minutes, animals were sacrificed and the diameter of dye extravasation around each site was measured with calipers on the inside surface of the skin. Each rat was injected in triplicate with each dose, and the results expressed as mean $\pm$ SEM.

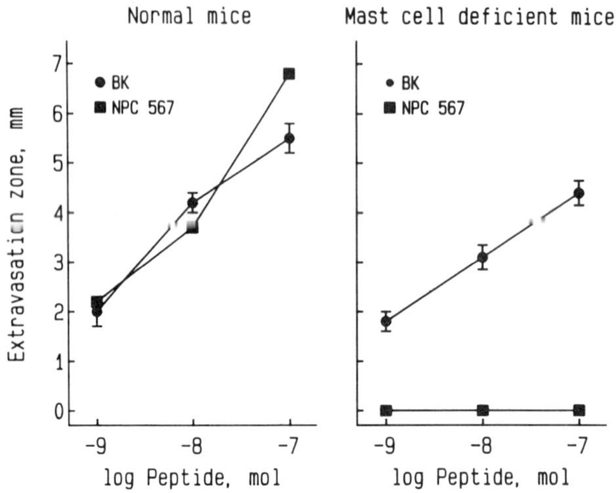

Figure 3 NPC 567 does not increase vascular permeability in mast cell-deficient mice. Mast cell-deficient mice (WBB6F1/J/W/W^v) and normal mice (CF-1) were injected intradermally with NPC 567 or bradykinin (10 μl). Each mouse received only a single injection. After 20 minutes, skin was prepared as in Figure 1 and dye leakage quantitated. Each point represents mean ± SEM from 4 animals.

However, when NPC 567 was administered to mast cell-deficient mice (WBB6F1/J/W/W^v), no increase in vascular permeability was observed (Fig. 3). In contrast, bradykinin caused increased vascular permeability in normal and mast cell-deficient mice (Fig. 3). The mast cell-deficient mice also exhibit other abnormalities in blood formed elements and plasma proteins, so lack of effect in these animals, while intriguing, did not prove participation of mast cell products. Thus, pharmacological inhibition of mast cell mediators was attempted in rats.

Rats were pretreated with cyproheptadine 20 minutes prior to administration of bradykinin at a dose (30 mg/kg i.p.) that blocked histamine and serotonin-induced plasma extravasation. Cyproheptadine only slightly affected bradykinin-induced plasma extravasation, but it nearly completely blocked NPC 567-induced plasma extravasation (Fig. 4). In cyproheptadine-pretreated rats, NPC 567 blocked bradykinin-elicited plasma extravasation (Fig. 5) at dose ratios of NPC 567:bradykinin of 100:1 and 10:1, but not 1:1.

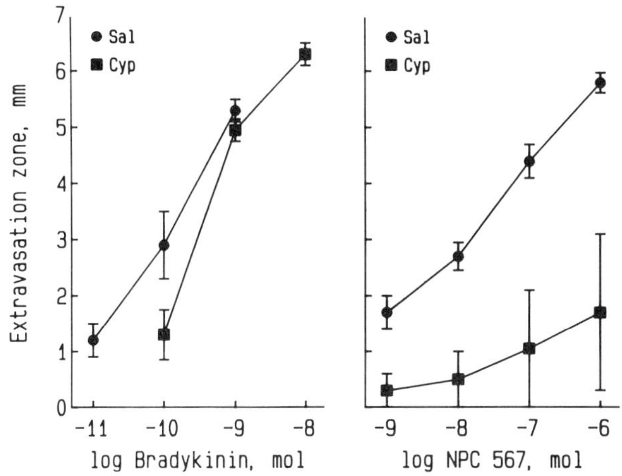

Figure 4 Cyproheptadine inhibits NPC 567-induced vascular leak, but not bradykinin-induced leak, in rats. Animals were injected intraperitoneally with saline or cyproheptadine, 10 mg/ml, 20 minutes prior to intradermal saline, bradykinin, or NPC 567. After 20 minutes, skin was processed as in Figure 1 and dye leakage quantitated. Each point represents mean ± SEM from 4-7 animals.

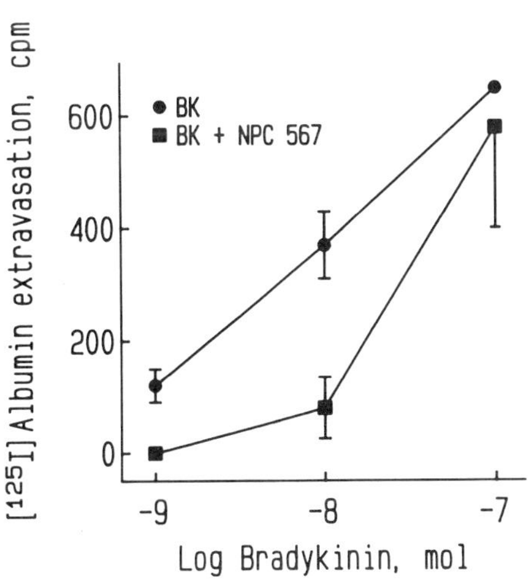

Figure 5 NPC 567 blocks bradykinin induced plasma extravasation in cyproheptadine-treated rats. To increase sensitivity of the assay, [^{125}I]-albumin was injected intravenously along with Evan's blue dye into animals that had been treated with cyproheptadine as in Figure 4. Bradykinin, or bradykinin plus NPC 567, 100 nM, were injected intradermally. Radioactivity was monitored in the extravasation zones. Results are mean ± SEM from 5 animals.

B. Carrageenan Paw Edema

Carrageenan is a polysaccharide seaweed component that is commonly used to elicit inflammation in animals when injected into the paw or pleural space. The inflammatory response to carrageenan injected into a rat paw consists of two phases (54). The first phase is characterized by edema, hyperemia, and hyperalgesia, followed by hypoalgesia. This phase is followed by phagocyte influx into the dermis associated with further edema accumulation and hyperalgesia and, later, influx of monocytes and proliferation of fibroblasts and vascular tissue. A role for bradykinin is readily suggested. The charged surface of carrageenan is known to activate kallikrein (55), and plasma immunoreactive bradykinin has been reported to be elevated following carrageenan injection into rat paws (20).

We injected rat hindpaws with carrageenan, then measured local immunoreactive kinin levels in the paws at various times (21). Immunoreactive kinin and its metabolic product, desArg^9-kinin, were found to be elevated 2 and 4 hours after carrageenan administration (Fig. 6), and the desArg^9-bradykinin product remained elevated at 6 hours.

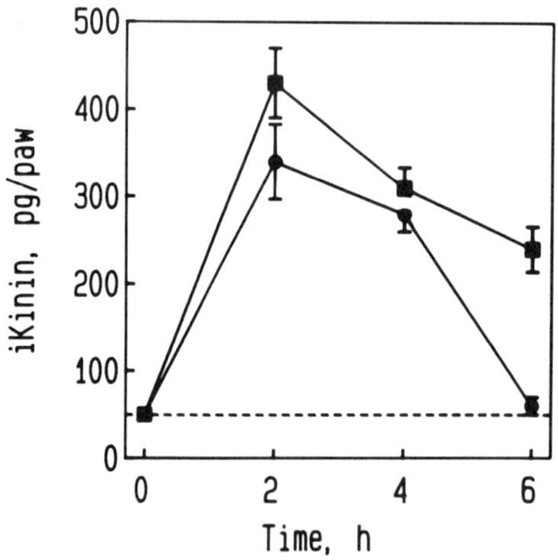

Figure 6 Carrageenan increases local concentrations of immunoreactive kinins. A hind paw was injected with carrageenan at time 0, then animals were sacrificed, paws rapidly removed, and homogenized in ice-cold 10% trichloroacetic acid (67). Kinins were quantitated using specific radioimmunoassays. Each point represents the mean ± SEM from 3 animals (From Ref. 21.)

When NPC 567 was constantly infused into the femoral artery, it significantly inhibited carrageenan-induced edema (Fig. 7). Since NPC 567 has been reported to inhibit kallikrein (56), the ability of NPC 567 to inhibit carrageenan-induced edema may have been due to inhibition of the enzyme, rather than receptor blockade. Thus, immunoreactive bradykinin was measured in paws 2 hours after carrageenan administration in control animals, and in animals receiving an infusion of NPC 567. The carrageenan-induced increase in immunoreactive bradykinin was not affected by NPC 567 (data not shown). Hargreaves and colleagues have also recently demonstrated that a bradykinin antagonist can inhibit carrageenan-induced paw edema after a single dose of antagonist administered to the paw (22).

C. Carrageenan-Induced Pleurisy

Injection of carrageenan into the pleural cavity of rats results in a dual component phagocytic inflammatory response in the diaphragmatic pleura followed by intrapleural exudation (57). In studies performed prior to the

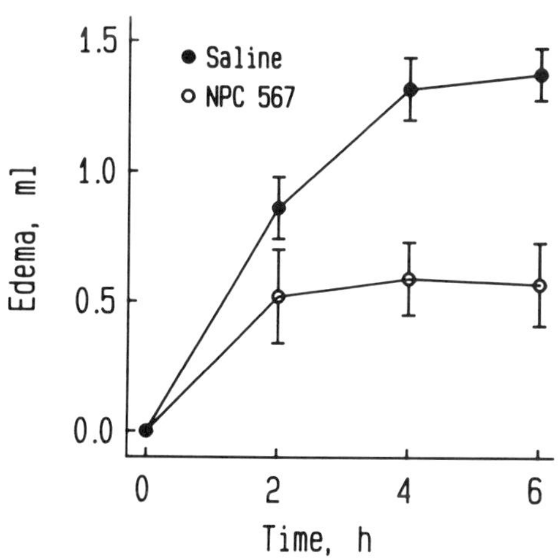

Figure 7 NPC 567 inhibits carrageenan-induced paw edema in rats. NPC 567 was loaded into mini-osmotic pumps (Alzet) and delivered into the common ileac artery at 100 nmol/h. Control rats received minipumps loaded with saline. Carrageenan was injected at time 0 and edema was monitored over time. Each point is mean ± SEM from 6 control or 7 NPC 567-treated animals. Edema volumes were significantly different at 2, 4, and 6 hours ($p < 0.05$ or less).

availability of bradykinin receptor antagonists, it was suggested that no evidence was obtained for a role for bradykinin in carrageenan-induced pleurisy (57). However, bromolein, a thiol protease from the stem of the pineapple, which activates Hageman factor to deplete prekallikrein and high molecular weight kininogen in the blood (58), has been reported to inhibit carrageenan pleurisy (59). Also, captopril, an inhibitor of kininase II, augments carrageenan-induced pleurisy in normal rats, but not in high molecular weight kininogen-deficient rats (60). In the only study reported thus far using a bradykinin antagonist, NPC 431 inhibited carrageenan-induced pleurisy (61).

D. Kaolin Inflammation

Kaolin administration leads to activation of plasma kallikrein (62) and increased vascular permeability. Inhibition of the enzyme with soybean trypsin inhibitor abrogated the increase in permeability (63). Bromelain, a thiol protease from the stem of the pineapple, activates Hageman factor resulting in depletion of prekallikrein and high molecular weight kininogen in the blood (58). Pretreatment of rats with bromolein blocked kaolin-induced increases in circulating bradykinin and vascular permeability (64).

E. Endotoxin Shock

Bradykinin has been implicated in both human sepsis and experimental endotoxin shock (65). Two studies have found that the D-Phe^7-BK antagonists NPC 413 (66) and NPC 567 (67) reduce the acute hypotensive effects of endotoxin in rats. In the latter study (67), NPC 567 was also found to reduce mortality in response to endotoxin. In that same study, two inflammatory mediators, thromboxane and prostacyclin, were also measured. Endotoxin increases the circulating levels of these two mediators. NPC 567 did not affect circulating thromboxane but did partially block circulating prostacyclin. The sources of circulating thromboxane and prostacyclin in endotoxin shock are not clear, but macropohages have been suggested as a significant source (68). Vascular tissue also synthesizes prostacyclin but not thromboxane, and bradykinin stimulates vascular prostacyclin synthesis (69). The authors suggested that endotoxin increases prostacyclin synthesis directly by stimulating macrophages and indirectly by increasing circulating bradykinin (demonstrated in the study (67)), which in turn stimulates vascular endothelium. Thus, that portion of endotoxin-elicited prostacyclin that was blocked by NPC 567 may represent that synthesized by vasculature, while the NPC 567-resistant portion may represent that synthesized by macrophages. That NPC 567 had no effect on endotoxin-stimulated thromboxane synthesis is consistent with thromboxane originating from macrophages.

F. Leukocyte Function

Several studies have implicated bradykinin in the regulation of white blood cell function. The studies that have been conducted suggest that the receptor subserving the actions of bradykinin on these cells are of the B1 type. Most existing studies were performed before the identification of lymphokines and are therefore difficult to interpret.

Using the murine macrophage-like line RAW264.7, it was found that bradykinin stimulates the release of tumor necrosis factor and interleukin 1 (40). The receptor responsible for bradykinin's actions seems to be of the B1 class, since desArg^9-BK was as potent as bradykinin in eliciting lymphokine release, and desArg^9[Leu^8]-BK blocked the effects of both kinins. NPC 567 also blocked the effects of the kinins. These studies are presently being extended to human monocytes. In preliminary studies it has been observed that bradykinin stimulates secretion of interleukin 6, and that stimulation is greatly augmented by pretreatment or cotreatment with small concentrations of lipopolysaccharide (F. DeBeer, unpublished observation).

G. Chondrocytes

Articular cartilage undergoes degradation in several chronic inflammatory diseases including rheumatoid arthritis and osteoarthritis. Among inflammatory mediators, certain cytokines, such as interleukin 1, have been shown to cause cartilage resorption and inhibition of collagen (70) and proteoglycan (71) synthesis. In pig articular cartilage explants bradykinin did not alter matrix metabolism, but receptors for bradykinin exist on chondrocytes, since bradykinin and kallidin both stimulated increases in inositol phosphate and intracellular free calcium concentrations, as well as PGE_2 synthesis (72). The receptor subtype was B2 since desArg^9-BK was without effect, while NPC 431 inhibited bradykinin-induced PGE_2 and calcium release. Bradykinin did not alter DNA synthesis in the cartilage explants.

H. Bone

Along with cartilage, bone is a target of inflammatory reactions in joint capsules. Bone destruction results from interactions between inflammatory cells and osteoclasts. In mouse calvarial bone in culture, bradykinin caused dose-dependent stimulation of bone mineral mobilization, matrix degradation, and lysosomal enzyme release (73,74). Bone destruction in response to bradykinin appears to be mediated by prostaglandins since the effect was inhibited by cyclooxygenase inhibitors and glucocorticoids. DesArg^9-bradykinin also stimulated bone degradation, suggesting that the receptor was of the B1 subtype (74). However, desArg^9[Leu^8]bradykinin did not affect bradykinin-induced effects. Curiously, the effects of desArg^9[Leu^8]-bradykinin on desArg^9-bradykinin-induced effects was not reported.

I. Human Studies

Few studies of kinin antagonists in human inflammatory diseases have yet been reported. The potential role of bradykinin in rhinitis and the effects of bradykinin antagonists are discussed in Chapter 10. Other human studies of the effects of NPC 567 in patients with rhinovirus infection have been concluded. The efficacy of this antagonist was considered to be insufficient to warrant further clinical development (Third Quarter Report, Nova Pharmaceutical Corporation). Assuming that bradykinin does play a role in the symptoms of this disease (Chapter 10), the reasons for the lack of effect of the kinin antagonist are unclear at present, but may be related to poor potency, poor metabolic stability (see Chapter 6), or novel bradykinin receptor (see Chapter 9).

The ability of bradykinin to elicit pain and inflammation has long been recognized. The present generation of bradykinin antagonists has allowed more direct demonstration of bradykinin's role in certain models. However, the metabolic lability of the available agents has limited the studies largely to models in which topical administration or infusion is possible. More detailed future studies will require antagonists with prolonged metabolic stability.

REFERENCES

1. Robbins, S. L., and R. S. Coltran. *Pathologic Basis of Disease*, 2nd ed. W. B. Saunders Co., Philadelphia, PA, 1979.
2. Collier, H. O., and I. R. Lee. Algesic actions of bradykinin. *Brit. J. Pharmacol.* **21**:151-158 (1963).
3. Clark, W. G., Pain, in: *Bradykinin, Kallidin, and Kallikrein*, vol. XXV, Supplement, *Handbook of Experimental Pharmacology* (E. G. Erdos, ed.). Springer-Verlag, New York, pp. 428-488 (1979).
4. Kellermeyer, R. W., and R. C. Graham. Kinins—possible physiologic and pathologic role in man. *New Eng. J. Med.* **279**:859-866 (1968).

5. Steranka, L. R., D. C. Manning, C. J. DeHaas, J. W. Ferkany, S. A. Borosky, J. R. Connor, R. J. Vavrek, J. M. Stewart, and S. H. Snyder. Bradykinin as a pain mediator: Receptors are localized to sensory neurons have analgesic actions. *Proc. Natl. Acad. Sci. USA* **85**:3245-3249 (1988).
6. Khan, A. A., S. N. Raja, J. N. Campbell, T. V. Hartke, and R. A. Meyer. Bradykinin in nociception. *Neurosci. Abstr.* **12**:219 (1986).
7. Szolcsanyi, J. Selective responsiveness of polymodal nociceptors of the rabbit ear to capsaicin, bradykinin and ultraviolet radiation. *J. Physiol.* **388**:9-23 (1987).
8. Franz, M., and S. Mense. Muscle receptors with group IV afferent fibres responding to application of bradykinin. *Brain Res.* **92**:369-383 (1975).
9. Meyer, R. A., and J. N. Campbell. Myelinated nociceptive afferents account for the hyperalgesia that follows a burn to the hand. *Science* **213**:1527-1529 (1981).
10. Deffenu, G., L. Pegrassi, and B. Lumachi. The use of bradykinin-induced effects in rats as an assay for analgesic drugs. *J. Pharm. Pharmacol.* **18**:135 (1966).
11. Sicuteri, F., M. Fanciullacci, and P. L. Del Bianco. Algesic effects of intra-arterial bradykinin in human subjects. *Life Sci.* **4**:309 (1965).
12. Burch, R. M., S. G. Farmer, and L. R. Steranka. Bradykinin receptor antagonists. *Med. Res. Rev.* **10**:237-269 (1990).
13. Griesbacher, T., and F. Lembeck. Effects of bradykinin antagonists on bradykinin-induced plasma extravasation, venoconstriction, prostaglandin E_2 release, and nociceptor stimulation and contraction of the iris sphincter muscle in the rabbit. *Br. J. Pharmacol.* **92**:333-340 (1987).
14. Walter, T., T. T. Chau, and B. M. Weichman. Effects of analgesics on bradykinin-induced writhing in mice presensitized with PGE_2. *Agents Actions* **27**:375-377 (1989).
15. Fujiyoshi, T., I. Hayaishi, S. Oh-ishi, M. Kuwashima, H. Iida, M. Dozen, N. Taniguchi, K. Ikeda, and H. Ohnishi. Kaolin-induced writhing in mice, a new model of possible bradykinin-induced pain for assessment of analgesic agents. *Agents Actions* **27**:332-334 (1989).
16. Steranka, L. R., C. J. DeHaas, R. J. Vavrek, J. M. Stewart, S. J. Enna, and S. H. Snyder. Antinociceptive effects of bradykinin antagonists. *Eur. J. Pharmacol.* **136**:261-262 (1987).
17. Haley, J. E., A. H. Dickenson, and M. Schacter. Electrophysiological evidence for a role of bradykinin in chemical nociception in the rat. *Neurosci. Lett.* **97**:198-202 (1989).
18. Kellermeyer, R. W. Inflammatory process in acute gouty arthritis. 3. Vascular permeability-enhancing activity in normal human synovial fluid; induction by Hageman factor activators; and inhibition by Hageman factor antiserum. *J. Lab. Clin. Med.* **70**:372-383 (1967).
19. Melmon, K. L., M. E. Webster, S. E. Goldfinger, and J. E. Seegmiller. The presence of a kinin in inflammatory synovial effusions from arthritides of varying etiologies. *Arth. Rheum.* **10**:13-20 (1967).

20. Hargreaves, K. M., E. S. Troullos, R. A. Dionne, E. A. Schmidt, S. C. Schafer, and J. L. Joris. Bradykinin is increased during acute and chronic inflammation: Therapeutic implications. *Clin. Pharmacol. Ther.* **44**:613-621 (1988).
21. Burch, R. M., and C. R. DeHaas. A bradykinin antagonist inhibits carrageenan edema in rats. *Naunyn-Schmiedeberg's Arch. Pharmacol.* (in press).
22. Costello, A. H., and k. M. Hargreaves. Suppression of carrageenan-induced hyperalgesia, hyperthermia and edema by a bradykinin antagonist. *Eur. J. Pharmacol.* **171**:259-263 (1989).
23. Whalley, E. T., S. Clegg, J. M. Stewart, and R. J. Vavrek. The effect of kinin agonists and antagonists on the pain response in the human blister base. *Naunyn-Schmeid. Arch. Pharmacol.* **336**:652-655 (1987).
24. Wang, J.-P., M.-F. Hsu, C. Ouyang, and C.-M. Teng. Edematous response caused by [$Thi^{5,8}$, D-Phe^7]bradykinin, a B_2 receptor antagonist, is due to mast cell degranulation. *Eur. J. Pharmacol.* **161**:143-149 (1989).
25. Lawrence, I. D., J. A. Warner, V. I. Cohan, L. M. Lichtenstein, A. Kagey-Sobotka, R. J. Vavrek, J. M. Stewart, and D. Proud. Induction of histamine release from human skin mast cells by bradykinin analogs. *Biochem. Pharmacol.* **38**:227-233 (1989).
26. Devillier, P., M. Renoux, G. Drapeau, and D. Regoli. Histamine release from rat peritoneal mast cells by kinin antagonists. *Eur. J. Pharmacol.* **149**: 137-140 (1988).
27. Devillier, P., G. Drapeau, M. Renoux, and D. Regoli. Role of the N-terminal arginine in the histamine-releasing activity of substance P, bradykinin and related peptides. *Eur. J. Pharmacol.* **168**:53-60 (1989).
28. Bonner, G., W. Niermann, R. Festage, and U. Bechsler. Changes in PMN-elastase in blood and in renal and plasma kallikrein-kinin systems after severe burn injury. *Adv. Exp. Med. Biol.* **240**:489-503 (1988).
29. Marceau, F., A. Lussier, D. Regoli, and J. P. Giroud. Pharmacology of kinins: Their relevance to tissue injury and inflammation. *Gen. Pharmacol.* **14**: 209-241 (1983).
30. Niewiaroski, S., E. Barkowski, and J. Rogowicka. Studies on the absorption and activation of Hageman factor (factor XII) by collagen and elastin. *Thromb. Diath. Hemorrhag.* **14**:387-400 (1965).
31. Moskowitz, R., H. Schwartz, B. Michel, O. Ratnoff, and T. Astrup. Generation of kinin-like agents by chondroitin sulfate, heparin, chitin sulfate, and articular cartilage: Possible pathophysiologic implications. *J. Lab. Clin. Med.* **76**:790-798 (1970).
32. Figuerosa, C. D., and K. D. Bhoola. The discovery of a tissue kallikrein in human neutrophils. *Brit. J. Pharmacol.* **97**:439P (1989).
33. Greenbaum, L. M. In: *Bradykinin, Kallidin and Kallikrein*, Vol. XXV, *Handbook of Experimental Pharmacology* (E. G. Erdos, ed.). Springer-Verlag, New York, pp. 91-102 (1979).
34. Kaplan, A., A. B. Kay, and K. F. Austen. A prealbumin activator of prekallikrein. III. Appearance of chemotactic activity for human neutrophils

by the conversion of human prekallikrein to kallikrein. *J. Exp. Med.* **135**: 81-97 (1972).
35. Lewis, G. P. Kinins in inflammatory and tissue injury. *Handbook of Experimental Pharmacology* **25**:516-530 (1970).
36. Graham, R. C., R. M. Erbert, O. D. Ratnoff, and J. M. Moses. Pathogenesis of inflammation. II. *In vivo* observations of inflammatory effects of activated Hageman factor and bradykinin. *J. Exp. Med.* **121**:807-818 (1965).
37. Roch-Arveiller, M., D. Regoli, and J. P. Giroud. Effect of bradykinin and various synthetic analogs on rat polymorphonuclear chemotaxis. *Agents Actions* **11**:499-502 (1981).
38. Fauve, R. M., and M. B. Hevin. Inflammation et resistance antitumorale. II. Effets antagonistes de la bradykinine et d'une fraction isolee d'un surnageant de culture de cellules malignes sur l'etalement des macrophages. *Ann. Immunol.* **128C**:1079-1083 (1977).
39. Eisen, V., and A. Noronha-Dutra. Effects of kallikrein and bradykinin on uptake and release of substances by peritoneal macrophages, in: *Kininogenases Kallikrein 4th Symposium* (G. L. Haberland, J. W. Rohen, and T. Suzuki, eds.). Schattauer Verlag, New York, pp. 304-319 (1977).
40. Tiffany, C. W., and R. M. Burch. Bradykinin stimulates tumor necrosis factor and interleukin 1 release from macrophages. *FEBS Lett.* **247**:189-192 (1989).
41. White, D. M., and M. Zimmermann. The bradykinin-induced release of substance P from nerve fibre endings in the rat saphenous nerve neuroma is not related to eletrophysiological excitiation. *Neurosci. Lett.* **92**:108-113 (1988).
42. Burch, R. M., J. R. Connor, and J. Axelrod. Interleukin 1 amplifies receptor-mediated activation of phospholipase A_2 in 3T3 fibroblasts. *Proc. Natl. Acad. Sci. USA* **85**:6306-6309 (1988).
43. Bathon, J. M., D. Proud, K. Krackow, and F. M. Wigley. Preincubation of human synovial cells with IL-1 modulates prostaglandin E_2 release in response to bradykinin. *J. Immunol.* **143**:579-586 (1989).
44. Burch, R. M., and C. W. Tiffany. Tumor necrosis factor causes amplification of arachidonic acid metabolism in response to interleukin 1, bradykinin, and other agonists. *J. Cell. Physiol.* **141**:85-89 (1989).
45. Burch, R. M., and J. Axelrod. Dissociation of bradykinin-induced prostaglandin formation from phosphatidylinositol turnover in Swiss 3T3 fibroblasts. Evidence for G protein regulation of phospholipase A_2. *Proc. Natl. Acad. Sci. USA* **84**:6374-6378 (1987).
46. Conklin, B. R., R. M. Burch, L. R. Steranka, and J. Axelrod. Distinct bradykinin receptors mediate stimulation of prostaglandin synthesis by endothelial cells and fibroblasts. *J. Pharmacol. Exp. Ther.* **244**:646-649 (1988).
47. Burch, R. M., J. R. Connor, and C. W. Tiffany. The kallikrein-kinin system in chronic inflammation. *Agents Actions* **27**:258-260 (1989).
48. Wood, D. D., E. J. Thrie, C. A. Dinarello, and P. L. Cohen. Isolation of an interleukin-1-like factor from human joint effusions. *Arthritis Rheum.* **26**: 975-983 (1983).

49. Keele, C. A., and V. Eisen. Components of the kallikrein-kinin system in joint effusions from patients with arthritis. *Adv. Exp. Med. Biol.* **8**:471-475 (1970).
50. Perris, A. D., and J. F. Whitfield, The mitogenic action of bradykinin on thymic lymphocytes and its dependence on calcium. *Proc. Soc. Exp. Biol.* 1198-1201 (1969).
51. Stachurska, J., W. Roszkowski, M. Kopec, and J. Ryzewski. Effects of bradykinin-induced stimulation of mitotic activity and DNA synthesis in thymocytes. *Proc. Soc. Exp. Biol.* **133**:1270-1274 (1976).
52. Whalley, E. T., I. A. Nwator, J. M. Stewart, and R. J. Vavrek. Analysis of the receptors mediating vascular actions of bradykinin. *Naunyn-Schmeid. Arch. Pharmacol.* **336**:430-433 (1987).
53. Steranka, L. R., R. Rodriguez, and C. J. DeHaas. Effects of bradykinin antagonists on rat skin. *Pharmacologist* A30 (1988).
54. Vinegar, R., J. F. Truax, J. L. Selph, P. R. Johnston, A. L. Venable, and K. K. McKenzie. Pathway to carrageenan-induced inflammation in the hind limb of the rat. *Fed. Proc.* **46**:118-126 (1987).
55. Schwartz, H., and R. Kellermeyer. Carrageenan and delayed hypersensitivity. II. Activation of Hageman factor by carrageenan and its possible significance. *Proc. Soc. Exp. Med. Biol.* **132**:1021-1024 (1969).
56. Spragg, J., R. J. Vavrek, and J. M. Stewart. The inhibition of glandular kallikrein by peptide analog antagonists of bradykinin. *Peptides* **9**:203-206 (1988).
57. Vinegar, R., J. F. Truax, J. L. Selph, and F. A. Voelker. Pathway of onset, development, and decay of carrageenan pleurisy in the rat. *Fed. Proc.* **41**: 2588-2596 (1982).
58. Ohishi, S., Y. Uchida, A. Ueno, and M. Katori. Bromelain, a thiolprotease from pineapple stem, depletes high molecular weight kininogen by activation of Hageman factor (Factor XII). *Thromb. Res.* **14**:665-670 (1979).
59. Katori, M., K. Ikeda, Y. Harada, Y. Uchida, K. Tanaka, and S. Ohishi. A possible role of prostaglandins and bradykinin as a trigger of exudation in carrageenan-induced rat pleurisy. *Agents Actions* **8**:108-110 (1978).
60. Dozen, M., K. Yamaki, and S. Oh-ishi. Captopril uncovers kinin-dependent release of arachidonic acid metabolites in carrageenin-induced rat pleurisy. *Japan. J. Pharmacol.* **51**:101-105 (1989).
61. Katori, M., M. Majima, Y. Uchida, and A. Ueno. In: *Kinins V*, in press.
62. Heimark, R. L., K. Kurachi, K. Fujikawa, and E. W. Davie. Surface activation of blood coagulation, fibrinolysis and kinin formation. *Nature* **286**:456-460 (1980).
63. Kumakura, S., S. Tsurufuji, S. Kurooka, and N. Sunahara. Role of bradykinin generating and degrading systems in the vascular permeability response induced with kaolin in rats. *J. Pharmacol. Exp. Ther.* **243**:1067-1073 (1987).
64. Kumakura, S., M. Yamashita, and S. Tsurufuji. Effect of bromelain on kaolin-induced inflammation in rats. *Eur. J. Pharmacol.* **150**:295-301 (1988).
65. Colman, R. W., and P. Y. Wong. Kallikrein-kinin system in pathologic conditions, in: *Bradykinin, Kallidin, and Kallikrein, Handbook of Experimental*

Pharmacology, vol. XXV (E. G. Erdos, ed.). Springer-Verlag, New York, pp. 584-586 (1979).
66. Weipert, J., H. Hoffmann, M. Siebeck, and E. T. Whalley. Attenuation of arterial blood pressure fall in endotoxin shock in the rat using the competitive bradykinin antagonist Lys-Lys-[Hyp^{2}, Thi^{5,8}, D-Phe^{7}]bradykinin (B4148). *Brit. J. Pharmacol.* **94**:282-284 (1988).
67. Wilson, D. D., L. de Garavilla, W. Kuhn, J. Togo, R. M. Burch, and L. R. Steranka. D-Arg-[Hyp^{3}-D-Phe^{7}]-bradykinin, a bradykinin antagonist, reduces mortality in a rat model of endotoxic shock. *Circ. Shock* **27**:93-101 (1989).
68. Rogers, T. S., P. V. Halushka, W. C. Wise, and J. A. Cook. Differential alteration of lipoxygenase and cyclooxygenase metabolism by rat peritoneal macrophages induced by endotoxin tolerance. *Prostaglandins* **31**:639-650 (1986).
69. Alexander, R. W., and M. A. Gimbrone, Jr. Stimulation of prostaglandin synthesis in cultured human umbilical vein smooth muscle cells. *Proc. Natl. Acad. Sci. USA* **73**:1617-1620 (1976).
70. Tyler, J. A., and H. P. Benton. Synthesis of type II collagen is decreased in cartilage cultured with interleukin 1 while the rate of intracellular degradation remains unchanged. *Collagen Relat. Res.* **8**:393-405 (1988).
71. Benton, H. P., and J. A. Tyler. Inhibition of cartilage proteoglycan synthesis by interleukin 1. *Biochem. Biophys. Res. Commun.* **154**:421-428 (1988).
72. Benton, H. P., T. R. Jackson, and M. R. Hanley. Identification of a novel inflammatory stimulant of chondrocytes. Early events in cell activation by bradykinin receptors on pig articular chondrocytes. *Biochem. J.* **258**:861-867 (1989).
73. Gustafson, G. T., and U. H. Lerner. Bradykinin stimulates bone resorption and lysosomal enzyme release in cultured mouse calvaria. *Biochem. J.* **219**: 329-332 (1984).
74. Lerner, U. H., I. L. Jones, and G. T. Gustafson. Bradykinin, a new potential mediator of inflammation-induced bone resorption. *Arth. Rheum.* **30**: 530-540 (1987).

9
Airway Pharmacology of Bradykinin

Stephen G. Farmer
Nova Pharmaceutical Corporation
Baltimore, Maryland

I. INTRODUCTION

A. Historical Perspective

Of the many mediators implicated in the pathophysiology of bronchial asthma, bradykinin was one of the earliest. Indeed, bradykinin was recognized as a potent bronchoconstrictor in guinea pigs over 30 years ago, before commercial sources were available, and investigators prepared the peptide from bovine serum or vespine venom glands. Collier and colleagues (1,2) reported the first studies of the pharmacological basis of bradykinin-induced bronchoconstriction. Indeed, nonsteroidal, anti-inflammatory drugs, such as aspirin, were perhaps the first drugs thought to be bradykinin antagonists (1,3).

Bradykinin-induced bronchoconstriction in guinea pigs was unaffected by antagonists of histamine, serotonin, or acetylcholine but was markedly inhibited by aspirin or phenylbutazone, although not by prior treatment with cortisone (2). In fact, it was suggested that the effect of anti-inflammatory drugs "raises the question whether suppression of a response to bradykinin or to a related peptide contributes to the antirheumatic action of nonsteroid agents" (2). Given current hypothesis for kinin involvement in inflammatory diseases, and the mediation of many kinin responses by prostaglandins, these were prophetic words indeed.

Observations in guinea pigs were soon extended to other species, and bradykinin and kallidin were also shown to be potent bronchospastic agents in rabbits and relatively weak or inactive in cats and rats (4-6). Interestingly, aspirin had little effect on the bradykinin response in these species. The first report of bradykinin's effect on isolated airway smooth muscle was also published by the same investigators. Bradykinin increased airway resistance in guinea pig perfused lungs (2) and contracted isolated trachea (2,5). In rabbit (7) and canine isolated airway smooth muscle as well as in human bronchus, however, bradykinin had little effect (5).

This study (5) was the earliest report of bradykinin's lack of effect on human airway smooth muscle, although it was also reported at around the same time that inhaled bradykinin was "very active" (8) as a bronchoconstrictor in asthmatic but not in nonasthmatic subjects (9-12). In several individuals, wheezing and cough also followed inhalation of bradykinin. Unlike guinea pigs, the constrictor effect of bradykinin in man was attenuated by atropine and mepyramine (8). These observations, which have since been substantiated and expanded upon by others, are discussed later. As with many pharmacological and nonpharmacological agents, therefore, asthmatic patients exhibit airway hyperresponsiveness to bradykinin.

These early studies preceded many publications on the airway effects of kinins, and in his elegant review, Collier provided an excellent description of the pulmonary effects of kinins as known in 1970 (13). The present chapter will attempt to review present knowledge of the pharmacology of bradykinin in the pulmonary airways. In addition, bradykinin is probably of importance in inflammatory diseases of the airways, and recent studies indicating the potential usefulness for bradykinin antagonists in the treatment of bronchial asthma will be addressed (see also Chapter 11).

II. AIRWAY EFFECTS OF BRADYKININ

A. Effects In Vivo

1. Effects on Pulmonary Function

Bradykinin-Induced Bronchoconstriction. Bradykinin is a potent bronchoconstrictor in guinea pigs (2,4,14-24), rabbits (5), dogs (25-28), and sheep (29,30). The mechanisms underlying bradykinin's actions in the airways exhibit species differences. In most species, including man, bradykinin has little direct effect on airway smooth muscle (5,31,32). Rather, it stimulates pulmonary sensory nerve endings (C-fibers), thereby initiating reflex bronchoconstriction via acetylcholine release from postganglionic vagal nerve endings in the bronchial smooth muscle. Thus, the bronchospastic effect of bradykinin in vivo is inhibited by muscarinic antagonists in man (31,32) and sheep (30). Similarly, bradykinin has no effect on isolated airway smooth muscle from dogs (25,28). Bradykinin does, however, stimulate canine bronchial, afferent C-fibers, and vagal sensory or reflex effects probably mediate bronchoconstriction in this species (26-28).

The mechanisms underlying bradykinin's airway effects in guinea pigs may also include sensory nerves (18,21,33). For example, intravenous bradykinin was reported to directly stimulate pulmonary afferent nerve endings, causing reflex activation of vagal efferent fibers and the onset of bronchoconstriction (33). Section of the vagus nerve trunks reduced, but did not abolish, the effect of bradykinin, although the effect of anticholinergic drugs was not determined (33). Drazen and Austen (18) demonstrated that atropine abolished bradykinin-induced increases in airway resistance, whereas the decrease in lung compliance was not altered. This suggests that airway resistance changes but not compliance changes, following intravenous bradykinin, are mediated by reflex release of acetylcholine. Conversely, others have shown that neither vagotomy nor anticholinergic drugs influence bradykinin-induced bronchoconstriction in guinea pigs (2,3,34), (S. G. Farmer, unpublished observations).

Contrary to observations in most species, bradykinin is a potent spasmogen of guinea pig isolated airway smooth muscle (see Section II.B.1). Its effects in cavine airways in vivo involve bradykinin receptor-mediated release of membrane-bound arachidonic acid, resulting in biosynthesis of eicosanoids such as thromboxane A_2 (TxA_2), which cause contraction of airway smooth muscle. Indeed, the earliest reports on the bronchopulmonary effects of bradykinin in the guinea pig found that the fatty acid cyclooxygenase inhibitor aspirin abolished bradykinin-induced bronchoconstriction (1-3,5). Indomethacin also substantially reduces bradykinin-induced bronchoconstriction in guinea pigs, confirming further the central role for products of arachidonic acid (35). Furthermore, bronchoconstriction to bradykinin, in anesthetized guinea pigs, is accompanied by elevations in circulating TxA_2 (21), which are abolished by pretreatment with aspirin (22). Effects of bradykinin on eicosanoid production in isolated airway preparations are discussed in Section II.B.2.

Bradykinin-induced bronchoconstriction in guinea pigs is potentiated by the β-adrenoceptor antagonist propranolol (16,35). Since bradykinin causes the release of epinephrine from the adrenal medulla in several species including the guinea pig (36-38), it was proposed that the constrictor effect of kinins in the airways was functionally antagonized by the bronchodilator action of catecholamines. Thus, inhibition of endogenous β-adrenoceptor responses to epinephrine may increase pulmonary responsiveness to bradykinin (35). Conversely, propranolol causes airway hyperreactivity to other bronchoconstrictors (39,40). In addition, the D-isomer of propranolol is equipotent with the racemic mixture in producing hyperreactivity, but the former is a very weak antagonist of β-adrenoceptors (41). Thus, propranolol-induced hyperreactivity to bradykinin may not involve antagonism of endogenous epinephrine.

In guinea pigs, pretreated with propranolol, the angiotensin-converting enzyme (ACE, EC 3.4.15.1) inhibitor captopril potentiates bradykinin-induced bronchoconstriction (35). Captopril, however, did not potentiate bradykinin in animals which did not receive propranolol. Moreover, the ACE inhibitor caused a marked, relatively long-lasting hypotensive response without affecting baseline airway resistance (35). In a preliminary report, treatment of guinea pigs with captopril, twice daily for 2 weeks, caused significant potentiation of bradykinin-induced bronchoconstriction (42). Treatment of hypertension with ACE inhibitors has recently been associated with airway hyperreactivity and cough in man, and the possible role of bradykinin in this phenomenon is discussed later (Section II.A.3).

Bradykinin-Induced Airway Hyperreactivity. In addition to causing bronchoconstriction, bradykinin has been reported to induce airway hyperresponsiveness to other bronchoconstrictor agents. In feline lungs, perfused via the bronchial circulation, bradykinin causes an approximately 10-fold increase in sensitivity to acetylcholine-induced bronchoconstriction and a 60% increase in the maximum effect of acetylcholine (43). Bradykinin itself has little effect on baseline resistance or on cat isolated airway smooth muscle tone, confirming previous observations (4,6). It was proposed that the effect of bradykinin is due to vasodilation and microvascular permeability changes and consequent thickening of the airway mucosa (43).

Bradykinin, at subthreshold constrictor doses (i.v.), also causes a transient potentiation of acetylcholine-induced bronchoconstriction in vivo in the guinea pig (44). Indomethacin did not influence this effect of the kinin, suggesting that the mechanisms (or possibly receptors) involved in bradykinin-induced contraction of airway smooth muscle are different than those mediating hyperreactivity. Bilateral vagotomy abolished the capacity of both bradykinin and substance P to increase airway responsiveness, suggesting a neuronal mechanism (44). Curiously though, bilateral vagotomy also reduced the bronchoconstrictor effect of acetylcholine itself, and higher doses had to be employed in order to elicit responses similar to those seen in control animals (44). This indicates that, following vagotomy, the animals were hyporeactive to acetylcholine. The effect of bradykinin on airway responses to the higher dose of acetylcholine were not examined in animals with intact vagi.

Bradykinin is a potent bronchoconstrictor in sheep, allergic animals exhibiting greater responsiveness to inhaled bradykinin than nonallergic sheep (30). Further, the bradykinin antagonist DArg[Hyp^3,DPhe^7]bradykinin (NPC 567) (45) inhibits the onset of allergen-induced airway hyperresponsiveness in *Ascaris*-sensitive sheep (29), although bradykinin by itself does not produce changes in airway reactivity in this species (30). The pulmonary pharmacology of bradykinin and bradykinin antagonists in allergic sheep are discussed in detail in Chapter 11.

Kinins and Anaphylaxis. Antigen challenge in sensitized guinea pigs is associated with elevations in blood levels of kinins, and application of antigen to sensitized guinea pig perfused lungs results in kallikrein production (46,47). Thus, bradykinin may contribute to allergen-induced bronchoconstriction. Conversely, the kinin antagonist NPC 567 does not inhibit allergic bronchoconstriction in guinea pigs (S. G. Farmer, unpublished observation) or sheep (29). Following inhalational challenge with *Ascaris suum* antigen, there is a dramatic increase in levels of immunoreactive kinins and of TAME-esterase in ovine bronchoalveolar fluid, and this also is discussed in Chapter 11.

2. Airway Effects on Bradykinin Antagonists in Animals

As discussed in the preceding section, there are many studies on the airway effects of bradykinin. Until recently, however, little was known concerning the nature of the receptors mediating pulmonary actions of kinins. Bradykinin receptors are classically divided into two subtypes, B1 and B2 (45,48) (see Chapter 1). In guinea pigs, NPC 567 and DArg[Hyp^3,Thi^{5,8},DPhe^7]bradykinin (NPC 349), B1 and B2 receptor antagonists (45,49), only partially inhibit bradykinin-induced bronchoconstriction (23). Moreover, the B1 receptor agonist desArg^9-bradykinin has no effect on airway resistance in this species (23,24). Studies in vitro also indicate that B1 and B2 receptor ligands have little or no effect on guinea pig airway smooth muscle, and a third bradykinin receptor, the B3, was proposed to mediate bradykinin-induced contraction of airway smooth muscle (23). These studies are delineated further below (Section II.B.1).

It was also reported recently that the B2 antagonist NPC 349 abolishes bradykinin-induced bronchoconstriction in the guinea pig (24). Nevertheless, this study used only a single dose of bradykinin (1 μg/kg) and a much higher dose of the antagonist (400 μg/kg). In our own studies, although we found that the bronchoconstrictor response to the same dose of bradykinin was abolished by NPC 567 (100 μg/kg), the effect of the antagonist diminished as the dose of bradykinin was increased (23). We also found NPC 349 (100 μg/kg) to be a poor inhibitor of higher doses of bradykinin-induced bronchoconstriction (23). Inhalation of an aerosolized solution of bradykinin causes dose-dependent bronchoconstriction in guinea pigs, although inhaled NPC 567 fails to influence the response to bradykinin at any dose tested (23).

The bradykinin antagonist NPC 567 has been shown to be a potent inhibitor of bradykinin-induced bronchoconstriction in sheep, suggesting that there are functional B2 receptors in the airways (30) (see Chapter 11).

3. Bradykinin in Human Airway Diseases

Kinins have been implicated in inflammatory conditions of the upper airways for several years (50-52). The role of kinins in allergic rhinitis and in the symptomatology of the common cold are discussed in detail in Chapter 10.

Bronchoalveolar Kinin Levels. As discussed earlier, it has long been known that inhaled bradykinin is a potent bronchoconstrictor in asthmatics but has very little or no activity in nonasthmatic individuals (8,9,11, 12,31,32,53,54). For many years bradykinin has been implicated in the pathogenesis of asthma, in that elevated kinin levels were detected in plasma of asthmatic patients (55,56), and a correlation between kinin levels and severity of symptoms was apparent (55). Bronchoalveolar kininogenase activity and levels of immunoreactive kinins increase, following allergen challenge, in allergic asthmatics (56). HPLC of the bronchoalveolar fluid showed the predominant kinin to be kallidin. Further, the major kininogenase activity was structurally, functionally, and antigenically compatible with tissue kallikreins. Thus, Christiansen et al. speculated that presence of tissue and plasma kallikrein activities in bronchoalveolar spaces of asthmatics could, via kinin generation, participate in a cascade of events leading to asthma (56).

Interestingly, one study found bradykinin to be an apparent *bronchodilator* in asthmatics (57). While intravenous injection of bradykinin has no effect on airway resistance or FEV_1 in nonasthmatic subjects, in asthmatics, bradykinin decreases airway resistance and increases FEV_1. It was suggested that bronchodilation in asthmatic subjects may be the result of higher intrinsic bronchial tone in these patients (57). It is puzzling that in most studies in asthmatics, bradykinin is a bronchoconstrictor, whereas bronchodilation was evident in this study. One major difference between the study by Newball and coworkers (57) was the route of administration of bradykinin. These investigators administered bradykinin intravenously, whereas an aerosolized mist of the kinin was inhaled in all of the other studies (8,31,32,53,54). It is possible that intravenous bradykinin may not have as ready access to airway luminal C-fibers, stimulation of which mediates bronchoconstriction in man (8,11,32), as bradykinin by inhalation. Moreover, catecholamines, released from the adrenal medulla (see above), may have mediated the bronchodilation following intravenous bradykinin (57). In a guinea pig preparation in vivo James (16) found that intravenous bradykinin caused tracheal relaxation, which was abolished by propranolol, in addition to increasing peripheral airway resistance. Bradykinin was also reported to be a mild bronchodilator in some aspirin-treated guinea pigs (3).

Pharmacology of Bradykinin-Induced Bronchoconstriction in Man. In asthmatic patients, inhalation of bradykinin aerosols results in cough, wheezing, and bronchoconstriction (8,11,12). Atropine and mepyramine were reported to inhibit these effects "in some experiments," (8) suggesting roles for both acetylcholine and histamine. Indeed, bradykinin is known to cause histamine release from mast cells by a mechanism which is probably independent of bradykinin receptors (58,59). The inhibitory effect of muscarinic receptor antagonists on bradykinin-induced bronchoconstriction in man has been confirmed with atropine (31) and ipratropium bromide (32). Thus, bradykinin-induced bronchoconstriction is mediated largely by a vagal reflex in asthmatics.

That bradykinin effects in human airways are largely neuronal is substantiated by the fact that the kinin also causes cough (8,32,54). Further evidence for a role of neuronal mechanisms is provided by the observation that both disodium cromoglycate and nedocromil sodium provide significant protection against bradykinin-induced bronchoconstriction and cough (32,54). Unlike the guinea pig, bradykinin-induced bronchoconstriction in man is not affected by prior treatment with a cyclooxygenase inhibitor (aspirin) (32), suggesting that prostaglandins are not involved. Also contrary to observations in cavine airways (35,42), bradykinin's effects in asthmatic airways are not influenced by the ACE inhibitors captopril or ramipril (32,60).

Cough. There are several recent reports of cough (61-63) and airway hyperreactivity (64,65) in hypertensive patients being treated with ACE inhibitors, and these effects have been attributed to inhibition of the catabolism of endogenous bradykinin (61,62,65). Indeed, bradykinin does cause cough in asthmatics (32,66) and nonasthmatics (54). However, administration of ramipril to human volunteers, while achieving adequate reductions in plasma activity of ACE, had no effect either on the incidence of cough or bronchoconstriction following inhalation of bradykinin (60).

An apparent lack of involvement for endogenous kinins in cough, induced by a variety of stimuli, has also been reported in guinea pigs. Thus, administration of captopril, twice a day for 2 weeks, had no effect on cough induced by capsaicin, citric acid, or cigarette smoke (42). That responses to exogenous bradykinin *were* potentiated suggests that endogenous substrates for ACE, including kinins, are not important in modulating airway sensitivity to irritants in this model (42).

B. Effects in Vitro

1. Airway Smooth Muscle

Mentioned previously is the fact that kinins have little direct effect on the airway smooth muscle from dogs, cats, rabbits, rats, and man (5-7, 25-27,31-32). Conversely, in trachea isolated from ferrets (67,68) or guinea pigs (5,23), bradykinin causes contraction. Alternatively, if guinea pig trachea is precontracted with histamine, bradykinin induces relaxation (69,70). In addition, some have reported that, in guinea pig trachea with basal tone, application of bradykinin causes relaxation, which is abolished by removal of the epithelial layer (23,71,72). Following epithelium removal bradykinin causes contraction, and it has been suggested that bradykinin may cause the release of smooth muscle inhibitory prostaglandins, such as PGE_2, which mediate the relaxation (71,72). Cultured tracheal epithelial cells from dogs also release an airway smooth muscle inhibitory prostaglandin (probably PGE_2) in response to bradykinin (73). Thus, indomethacin abolishes bradykinin-induced, epithelium-dependent tracheal relaxation in both species (71-73).

The airway epithelium has an inhibitory influence on the spasmogenic effects of other bronchoconstrictors, in addition to bradykinin (74,75). The stimulatory effect of removing the epithelium on airway responses to bradykinin may be relevant to the known disruption and sloughing of airway epithelium during asthma (76), in addition to the fact that bradykinin is a bronchoconstrictor in asthmatics but not nonasthmatics (see above). However, the exquisite hyperreactivity of the asthmatic airways, not only to bradykinin, but to many other pharmacological and nonpharmacological stimuli, probably has several contributing factors (77-79).

Unlike the guinea pig trachea, contractile responses of ferret trachea to bradykinin are unaffected by removing the epithelium (68). On the other hand, inhibitors of ACE or neutral endopeptidase (NEP, 3.4.24.11) cause sinistral shifts in bradykinin and kallidin concentration-response curves in ferret trachea, suggesting that these enzymes are important to kinin degradation in vitro (68). It was also demonstrated that the metabolic products of bradykinin degradation by ACE and NEP, the C-terminal dipeptide bradykinin-(8-9), and the N-terminal heptapeptide bradykinin-(1-7), were inactive or very weak in their respective abilities to contract ferret trachea (68). We have also found that, in the presence of a cocktail of inhibitors of ACE, NEP, and kininase I, there is a small, approximately threefold sinistral shift in the concentration-response curve for bradykinin-induced contractions in guinea pig epithelium-denuded trachea (23) (S. G. Farmer, unpublished observations). Minor enzymatic degradation of bradykinin, therefore, may also have some importance in this tissue.

Contractions of guinea pig trachea, induced by low concentrations of bradykinin ($\leqslant 0.1\ \mu M$), are inhibited by cyclooxygenase inhibitors such as aspirin (5) and indomethacin (23,72), suggesting they are mediated by excitatory prostaglandins. Even in the presence of indomethacin though, higher concentrations of bradykinin ($\geqslant 0.1\ \mu M$) elicit tracheal contraction (23) (S. G. Farmer and R. M. Burch, unpublished observations). Bradykinin, therefore, seems to cause prostaglandin-dependent and -independent contraction of this tissue. In guinea pig tracheal smooth muscle cells in culture, bradykinin causes concentration-dependent release of PGE_2 and the stable prostacyclin metabolite 6-keto-$PGF_{1\alpha}$ (R. M. Burch and S. G. Farmer, unpublished observations). Release of these eicosanoids was abolished by indomethacin. Interestingly, we could not detect the release of TxA_2. Nevertheless, and unlike most smooth muscle tissues, prostacyclin causes contraction of guinea pig trachea (80) (S. G. Farmer, unpublished observations).

In guinea pig trachea which has been precontracted with histamine, bradykinin and its stable analog [Tyr(Me^8)]bradykinin cause concentration-dependent relaxations which are abolished by indomethacin (69) and several other cyclooxygenase inhibitors (70). Bradykinin-induced relaxation of guinea pig trachea, then, is dependent upon prostaglandin biosynthesis.

Airway Bradykinin Receptors. While there are several reports of the pulmonary effects of bradykinin on airways in vivo and in vitro, there is a paucity of information on the nature of bradykinin receptors mediating those effects. In precontracted guinea pig trachea, bradykinin causes concentration-dependent relaxations, as discussed above. DesArg^9-bradykinin, a B1 receptor agonist, is inactive in this tissue, and bradykinin-induced relaxation is not blocked by desArg^9[Leu^8]bradykinin (a B1 receptor antagonist) or by NPC 567 or [Thi^{6,9},DPhe^8]kallidin (B2 antagonists) (70,81). The lack of effect of the B1 or B2 receptor antagonists indicate that bradykinin-induced, eicosanoid-dependent relaxation of guinea pig trachea is not mediated by either the B1 or B2 receptor subtype (69,70). Indeed, it was suggested that bradykinin-induced tracheal relaxation may not be mediated by bradykinin receptors (70).

Recently, we examined the effect of several B1 and B2 receptor antagonists on bradykinin-induced contraction of guinea pig airway smooth muscle in vitro, as well as on bradykinin-induced bronchoconstriction in vivo. The relative ineffectiveness of B1 and B2 antagonists to inhibit bradykinin-induced bronchoconstriction in anesthetized guinea pigs is described above (see Section II.A.2). As bradykinin is a bronchoconstrictor in asthmatic patients, we were interested in the nature of receptors mediating its excitatory effects.

Membranes prepared from guinea pig lungs and tracheal smooth muscle contain saturable, specific binding sites for bradykinin, but not desArg^9-bradykinin (23). Neither desArg^9[Leu^8]-bradykinin nor NPC 567 displace bradykinin from the tracheal binding site, and in lung membranes NPC 567 displaced only 60% of total specifically bound bradykinin. Furthermore, sheep trachea and lung also contain binding sites for bradykinin from which NPC 567 displaces only 28% and 73% of [^{3}H]-bradykinin binding, respectively (23). DesArg^9[Leu^8]bradykinin was without effect in sheep airway tissue. Thus, pulmonary tissue appears to contain a novel bradykinin binding site for which the designation "B3 receptor" has been proposed (23).

In functional studies, desArg^9-bradykinin was without effect on tracheal tone, and bradykinin-induced contraction was not affected by desArg^9 [Leu^8]-bradykinin, a B1 antagonist (23). In addition, several B2 receptor antagonists, including NPC 349 and NPC 567, had minimal effects on bradykinin-induced contraction, providing further evidence for a novel receptor mediating tracheal contraction (23).

Evidence for the existence of the B3 receptor will only be conclusive when specific antagonists become available. Nevertheless, recent findings provide further confirmation for B3 receptors, mediating efflux of $^{45}Ca^{2+}$ in guinea pig trachealis. In guinea pig tracheal smooth muscle cells, grown in culture, bradykinin causes prostaglandin synthesis (see above) and stimulates the efflux of $^{45}Ca^{2+}$ (R. M. Burch and S. G. Farmer, unpublished observations). Whereas indomethacin abolishes prostaglandin production, in response to bradykinin, the cyclooxygenase inhibitor is completely without effect on $^{45}Ca^{2+}$ efflux. In addition, NPC 567 inhibits bradykinin-induced prostaglandin synthesis in these cells, indicating that there are, in fact, B2 receptors present. The biological observations are supported by the ability of NPC 567 to compete for binding of [^{3}H]bradykinin to membranes prepared from these cells. The efflux of $^{45}Ca^{2+}$, however, is completely resistant to NPC 567 and is not stimulated by desArg^9-bradykinin.

The physiological relevance of this novel bradykinin receptor is unclear at present, as is the nature of bradykinin receptors mediating the airway effects in man. NPC 567, although weak, did partially inhibit bradykinin-induced bronchoconstriction in guinea pigs, suggesting that the B2 receptors detected in lung binding may have some functional significance (23). Furthermore, NPC 567 is a relatively potent antagonist of bradykinin-induced bronchoconstriction in sheep (82,83) suggesting that there are functional B2 receptors, as has also been suggested from ligand binding studies in sheep trachea and lung (23). These receptors appear to be located throughout the airways with the greatest distribution found in the distal airways (lung parenchyma) as compared to proximal airways (tracheal smooth muscle).

Based on observations that the pulmonary effects of bradykinin in sheep are blocked by nedocromil sodium or atropine (30), one possibility is that the B2 receptors in the airways are associated with sensory nerves, whereas the B3 receptors are located on airway smooth muscle cells. As discussed by Abraham (Chapter 11), NPC 567 inhibits allergen-induced airway hyperresponsiveness and late asthmatic responses in allergic sheep, indicating not only that bradykinin is involved in these phenomena but also that its effects are mediated largely by B2 receptors.

2. *Bradykinin Signal Transduction in the Airways*

Activation of B2 receptors in virtually all tissues so far described leads to stimulation of phosphatidylinositol-specific phospholipase C activity, resulting in the formation of inositol phosphates and diacylglycerol (49,84-89). Eicosanoid synthesis may also be enhanced, possibly by release of arachidonic acid from the diacylglycerol generated during inositol lipid hydrolysis. In several tissues, however, inositol lipid hydrolysis is pharmacologically independent of arachidonate release and has been proposed to result from activation of phospholipase A_2 (88,90,91).

In addition, B2 receptor activation, in tissues including the lungs, may lead to enhanced cellular accumulation of cyclic AMP (92,93). This is due to stimulation of the biosynthesis of eicosanoids, which subsequently bind to their receptors and activate adenylate cyclase (93). In guinea pig lung slices, for example, bradykinin produces a rapid rise in the concentrations of both cyclic AMP and cyclic GMP (92). Bradykinin-induced increases in cAMP levels, but not cGMP levels, were inhibited by aspirin and indomethacin. Since PGE_1 and PGE_2 activate adenylate cyclase in guinea pig lung tissue, the authors suggested that bradykinin induced prostaglandin production as a consequence of stimulating guanylate cyclase. Increased cellular levels of cAMP, in turn, are mediated by prostaglandins (92).

In perfused lungs, several studies have demonstrated that bradykinin stimulates the release of eicosanoids. In guinea pig lungs, bradykinin causes indomethacin- and aspirin-sensitive release of TxA_2 and other prostaglandins, as determined by bioassay on several smooth muscle preparations (94). Interestingly, a later study demonstrated that the release of TxA_2 from guinea pig lungs, provoked by histamine and serotonin, but *not* by bradykinin, is inhibited by dexamethasone (95). This may be related to the earlier report that bradykinin-induced bronchoconstriction is inhibited by aspirin but not by cortisone (2). Since glucocorticosteroids, via production of lipocortin, inhibit phospholipase A_2 (96), it appears that bradykinin-induced release of arachidonic acid in guinea pig lungs is independent of this enzyme and may involve a phospholipid-phospholipase C.

Bakhle and colleagues have shown that bradykinin releases 6-oxo-$PGF_{1\alpha}$ and thromboxane from guinea pig perfused lungs (97). The eicosanoids were analyzed both by radioimmunoassay and by bioassay on strips of trachea. The effects of bradykinin were abolished by indomethacin, and no evidence for bradykinin-induced release of leukotriene-like substances was seen (97). A selective and potent LTD_4 receptor antagonist, SK&F-104353 (98), does not influence bradykinin-induced contraction of guinea pig trachea (S. G. Farmer and R. M. Burch, unpublished observations), indicating further that peptidoleukotrienes are not involved in this response.

In human cultured tracheal smooth muscle cells, bradykinin receptors are coupled to changes in cytosolic Ca^{2+}, causing concentration-dependent increases (99). β-Adrenoceptor activation in these cells stimulated adenylate cyclase activity, but the effect of bradykinin was not examined (99).

3. Neurogenic Inflammation and Pulmonary Microvascular Effects of Kinins

Bradykinin increases microvascular permeability, contributing to the acute inflammatory response (see Chapter 1). Thus, kinins may bring about many physiological responses, including pain and hyperalgesia by stimulating C- and A-fibers in the periphery (45,100-105). As discussed in Chapters 4 and 8, there is also considerable evidence that kinins contribute to the inflammatory response (48,51).

Airway neurogenic inflammation is the process whereby vasoactive and bronchoconstrictor neuropeptides, such as substance P and neurokinin A, are released from sensory nerve endings (106-111). There has been a great deal of interest in the potential involvement of neurogenic inflammation in the pathophysiology of asthma in recent years. Kinins, by virtue of their ability to sensitize and stimulate afferent nerve endings in the airway, probably contribute to airway neurogenic inflammation.

For example, local injection of bradykinin into the trachea of anesthetized rats causes protein extravasation that was dramatically reduced by neonatal treatment with capsaicin, which abolishes sensory nerve release of neuropeptides (112). Intravenous bradykinin also causes increased microvascular permeability changes in the airways of guinea pigs (113). Recently, it was shown that several putative mediators of pulmonary inflammation, including bradykinin, cause a significant release of immunoreactive tachykinins in rat superfused trachea (114) and guinea pig perfused lungs (115). Similar release could also be achieved by vagal nerve stimulation, presumably due to antidromic stimulation of afferent C-fibers (115). Finally, bradykinin-induced microvascular leakage in the guinea pig may also involve eicosanoids and platelet-activating factor (PAF), since WEB 2086, a PAF antagonist, or indomethacin inhibited the effect of bradykinin (116).

4. Airway Secretion

Bradykinin is one of several mediators that stimulate airway mucosal electrolyte secretion (117,118). For instance, in canine isolated tracheal mucosa, bradykinin stimulates Cl^- ion secretion and PGE_2 release (119). Autoradiographical studies showed specific bradykinin binding sites in this tissue, located on the epithelial cells (119). Indomethacin abolished bradykinin-induced Cl^- secretion and PGE_2 synthesis, indicating that its effect on secretion is mediated indirectly by prostaglandin (119).

In canine isolated tracheal mucosa, bradykinin and kallidin both induce increases in transmembrane ion conductance, effects which are reversibly inhibited by the B1 and B2 receptor antagonist NPC 349 (120). That desArg^9-bradykinin was inactive implies that the receptors mediating kinin effects, and which are on the luminal membrane in this tissue, are of the B2 subtype. In contrast to canine airway, Kyle and Widdicombe found that neither bradykinin nor kallidin stimulate mucus secretion in ferret trachea (67).

In dog tracheal explants, rather large concentrations of kallidin and Met,Lys-bradykinin both enhance the incorporation of radiolabeled glucosamine into high molecular weight molecules, probably mucin-type glycoproteins, implying further that kinins are involved in airway mucus production (121). It is interesting that bradykinin was without effect in this report, suggesting that, under some circumstances, bradykinin and kallidin activate different receptors.

The potential interactions between cyclic AMP and intracellular Ca^{2+} in regulating airway epithelial Cl^- secretion, induced by isoproterenol and bradykinin, were recently examined (122). Both agonists increased intracellular cAMP, but only bradykinin was inhibited by indomethacin, providing further evidence for the mediation by prostaglandins of the bradykinin effect. Whereas isoproterenol and bradykinin both caused transient increases in cytosolic Ca^{2+}, from intracellular stores, only bradykinin stimulated accumulation of inositol phospholipids. The latter effect of the kinin was unaffected by indomethacin, but the cyclooxygenase inhibitor reduced the peak increase in Ca^{2+} (122). It was proposed that β-adrenoceptor activation increases cytosolic Ca^{2+} via cAMP independently of phosphoinositides. Conversely, bradykinin increases intracellular Ca^{2+} directly, via receptor-mediated stimulation of phospholipase C, and indirectly via prostaglandin-induced elevations in cellular cAMP (122).

5. Ciliary Function

In addition to secreting mucus and electrolytes, mucociliary clearance by the pulmonary epithelium plays a vital role in clearing inhaled debris and bacteria from the airways. A few studies have examined possible effects of kinins on airway ciliary function. Inhalation of aerosolized bradykinin increased ciliary beat frequency in the tracheae of anesthetized dogs, an effect which was abolished by the autonomic ganglion blocker, hexamethonium, or by indomethacin (123). It was proposed that bradykinin-induced stimulation of airway ciliary beat frequency is prostaglandin- and nerve-mediated.

These preliminary findings were recently extended in rabbit tracheal epithelial cells in culture, wherein bradykinin elicited a rapid, 35% transient increase in ciliary beat frequency (124). The effect of bradykinin was inhibited, in a concentration-dependent fashion, by the B1 and B2 receptor antagonist NPC 349 but was unaffected by desArg^9[Leu^8]bradykinin, a B1 antagonist. Ciliary stimulation by bradykinin was also inhibited by removing calcium from the buffer, by the voltage-operated Ca^{2+} channel blocker, nifedipine, by indomethacin, and by the rather nonspecific phospholipase A_2 inhibitor, mepacrine (124). In addition, bradykinin increased PGE_2 release and this, too, was abolished by calcium removal or indomethacin. The ACE inhibitor captopril was without effect, whereas phosphoramidon, an NEP inhibitor, potentiated the effect of bradykinin. It was suggested, therefore, that bradykinin-induced stimulation of airway cilia is mediated by activation of epithelial B2 receptors, Ca^{2+} influx, and PGE_2 production. Further, NEP may play a role in modulating the effect of endogenous kinins (124).

III. CONCLUDING REMARKS

Bradykinin is only one of several mediators, including peptidoleukotrienes, PAF, various neuropeptides and neurotransmitters, implicated in the pathophysiology of bronchial asthma. While it is unlikely that asthma is a "single mediator disease," the pharmaceutical industry has, particularly in recent years, been consuming vast resources in the search for antagonists of the receptors of these mediators. The potential role of each of these substances, including kinins, in airway inflammatory disease will only become apparent with the clinical use of specific antagonists. Indeed, the ideal therapy for asthma may lie in the use of two or more drugs simultaneously.

As alluded to in previous pages, although the bronchospastic effect of bradykinin is inhibited by nonsteroidal, anti-inflammatory drugs in guinea pigs, aspirin is neither an inhibitor of bradykinin-induced bronchoconstriction, nor is it a useful antiasthmatic in man. Caution should, as always, therefore, be used in extrapolating results obtained in animals to potential effects in the clinic.

Conversely, the bronchoconstrictor effect per se of endogenous kinins may not be important in the asthmatic airways. Indeed, antigen-induced bronchoconstriction in guinea pigs or sheep is unaltered by NPC 567. Rather, kinins, which stimulate and sensitize airway sensory nerve endings, and which can lead to the production of other inflammatory substances, may be involved in airway hyperreactivity. A hallmark feature of asthma is the nonspecific airway hyperreactivity, which manifests itself as an extreme sensitivity, or "twitchiness" of the asthmatic airways to many stimuli (77-79). Thus, data in an animal model of allergen-induced airway hyperresponsiveness, inflammation, and late onset reactions (see Chapter 11) suggest that a bradykinin antagonist may represent a potentially novel approach for the prophylaxis of bronchial asthma.

It is clear that in the past few years our understanding of the role played by bradykinin, both in normal animals and during pathological states, has developed considerably. This is due, to an extent, to the discovery of specific antagonists of kinin receptors. In addition to being of limited pharmacological potency, however, all of the currently available agents are peptides and, as such, metabolically labile. There are indications, nevertheless, that the peptide antagonists have clinical potential. NPC 567 is anticipated to enter clinical development in 1990 as an inhalational, prophylactic treatment for bronchial asthma. As more stable, nonpeptide bradykinin antagonists become available, hopefully in the not too distant future, novel, potentially orally active drugs will augment our current armamentarium for treating many airway inflammatory diseases.

REFERENCES

1. Collier, H. O. J., J. A. Holgate, M. Schachter, and P. G. Shorley. An apparent bronchoconstrictor action of bradykinin and its suppression by some anti-inflammatory agents. *J. Physiol.* **149**:54P (1959).
2. Collier, H. O. J., J. A. Holgate, M. Schachter, and P. G. Shorley. The bronchoconstrictor action of bradykinin in the guinea-pig. *Br. J. Pharmacol.* **15**: 290-297 (1960).
3. Collier, H. O. J., and P. G. Shorley. Analgesic antipyretic drugs as antagonists of bradykinin. *Br. J. Pharmacol.* **15**:601-610 (1960).
4. Konzett, H., and Stürmer, E. Biological activity of synthetic polypeptides with bradykinin-like properties. *Br. J. Pharmacol.* **15**:544-551 (1960).
5. Bhoola, K. D., H. O. J. Collier, M. Schachter, and P. G. Shorley. Action of some peptides on bronchial muscle. *Br. J. Pharmacol.* **19**:190-197 (1962).
6. Greeff, K., and E. Moog. Vergleichende Untersuchungen über die bronchokonstrictorische und gefäßkonstrictorische Wirkung des Bradykinins, Histamins und Serotonins an isolierten Lungenpräparaten. *Naunyn-Schmiedeberg's Arch. Exp. Pathol. Pharmakol.* **248**:204-215 (1964).
7. Hauge, A., P. K. M. Lunde, and B. A. Waaler. The effect of bradykinin, kallidin and eledoisin upon the pulmonary vascular bed of an isolated blood-perfused rabbit lung preparation. *Acta Physiol. Scand.* **66**:269-277 (1966).
8. Herxheimer, H., and E. Stresemann. The effect of bradykinin aerosol in guinea-pigs and in man. *J. Physiol.* **158**:38P (1961).
9. Lecomte, J., J. M. Petit, J. Mélon, J. Troquet, and R. Marcelle. Propriétés bronchoconstrictrices de la bradykinine chez l'homme asthmatique. *Arch. Int. Pharmacodyn. Ther.* **137**:232-235 (1962).
10. Girard, J. P., and P. Moret. Action de la sérotonine et de la bradykinine en aérosols chez les asthmatiques. *Helv. Med Acta* **30**:520-526 (1963).
11. Stresemann, E. Die Wirkung von Bradykinin-Aerosol auf die Atmung des Menschen und des Meerschweinchens und der Einfluß verschiedener Substanzen auf den experimentellen Bradykinin-Bronchospasmus. *Acta Allergol.* (Kbh.) **18**:235-255 (1963).
12. Herxheimer, H., and E. Stresemann. Bradykinin and ethanol in bronchial asthma. *Arch. Int. Pharmacodyn. Ther.* **144**:315-318 (1963).
13. Collier, H. O. J. Kinins and ventilation of the lungs, in: *Handbook of Experimental Pharmacology*, Volume XXV (E. G. Erdös, ed.). Springer-Verlag, Berlin, Heidelberg, New York, pp. 409-420 (1970).
14. Elliott, D. F., E. W. Horton, and G. P. Lewis. Actions of pure bradykinin. *J. Physiol.* **153**:473-480 (1960).
15. Gjuris, V., and E. Westermann. Bronchoconstrictor action of bradykinin, kallidin and eledoisin. *Nature* **205**:402-404 (1965).
16. James, G. W. L. The use of an *in vivo* trachea preparation of the guinea-pig to assess drug action on the lung. *J. Pharm. Pharmacol.* **21**:379-386 (1969).
17. Drazen, J. M., and K. F. Austen. Effects of intravenous administration of slow-reacting substance of anaphylaxis, histamine, bradykinin and prosta-

glandin $F_{2\alpha}$ on pulmonary mechanics in the guinea pig. *J. Clin. Invest.* **53**: 1679-1685 (1974).
18. Drazen, J. M., and K. F. Austen. Atropine modification of the pulmonary effects of chemical mediators in the guinea-pig. *J. Appl. Physiol.* **38**:834-838 (1975).
19. Lefort, J., and B. B. Vargaftig. Role of platelets in aspirin-sensitive bronchoconstriction in the guinea-pig; interactions with salicyclic acid. *Br. J. Pharmacol.* **63**:35-42 (1978).
20. Altinkurt, O., and I. Kanzik. Effects of vitamin K_3 on the hypotensive and bronchoconstrictive responses to bradykinin and histamine in the guinea pig. *Arzneim. -Forsch.* **30**:286-287 (1980).
21. Folco, G., C. Omini, G. Rossoni, T. Vigano, and F. Berti. Anticholinergic agents prevent guinea-pig airway constriction induced by histamine, bradykinin and leukotriene C_4; relationship to circulating TXA_2. *Eur. J. Pharmacol.* **78**:159-165 (1982).
22. Rossoni, G., C. Omini, T.Uigano, V. Mandelli, G. C. Follo, and F. Berti. Bronchoconstriction by histamine and bradykinin in guinea pigs: Relationship to thromboxane A_2 generation and the effect of aspirin. *Prostaglandins* **20**:547-557 (198;6).
23. Farmer, S. G., R. M. Burch, S. N. Meeker, and D. E. Wilkins. Evidence for a pulmonary bradykinin B_3 receptor. *Mol. Pharmacol.* **36**:1-8 (1989).
24. Jin, L. S., E. Seeds, C. P. Page, and M. Schachter. Inhibition of bradykinin-induced bronchoconstriction in the guinea-pig by a synthetic B_2 receptor antagonist. *Br. J. Pharmacol.* **97**:598-602 (1989).
25. Waaler, B. A. The effect of bradykinin in an isolated perfused dog lung preparation. *J. Physiol.* **157**:475-483 (1961).
26. Kaufman, M. P., H. M. Coleridge, J. C. G. Coleridge, and D. G. Baker. Bradykinin stimulates afferent vagal C-fibers in intrapulmonary airways of dogs. *J. Appl. Physiol.* **48**:511-517 (1980).
27. Roberts, A. M., M. P. Kaufman, D. G. Baker, J. K. Brown, H. M. Coleridge, and J. C. G. Coleridge. Reflex tracheal contraction induced by stimulation of bronchial C-fibers in dogs. *J. Appl. Physiol.* **51**:485-493 (1981).
28. Coleridge, H. M., J. C. G. Coleridge, and H. D. Schultz. Afferent pathways involved in reflex regulation of airway smooth muscle. *Pharmacol. Ther.* **42**:1-63 (1989).
29. Soler, M., M. Sielczak, and W. M. Abraham. A bradykinin antagonist blocks antigen-induced airway hyperresponsiveness and inflammation in sheep. *Pulm. Pharmacol.* **3**:9-15.
30. Abraham, W. M., A. Ahmed, A. Cortes, M. Soler, S. G. Farmer, L. E. Baugh, and S. L. Harbeson. Airway effects of inhaled bradykinin, substance P and neurokinin A in sheep (submitted).
31. Simonsson, B. G., B.-E. Skoogh, N. P. Bergh, R. Andersson, and N. Svedmyr. *In vivo* and *in vitro* effect of bradykinin on bronchial motor tone in normal subjects and patients with airways obstruction. *Respiration* **30**:378-388 (1973).

32. Fuller, R. W., C. M. S. Dixon, F. M. C. Cuss, and P. J. Barnes. Bradykinin-induced bronchoconstriction in humans: Mode of action. *Am. Rev. Respir. Dis.* **135**:176-180 (1987).
33. Della Bella, D., G. Benelli, E. Pajola, and P. Valli. Bronchial motility regulation and bradykinin. *Adv. Exp. Med. Biol.* **21**:277-283 (1972).
34. Berry, P. A., and H. O. J. Collier. Bronchoconstrictor action and antagonism of a slow-reacting substance from anaphylaxis of guinea-pig lung. *Br. J. Pharmacol.* **23**:201-216 (1964).
35. Greenberg, R., G. H. Osman, E. H. O'Keefe, and M. J. Antonaccio. The effects of captopril (SQ 14,225) on bradykinin-induced bronchoconstriction in the anesthetized guinea pig. *Eur. J. Pharmacol.* **57**:287-294 (1979).
36. Piper, P. J., H. O. J. Collier, and J. R. Vane. Release of catecholamines in the guinea-pig by substances involved in anaphylaxis. *Nature* **213**:838-840 (1967).
37. Staszewska-Barczak, J., and J. R. Vane. The release of catecholamines from the adrenal medulla by peptides. *Br. J. Pharmacol.* **30**:;655-667 (1967).
38. Terragno, N. A., and A. Terragno. Release of vasoactive substances by kinins, in: *Bradykinin, Kallidin and Kallikrein, Handbook of Experimental Pharmacology*, Volume XXV, Supplement (E. G. Erdös, ed.). Springer-Verlag, Berlin, Heidelberg, New York, pp. 401-426 (1979).
39. Mazzoni, L., J. Morley, S. Sanjar, and E. Schaueblin. An anomalous interaction between propranolol and isoprenaline. *Br. J. Pharmacol.* **91**:326P (1987).
40. Dixon, E. J. A., P. Wilsoncroft, D. N. Roberson, and C. P. Page. The effect of Paf antagonists on bronchial hyperresponsiveness induced by Paf, propranolol or indomethacin. *Br. J. Pharmacol.* **97**:717-722 (1989).
41. Ney, U. M. Propranolol-induced airway hyperreactivity in guinea-pigs. *Br. J. Pharmacol.* **79**:1003-1009 (1983).
42. Karlsson, J.-A., C. Zackrisson, and K. Forsberg. Effect of prolonged inhibition of angiotensin converting enzyme on MK-447. Studies on the irritant induced cough and bronchoconstriction in guinea-pigs. *Am. Rev. Respir. Dis.* **137** (Suppl.):508 (1988).
43. Kimura, K., M. Miura, U. Katsumata, H. Inoue, and T. Takishima. Bradykinin-induced airway hyperreactivity in a perfused bronchial artery preparation. *Am. Rev. Respir. Dis.* **139**:A106 (1989).
44. Omini, C., G. Brunelli, A. Hernandez, and L. Daffonchio. Bradykinin and substance P potentiate acetylcholine-induced bronchoconstriction in guinea pig. *Eur. J. Pharmacol.* **163**:195-197 (1989).
45. Steranka, L. R., S. G. Farmer, and R. M. Burch. Antagonists of B_2 bradykinin receptors. *FASEB J.* **3**:2019-2025 (1989).
46. Brocklehurst, W. E., and S. C. Lahiri. The production of bradykinin during anaphylaxis. *J. Physiol.* **160**:15-16P (1962).
47. Jonasson, O., and E. L. Becker. Release of kallikrein from guinea-pig lung during anaphylaxis. *J. Exp. Med.* **123**:509-522 (1966).

48. Marceau, F., A. Lussier, D. Regoli, and J. P. Giroud. Pharmacology of kinins: Their relevance to tissue injury and inflammation. *Gen. Pharmacol.* **14**: 209-229 (1983).
49. Burch, R. M., S. G. Farmer, and L. R. Steranka. Bradykinin receptor antagonists. *Med. Res. Rev.* **10**:237-269.
50. Proud, D., A. Togias, R. M. Naclerio, S. A. Crush, P. S. Norman, and L. M. Lichtenstein. Kinins are generated *in vivo* following nasal airway challenge of allergic individuals with allergen. *J. Clin. Invest.* **72**:1678-1685 (1983).
51. Proud, D., and A. P. Kaplan. Kinin formation: Mechanisms and role in inflammatory disorders. *Annu. Rev. Immunol.* **6**:49-84 (1988).
52. Proud, D., C. J. Reynolds, S. Lacapra, A. Kagey-Sobotka, L. M. Lichtenstein, and R. M. Naclerio. Nasal provocation with bradykinin induces symptoms of rhinitis and a sore throat. *Am. Rev. Respir. Dis.* **137**:613-616 (1988).
53. Varonier, H. S., and R. Panzani. The effect of inhalations of bradykinin on healthy and atopic (asthmatic) children. *Int. Arch. Allergy* **34**:293-296 (1968).
54. Dixon, C. M. S., and P. J. Barnes. Bradykinin-induced bronchoconstriction: Inhibition by nedocromil sodium and sodium cromoglycate. *Br. J. Clin. Pharmacol.* **27**:831-836 (1989).
55. Abe, K., N. Watanabe, N. Kumagai, T. Mouri, T. Seki, and K. Yoshinaga. Circulating plasma kinin in patients with bronchial asthma. *Experientia* **23**: 626-627 (1967).
56. Christiansen, S. C., D. Proud, and C. G. Cochrane. Detection of tissue kallikrein in the bronchoalveolar lavage fluid of asthmatic subjects. *J. Clin. Invest.* **79**:188-197 (1987).
57. Newball, H. H., H. R. Keiser, and J. J. Pisano. Bradykinin and human airways. *Respir. Physiol.* **24**:139-146 (1975).
58. Devillier, P., M. Renoux, G. Drapeau, and D. Regoli. Histamine release from rat peritoneal mast cells by kinin antagonists. *Eur. J. Pharmacol.* **149**: 137-140 (1988).
59. Lawrence, I. D., J. A. Warner, V. L. Cohan, L. M. Lichtenstein, A. Kagey-Sobotka, R. J. Vavrek, J. M. Stewart, and D. Proud. Induction of histamine release from human skin mast cells by bradykinin analogs. *Biochem. Pharmacol.* **38**:227-233 (1989).
60. Dixon, C. M. S., R. W. Fuller, and P. J. Barnes. The effect of an angiotensin converting enzyme inhibitor, ramipril, on bronchial responses to inhaled histamine and bradykinin in asthmatic subjects. *Br. J. Clin. Pharmacol.* **23**: 91-93 (1987).
61. Morice, A. H., R. Lowry, M. J. Brown, and T. Higenbottam. Angiotensin-converting enzyme and the cough reflex. *Lancet* **Nov. 14**:1116-1118 (1987).
62. Stoller, J. K., A. C. Mehta, and D. G. Vidt. Captopril-induced cough. *Chest* **93**:659-661 (1988).
63. Morice, A. H., M. J. Brown, and T. Higenbottam. Cough associated with angiotensin converting enzyme inhibition. *J. Cardiovasc. Pharmacol.* **13 Suppl. 3**:S59-S62 (1989).

64. Cough and wheeze in asthma: Are they interdependent? *Lancet* **Feb. 27**:447-448 (1988).
65. Bucknall, C. E., J. B. Neilly, R. Carter, R. D. Stevenson, and P. F. Semple. Bronchial hyperreactivity in patients who cough after receiving angiotensin converting enzyme inhibitors. *Br. Med. J.* **296**:86-88 (1988).
66. Choudry, N. B., R. W. Fuller, and N. B. Pride. Sensitivity of the human cough reflex: Effect of inflammatory mediators prostaglandin E_2, bradykinin and histamine. *Am. Rev. Respir. Dis.* **140**:137-141 (1989).
67. Kyle, H., and J. G. Widdicombe. The effects of peptides and mediators on mucus secretion and smooth muscle tone in the ferret trachea. *Agents Actions* **22**:86-90 (1987).
68. Dusser, D. J., J. A. Nadel, K. Sekizawa, P. D. Graf, and D. B. Borson. Neutral endopeptidase and angiotensin converting enzyme inhibitors potentiate kinin-induced contraction of ferret trachea. *J. Pharmacol. Exp. Ther.* **244**: 531-536 (1988).
69. Mizrahi, J., P. D'Orléans-Juste, S. Caranikas, and D. Regoli. Effects of peptides and amines on isolated guinea pig tracheae as influenced by inhibitors of the metabolism of arachidonic acid. *Pharmacol.* **25**:320-326 (1982).
70. Rhaleb, N.-E., S. Dion, P. D'Orléans-Juste, G. Drapeau, D. Regoli, and R. G. Browne. Bradykinin antagonism: Differentiation between peptide antagonists and inflammatory agents. *Eur. J. Pharmacol.* **151**:275-279 (1988).
71. Bewley, J., K. D. Bhoola, D. M. Crothers, and M. I. Cingi. Biphasic responses of the isolated guinea-pig tracheal muscle strip to kallidin and bradykinin. *Br. J. Pharmacol.* **92**:597P (1988).
72. Bramley, A. M., M. N. Samhoun, and P. J. Piper. Modulation of bradykinin-induced responses by indomethacin and removal of the epithelium in guinea pig trachea *in vitro*. *Br. J. Pharmacol.* **95**:774P (1988).
73. Barnett, K., D. B. Jacoby, J. A. Nadel, and S. C. Lazarus. The effects of epithelial cell supernatant on contractions of isolated canine tracheal smooth muscle. *Am. Rev. Respir. Dis.* **138**:780-783 (1988).
74. Farmer, S. G. Airway smooth muscle responsiveness: Modulation by the epithelium. *Trends Pharmacol. Sci.* **8**:8-10 (1987).
75. Goldie, R. G., L. B. Fernandes, S. G. Farmer, and D. W. P. Hay. Epithelium-derived inhibitory factor. *Trends Pharmacol. Sci.* **11**:67-70.
76. Laitinen, L. A., M. Heino, A. Laitinen, and T. Haahtela. Damage of the airway epithelium and bronchial reactivity in patients with asthma. *Am. Rev. Respir. Dis.* **131**:599-606 (1985).
77. Boushey, H. A., M. J. Holtzman, J. R. Sheller, and J. A. Nadel. State of the art: Bronchial hyperreactivity. *Am. Rev. Respir. Dis.* **121**:389-413 (1980).
78. Garland, L. G. The pharmacology of airway hyperreactivity. *Trends Pharmacol. Sci.* **5**:338-340 (1984).
79. Murlas, C. G. Pathogenesis of airway hyperreactivity. *Chest* **93**:1278-1280 (1988).

80. Dong, Y. J., R. L. Jones, and N. H. Wilson. Prostaglandin E receptor subtypes in smooth muscle: Agonist activities of stable prostacyclin analogues. *Br. J. Pharmacol.* **87**:97-107 (1986).
81. Regoli, D. Peptide receptors in the airways. *Am. Rev. Respir. Dis.* **136**:35S-39S (1987).
82. Abraham, W. M., L. E. Baugh, S. L. Harbeson, A. Cortes, and A. Ahmed. Airway effects of inhaled bradykinin and neurokinin A in allergic sheep. *Am. Rev. Respir. Dis.* **139**:A239 (1989).
83. Abraham, W. M., M. Soler, A. Ahmed, and A. Cortes. Pharmacology of bradykinin-induced bronchoconstriction in allergic sheep. *FASEB J.* **3**:282 (1989).
84. Higashida, H., and D. A. Brown. Ca^{2+}-dependent K^+ channels in neuroblastoma hybrid cells activated by intracellular inositol trisphosphate and extracellular bradykinin. *FEBS Lett.* **238**:395-400 (1988).
85. Portilla, D., J. Morrissey, and A. R. Morrison. Bradykinin-activated membrane-associated phospholipase C in Madin-Darby canine kidney cells. *J. Clin. Invest.* **81**:1896-1902 (1988).
86. Volonté, C., G. S. Parries, and E. Racker. Stimulation of inositol incorporation into lipids of PC12 cells by nerve growth factor and bradykinin. *J. Neurochem.* **51**:1156-1162 (1988).
87. Chuang, D.-M. Neurotransmitter receptors and phosphoinositide turnover. *Annu. Rev. Pharmacol. Toxicol.* **29**:71-110 (1989).
88. Kaya, H., G. M. Patton, and S. L. Hong. Bradykinin-induced activation of phospholipase A_2 is independent of the activation of polyphosphoinositide-hydrolyzing phospholipase C. *J. Biol. Chem.* **264**:4972-4977 (1989).
89. Perney, T. M., and R. J. Miller. Two different G-proteins mediate neuropeptide Y and bradykinin- stimulated phospholipid breakdown in cultured rat sensory neurons. *J. Biol. Chem.* **264**:7317-7327 (1989).
90. Burch, R. M., and J. Axelrod. Dissociation of bradykinin-stimulated arachidonic acid release from inositol phosphate formation in Swiss 3T3 fibroblasts. Evidence for a G protein-dependent coupled phospholipase A_2. *Proc. Natl. Acad. Sci. USA* **84**:6374-6378 (1987).
91. Slivka, S. R., and P. A. Insel, Phorbol ester and neomycin dissociate bradykinin receptor- mediated arachidonic acid release and polyphosphoinositide hydrolysis in Madin-Darby canine kidney cells. Evidence that bradykinin mediates noninterdependent activation of phospholipases A_2 and C. *J. Biol. Chem.* **263**:14640-14647 (1988).
92. Stoner, J., V. C. Maganiello, and M. Vaughan. Effects of bradykinin and indomethacin on cyclic GMP and cyclic AMP in lung slices. *Proc. Natl. Acad. Sci. USA* **70**:3830-3833 (1973).
93. Brunton, L. L., R. A. Wiklund, P. M. Van Arsdale, and A. G. Gilman. Binding of [^{3}H]prostaglandin E_1 to putative receptors linked to adenylate cyclase of cultured cell clones. *J. Biol. Chem.* **251**:3037-3044 (1976).

94. Palmer, M. A., P. J. Piper, and J. R. Vane. Release of rabbit aorta contracting substance (RCS) and prostaglandins induced by chemical or mechanical stimulation of guinea-pig lungs. *Br. J. Pharmacol.* **49**:226-242 (1973).
95. Blackwell, G. J., R. J. Flower, F. P. Nijkamp, and J. R. Vane. Phospholipase A_2 activity of guinea-pig isolated perfused lungs: Stimulation and inhibition by antiinflammatory steroids. *Br. J. Pharmacol.* **62**:79-89 (1978).
96. Flower, R. J. Lipocortin and the mechanism of action of the glucocorticoids. *Br. J. Pharmacol.* **94**:987-1013 (1988).
97. Bakhle, Y. S., S. Moncada, G. De Nucci, and J. A. Salmon. Differential release of eicosanoids by bradykinin, arachidonic acid and calcium ionophore A23187 in guiena-pig isolated perfused lung. *Br. J. Pharmacol.* **86**: 55-62 (1985).
98. Hay, D. W. P., R. M. Muccitelli, S. S. Tucker, L. M. Vickery-Clark, K. A. Wilson, J. G. Gleason, R. F. Hall, M. A. Wasserman, and T. J. Torphy. Pharmacologic profile of SK&F 104353: a novel, potent and selective peptidoleukotriene receptor antagonist in guinea pig and human airways. *J. Pharmacol. Exp. Ther.* **243**:474-481 (1987).
99. Panettieri, R. A., R. K. Murray, L. R. DePalo, P. A. Yadvish, and M. I. Kotlikoff. A human airway smooth muscle cell line that retains physiological responsiveness. *Am. J. Physiol.* **256**:C329-C335 (1989).
100. Clark, W. G. Kinins and peripheral and central nervous system, in: *Bradykinin, Kallidin and Kallikrein. Handbook of Experimental Pharmacology*, Volume XXV, Supplement (E. G. Erdös, ed.). Springer-Verlag, New York, pp. 311-356 (1979).
101. Griesbacher, T., and F. Lembeck. Effect of bradykinin antagonists on bradykinin-induced plasma extravasation, venoconstriction, prostaglandin E_2 release, and nociceptor stimulation and contraction of the iris sphincter muscle in the rabbit. *Br. J. Pharmacol.* **92**:333-340 (1987).
102. Taiwo, Y. O., and J. D. Levine. Characterization of the arachidonic acid metabolites mediating bradykinin and noradrenaline hyperalgesia. *Brain Res.* **458**:402-406 (1988).
103. Steranka, L. R., D. C. Manning, C. J. Dehaas, J. W. Ferkany, S. A. Borosky, J. R. Connor, R. J. Vavrek, J. M. Stewart, and S. H. Snyder. Bradykinin as a pain mediator: receptors are localized to sensory neurons, and antagonists have analgesic actions. *Proc. Natl. Acad. Sci. USA* **85**:3245-3249 (1988).
104. Dray, A., J. Bettaney, P. Forster, and M. N. Perkins. Bradykinin-induced stimulation of afferent fibres is mediated through protein kinase C. *Neurosci. Lett.* **91**:301-307 (1988).
105. Haley, J. E., A. H. Dickenson, and M. Schachter. Electrophysiological evidence for a role of bradykinin in chemical nociception in the rat. *Neurosci. Lett.* **97**:198-202 (1989).
106. Martling, C.-R. Sensory nerves containing tachykinins and CGRP in the lower airways. *Acta Physiol. Scand.* **130 (Suppl. 563)**:1-57 (1987).

107. McDonald, D. M. Neurogenic inflammation in the respiratory tract: Actions of sensory nerve mediators on blood vessels and epithelium of the airway mucosa. *Am. Rev. Respir. Dis.* **136 (Suppl.)**:S65-S72 (1987).
108. McDonald, D. M. Neurogenic inflammation in the rat trachea. I. Changes in venules, leucocytes and epithelial cells. *J. Neurocytol.* **17**:583-603 (1988).
109. McDonald, D. M., R. A. Mitchell, G. Gabella, and A. Haskell. Neurogenic inflammation in the rat trachea. II. Identity and distribution of nerves mediating the increase in vascular permeability. *J. Neurocytol.* **17**:605-628 (1988).
110. Kowalski, M. L., A. Didier, and M. A. Kaliner. Neurogenic inflammation in the airways. I. Neurogenic stimulation induces plasma protein extravasation into the rat airway lumen. *Am. Rev. Respir. Dis.* **140**:101-109 (1989).
111. Payan, D. G. Neuropeptides and inflammation: The role of substance P. *Annu. Rev. Med.* **40**:341-352 (1989).
112. Lundberg, J. M., and A. Saria. Capsaicin-induced desensitization of airway mucosa to cigarette smoke, mechanical and chemical irritants. *Nature* **302**:251-253 (1983).
113. Saria, A., J. M. Lundberg, G. Skofitsch, and F. Lembeck. Vascular protein leakage in various tissues induced by substance P, capsaicin, bradykinin, serotonin, histamine and by antigen challenge. *Naunyn-Schmiedeberg's Arch. Pharmacol.* **324**:212-218 (1983).
114. Ray, N. J., A. J. Jones, and P. Keen. Evidence that $GABA_B$ receptors can modulate release of substance P from capsaicin-sensitive neurons in rat trachea. *Br. J. Pharmacol.* **97**:562P (1989).
115. Saria, A., C.-R. Martling, Z. Yan, E. Theodorsson-Norheim, R. Gamse, and J. M. Lundberg. Release of multiple tachykinins from capsaicin-sensitive sensory nerves in the lung by bradykinin, histamine, dimethylphenyl piperazinium, and vagal nerve stimulation. *Am. Rev. Respir. Dis.* **137**:1330-1335 (1988).
116. Rogers, D. F., S. Dijk, and P. J. Barnes. Bradykinin induced microvascular leakage in guinea-pig airways *in vivo*: Involvement of platelet activating factor. *Am. Rev. Respir. Dis.* **137**:236 (1988).
117. Marin, M. G. Pharmacology of airway secretion. *Pharmacol. Rev.* **38**:273-289 (1986).
118. Welsh, M. J. Electrolyte transport by airway epithelia. *Physiol. Rev.* **67**: 1143-1184 (1987).
119. Leikauf, G. D., I. F. Ueki, J. A. Nadel, and J. H. Widdicombe. Bradykinin stimulates Cl^- secretion and prostaglandin E_2 release by canine tracheal epithelium. *Am. J. Physiol.* **248**:F48-F55 (1985).
120. Rangachari, P. K., D. McWade, and B. Donoff. Luminal receptors for bradykinin on the canine tracheal epithelium: functional subtyping. *Regul. Pept.* **21**:237-244 (1988).
121. Baker, A. P., L. M. Hillegass, D. A. Holden, and W. J. Smith. Effect of kallidin, substance P and other basic polypeptides on the production of respiratory macromolecules. *Am. Rev. Respir. Dis.* **115**:811-817 (1972).

122. McCann, J. D., R. C. Bhalla, and M. J. Welsh. Release of intracellular calcium by two different second messengers in airway epithelium. *Am. J. Physiol.* **257**:L116-L124 (1989).
123. Wong, L. B., I. F. Miller, and D. B. Yeates. Ciliary beat frequency stimulation by bradykinin requires activation of both neural and cyclooxygenase pathways. *Am. Rev. Respir. Dis.* **137**:8 (1988).
124. Tamaoki, J., K. Kobayashi, N. Sakai, A. Chiyotani, T. Kanemura, and T. Takizawa. Effect of bradykinin on airway ciliary motility and its modulation by neutral endopeptidase. *Am. Rev. Respir. Dis.* **140**:430-435 (1989).

10
Kinins in Rhinitis

Jacqueline A. Pongracic, Laurie Churchill, and David Proud
The Johns Hopkins University School of Medicine
Baltimore, Maryland

I. INTRODUCTION

The concept that kinins may be important mediators of inflammatory events in humans is by no means new. Virtually as soon as bradykinin was purified and sequenced, it was suggested that this peptide may play a crucial role in the inflammatory response to tissue injury (1). Since that time, several investigators (2-4) have reiterated the suggestion that kinins may be important mediators of inflammation, prompted, in each case, by an awareness of the known pharmacological properties of these peptides. In addition to their ability to contract most smooth muscle preparations and to cause pain, low doses of kinins cause vasodilatation and increased capillary blood flow (5). On a weight basis, kinins are also 100-fold more potent than histamine in causing increased vascular permeability and, as a result of this property, are extremely effective in inducing edema (4). Moreover, it is now firmly established that kinins can stimulate the release of additional proinflammatory mediators, such as prostaglandins and platelet activating factor, from several cell types (6-8). Unfortunately, while it is clear that this spectrum of properties would appear to make kinins prime candidates to be mediators of human inflammatory reactions, by the early 1980s the evidence documenting that kinin generation occurred during inflammatory events in man was weak and largely circumstantial.

At first glance, the report of increased systemic plasma kinins during asthmatic attacks in man (9) would appear to provide direct evidence that kinins can be produced during inflammatory reactions in humans. However, these data are now viewed with skepticism. This is due largely to the more recent awareness of the technical difficulties of performing reliable measurements of plasma kinins. Thus, as technology has improved, and as more stringent methods of collection have been used to prevent spontaneous kinin formation, the resting plasma kinin levels of 2-3 ng/ml reported by these earlier workers have been superseded by values of less than 20 pg/ml (10,11). Because of these technical problems the only remaining evidence to support systemic generation of kinins during inflammatory events is circumstantial. For example, the observation that high molecular weight kininogen is consumed during human anaphylaxis has been presumed to reflect systemic kinin formation (12).

Although circumstantial evidence of the type described above leaves open the potential for an increase in circulating kinins during systemic inflammatory events, it is generally accepted that kinins normally function as local autacoids. Even fewer studies existed, however, to support a role for kinins in local inflammatory events in man. It had been reported that a kinin-like material was present in the nasal secretions of allergic individuals challenged with allergen (13). Unfortunately, this study was limited by the inability to obtain adequate samples from nonallergic controls or from allergic subjects prior to challenge. In addition, kinin-like activity was detected in only half of the allergic subjects tested after challenge and was not definitively identified as a kinin.

In view of the criticisms that could be raised about existing data, we decided to reexamine the potential for kinin involvement during local inflammatory reactions in man. The nasal airways seemed to provide an ideal model for our studies, since our group had just developed a model of nasal provocation with allergen in which it was possible to examine the presence of inflammatory mediators in nasal secretions recovered by lavage (14). Since 1983, we have performed numerous studies to evaluate the role of kinins in a variety of types of airway inflammation. Although we have examined both the upper and lower airways, data regarding the latter is reviewed in Chapter 9. The present chapter, therefore, will focus on the potential role of kinins in the pathogenesis of rhinitis.

II. ALLERGIC RHINITIS

A. The Immediate Allergic Response

Insufflation of an appropriate allergen into the nasal cavity of an allergic individual results in the rapid manifestation of sneezing, nasal congestion, and rhinorrhea. To examine the profile of inflammatory mediators that are generated in nasal secretions during this immediate allergic response, our nasal provocation model uses a three-stage protocol. Because it is not uncommon to find significant "resting" levels of certain mediators in nasal lavages performed on unstimulated subjects, regardless of their atopic status, the first stage of the protocol consists of performing a series of nasal lavages to establish a stable baseline. To control for nonspecific irritation, the second stage of the protocol consists of administering a placebo challenge using either the diluent used for the preparation of allergen extract or (if pollen grains are used for the specific allergen challenge) lactose powder. A nasal lavage is performed 10 minutes after challenge. In the final stage of the protocol, increasing doses of allergen extract (or pollen grains) are insufflated into the nose with a lavage being performed 10 minutes after administration of each dose. Symptom scores and the number of sneezes are recorded at each stage of the experiment and recovered nasal lavages are analyzed for their mediator content. Typically, no increase in mediators or clinical symptoms is observed following diluent challenge, while the concentrations of a range of inflammatory mediators increase in a dose-dependent fashion upon antigen provocation. In a controlled study comparing 8 allergic individuals to 8 nonallergic controls (15), allergen challenge resulted in striking increases in kinin generation in the nasal washes of allergic subjects (5.6 ± 1.7 ng/ml) but not in the controls (0.04 ± 0.02 ng/ml). The presence of kinins was highly correlated with that of histamine and TAME-esterase activity, and with the onset of symptoms ($p < 0.001$ in each case). In additional studies (16,17) it has been demonstrated that kinin generation during the immediate allergic response is also associated with the production of prostaglandin D_2 and of sulfidopeptide leukotrienes. The specificity of this response was further demonstrated by showing that provocation of allergic subjects with a nonrelevant allergen failed to induce a clinical response or increased production of kinins and other mediators. Moreover, in contrast to the problems associated with plasma kinin measurements, it was possible to rigorously validate the accuracy of kinin measurements in nasal lavages and, by using HPLC analysis, to definitively identify the kinins produced during the immediate allergic response as a mixture of bradykinin and Lys-bradykinin (15).

Having provided the first demonstration of kinin formation during a local inflammatory event in man, we were interested in elucidating the mechanisms regulating kinin generation and metabolism during this reaction. The nasal challenge model lent itself particularly well to such biochemical studies, in part because the lavage procedure employed dilutes many enzyme-substrate interactions below K_m and essentially "freezes" many reactions. One important parameter that can regulate the generation of kinins is the availability of substrate for kinin-forming enzymes. Two such substrates exist in man. High molecular weight kininogen has been reported to exist only in plasma, with lower amounts being associated with bloodborne cells such as platelets, endothelial cells and neutrophils (18-20). In contrast, low molecular weight kininogen has been detected extravascularly in the distal nephron of the human kidney (21). To determine if kininogens could be produced locally in the upper airways, or if they were derived from plasma, we used specific radioimmunoassays for high molecular weight kininogen (22), total kininogen (21), and albumin to study the availability of kininogens during the immediate allergic response (23). These studies clearly demonstrated that both high and low molecular weight kininogens entered nasal secretions by transudation from plasma. Since each milliliter of blood contains sufficient kininogens to yield 3 μg of kinin, it is clear that, as long as this transduction is maintained, an enormous pool of available substrate for kinin-forming enzymes could be provided to permit chronic kinin formation.

The presence of both bradykinin and Lys-bradykinin in nasal secretions during the immediate allergic reaction strongly suggested that more than one enzyme was involved in the generation or conversion of kinins. Since human plasma prekallikrein circulates in plasma as a complex with high molecular weight kininogen (24), and since this kininogen enters nasal secretions from plasma, it was not surprising that an antibody that recognizes plasma prekallikrein and kallikrein detected increased immunoreactive plasma (pre)kallikrein in nasal secretions during the allergic reaction (25). Biochemical analysis revealed, however, that prekallikrein activation occurs during this process and that the activated kallikrein produced can generate bradykinin from its specific substrate, high molecular weight kininogen (26), prior to inactivation by the plasma protease inhibitors, C1 inactivator and α_2-macroglobulin (25). Unlike the passive diffusion of kininogens and prekallikrein from plasma, the conversion of prekallikrein to kallikrein is an active enzymatic process. The presence of C1 inactivator-Hageman factor complexes in nasal secretions (D. Proud and A. P. Kaplan, unpublished observations) indicates that the generation of kallikrein occurs as a result of contact activation of Hageman factor. This contact activation is, presumably, initiated by interaction with a negative surface exposed by the initial inflammatory event or by interaction with some negatively charged macromolecule, such as mucus glycoproteins or mast cell heparin (27). Although activation of plasma kallikrein undoubtedly contributes to the generation of bradykinin during the immediate allergic reaction, this enzyme generates exclusively bradykinin (28) and cannot, therefore, explain the production of Lys-bradykinin. This latter peptide is generated by tissue kallikrein that has been shown, for the first time, to be present in the upper airways. Immunoreactive tissue kallikrein is present even in "resting" nasal secretions, but concentrations of this material increase significantly in allergic subjects in response to allergen challenge (29). The identity of this material as authentic tissue kallikrein was established by both immunological and physicochemical criteria as well as by its ability to generate Lys-bradykinin from purified human kininogens. Although present in nasal secretions in considerably lower concentrations than immunoreactive plasma kallikrein, virtually all of the kininogenase activity in postchallenge lavages can be attributed to tissue kallikrein (29), presumably due to its resistance to inhibition by plasma protease inhibitors. This resistance to inhibition, together with the fact that, while plasma kallikrein releases kinin in vivo only from high molecular weight kininogen, tissue kallikrein can generate kinin from both high and low molecular weight kininogens (and, thereby, has a larger available source of substrate), probably explains the observation that as much as 45% of the kinin detected during the immediate allergic response is Lys-bradykinin (15,30). Indeed, since postchallenge nasal lavages also contain elevated levels of an aminopeptidase M-like enzyme capable of converting Lys-bradykinin to bradykinin (31), it is likely that an even higher percentage of the total kinin originally generated may be Lys-bradykinin, suggesting an important role for tissue kallikrein in kinin formation during the immediate allergic response.

Metabolic destruction of kinins is a major mechanism for the regulation of their actions and virtually all tissues and biological fluids contain enzymes that are capable of degrading these peptides. In nasal secretions recovered by lavage, the profile of peptidases is quite simple. In addition to the aminopeptidase mentioned above, which converts Lys-bradykinin to bradykinin but does not cause the loss of biological activity, the major kinin degrading enzyme is a carboxypeptidase N-like enzyme that removes the C-terminal arginine residue. Lower levels of angiotensin converting enzyme (kininase II) activity can also be detected (31). It must be realized, however, that this profile does not reflect the activity of cell membrane peptidases that are not recovered in lavage. Thus, within the nasal cavity, it is likely that other peptidases, such as epithelial cell surface neutral endopeptidase or endothelial cell surface angiotensin converting enzyme may play a more significant role in regulating kinin activity.

B. The Late Phase Response

In studying allergic rhinitis, it is clear that the immediate response to allergen provocation does not completely reflect the pathophysiology of the clinical entity. It has been known since the pioneering studies of Blackley in 1873 that, following provocation with allergen, many individuals experience not only an immediate response but also a recurrence of symptoms some several hours after the initial allergen exposure (32). In recent years, this so-called "late phase response" has attracted a resurgence of interest because it has been suggested by several investigators that it may be a better model of chronic disease than is the immediate response (33-35). This is based upon several features, including the much longer duration of the late response compared to the immediate reaction, the histopathology of the late response, which is characterized by edema and by an influx of inflammatory cells, including eosinophils, neutrophils, and mononuclear cells, and upon the observation that oral steroids, which are extremely effective in the treatment of chronic allergic disease, inhibit the late phase but not the immediate response to allergen challenge. In light of these parallels between the late response and chronic allergic disease, we were interested in knowing if kinin formation occurred during the late phase reaction. We examined the profile of inflammatory mediators produced in nine individuals experiencing both an immediate response and a late phase reaction (dual responders). A control group consisting of three allergic subjects who experienced only an immediate response and two of the dual responders who were challenged only with diluent was also examined. The protocol involved the same baseline and placebo stages described above. A single dose of allergen was then administered and nasal lavages were collected 10 and 20 minutes postchallenge and then at hourly intervals up to 11 hours. Subjects kept hourly symptom diaries of sneezing, rhinorrhea, and congestion. Although individual temporal variations were observed in the responses of those subjects experiencing a late phase reaction, several common features were noted (36). In each patient, the immediate response was associated with increased levels of histamine, PGD_2, TAME-esterase activity, and, of course, kinins in nasal lavages. This initial response usually abated within an hour and was followed by a quiescent period lasting 1-3 hours. During this period, mediator concentrations were essentially at baseline levels. Over the next several hours there was a recurrence of symptoms that was associated with a second increase in the levels of histamine. TAME-esterase activity and kinins, but not PGD_2, in recovered lavages. The absence of PGD_2, the major cyclooxygenase product of the human mast cell (37), during the late response raised the possibility that the basophil, rather than the mast cell, may be the source of the histamine seen during this reaction, since, while both the mast cell and the basophil contain histamine, the basophil does not produce PGD_2. This was supported by the subsequent demonstration that basophil influx into the nose occurs during the late phase (38). Of particular interest with regard to the late phase response were our observations on kinins. Although the levels of histamine and TAME-esterase activity detected during the late response were similar to those seen during the immediate reaction, this was not the case for kinins. The levels of kinins seen during the late response (6.3 ± 3.5 ng/ml; mean ± SEM) were increased significantly ($p = 0.02$) over values noted for baseline and quiescent periods but were significantly ($p < 0.05$) less than the concentrations seen during the immediate response (14.1 ± 3.4 ng/ml). Interestingly, symptom scores during the late response (5.7 ± 0.9) were also lower than during the immediate response (9.3 ± 1.1). The reason for the lower levels of kinins during the late response is unknown, but several possibilities exist. It may be that there is a less marked increase in vascular transudation such that lower levels of kininogens and of plasma kallikrein are available to support kinin formation. Alternatively, it may be that the secretion of glandular components such as tissue kallikrein is reduced. Finally, it is possible that an increased rate of kinin degradation is associated with the late phase, perhaps as a result of the influx of neutrophils that are known to contain several kinin-degrading enzymes (39) and to express neutral endopeptidase on their surfaces (40). Whatever the explanation, HPLC analysis of the kinins generated during the late response shows that, as for the immediate reaction, both bradykinin and Lys-bradykinin are produced (36).

Not only are kinins generated during the late allergic response, but pharmacological interventions that have been shown to affect this response have also altered the production of these peptides. Administration of oral prednisone inhibits the late response without significantly inhibiting the immediate response. Inhibition of the late response by oral steroids is associated with decreased production of kinins and of other mediators (41). In contrast, topical flunisolide inhibited symptoms and the generation of mediators (including kinins) during both the immediate and late responses (42). To date, no medication that inhibits the symptomatic response to allergen challenge has failed to significantly inhibit kinin generation.

III. COLD, DRY AIR-INDUCED RHINITIS

In evaluating the role of kinins in experimentally induced rhinitis, we have also examined a model of cold, dry air provocation. Some individuals report a history of symptoms of rhinitis upon exposure to cold, dry environments. It is possible to experimentally induce symptoms in such individuals. The protocol, and an example of the results obtained, are illustrated in Figure 1. In brief, a series of lavages are performed to ensure a low stable baseline of mediators. Subjects then breath warm, moist air (WMA, at 37 °C, 98% relative humidity) for 15 minutes via a pediatric face mask placed over the nose. Lavages are performed 10 and 20 minutes postchallenge and subjects then inhale cold, dry air (CDA, at −4 °C, 10% relative humidity). Lavages are, again, performed 10 and 20 minutes postchallenge. As can be seen in Figure 1, no significant symptomatic response or mediator generation occurs after challenge with WMA, while CDA provocation leads to congestion and rhinorrhea accompanied by increases in the levels of histamine, PGD_2, LTC_4, kinins, and TAME-esterase activity in nasal lavages. These data were confirmed in a controlled study comparing 12 subjects with a clinical history of rhinitis upon exposure to cold and dry environments with 5 subjects who had no such history (43). In the group with positive clinical histories, kinins were one of the most sensitive indices of a response. Kinins were significantly elevated after CDA challenge (2.9 ± 0.07 ng/ml) and correlated with increases in histamine and TAME-esterase activity ($p < 0.001$) and with increases in PGD_2 and symptom scores ($p < 0.05$). There was no significant increase in any parameter upon challenge of the asymptomatic group.

Since histamine is derived only from mast cells and basophils, and since the mediator profile observed after CDA challenge is essentially identical to that observed during the immediate response to allergen provocation, it seems likely that mast cell activation occurs during the response to CDA. This suggests that it is possible to activate mast cells in vivo using a physical stimulus. We have hypothesized that evaporative water loss causes an increase in the osmolarity of the nasal mucosa (44). Since hyperosmolar stimuli can activate mast cells in vitro (45,46), the increased osmolarity of the nasal mucosa may provide an environment for mast cell activation in vivo. Presumably, those subjects who show no response to provocation with CDA are able to compensate for changes in osmolarity and maintain the nasal mucosa under isomolar conditions. Measurements of the osmolarity of recovered lavages support this hypothesis (44).

Using the three model systems described above, we have performed several thousand challenge experiments and have never observed a positive response, in terms of symptoms or the generation of other mediators, that was not accompanied by kinin production. The profile of mediators detected in these challenge systems strongly suggests that, in each case, kinin generation is associated with mast cell or basophil activation. It is tempting to speculate, therefore, that the release of cellular products, such

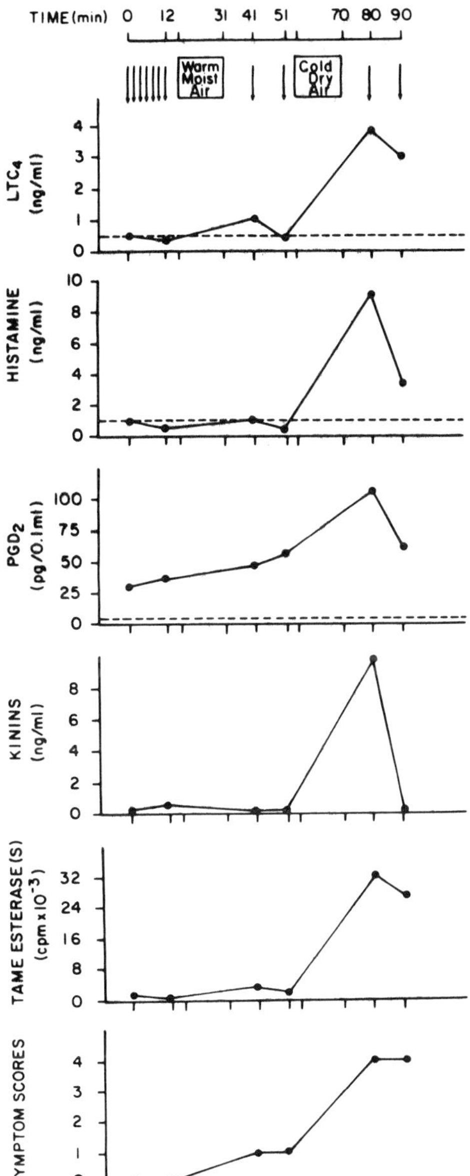

Figure 1 The response of a sensitive individual to provocation with cold, dry air. Downward arrows indicate the performance of nasal lavages.

as histamine or PGD_2, triggers an increase in vascular permeability that permits the initial influx of kininogens from plasma and allows subsequent kinin generation. Once kinin generation is initiated, these peptides could stimulate more pronounced vascular permeability changes and contribute to chronic inflammation. This relationship between mast cell/basophil activation and kinin generation does not always hold, however. In an attempt to corroborate our hypothesis that cold, dry air initiates mast cell mediator release by increasing the osmolarity of the nasal mucosa, we examined the effects of nasal provocation with hyperosmolar mannitol. Although a brief (10-s) exposure to hyperosmolar fluid is obviously not the same as prolonged exposure to cold, dry air, it was interesting to note that this stimuli did, indeed, result in increased levels of histamine in nasal lavages but did not result in kinin generation or in the onset of a significant symptomatic response (47). Furthermore, we will now describe a situation in which kinin generation is associated with rhinitis in the apparent absence of mast cell/basophil involvement.

IV. RHINOVIRUS COLDS

As its name implies, the common cold is the most prevalent acute respiratory illness experienced by humans. In the United States, an adult will experience an average of 2 to 4 colds per year. Over 250 strains of virus can induce colds, but over a third of the colds experienced each year are caused by the 100 or so strains of rhinovirus (48). Although the central role of viral infection in the development of a cold is undisputed, little is known regarding the subsequent events that lead to the manifestation of symptoms. Unlike influenza virus, rhinovirus infections produce no discernable damage to the respiratory epithelium (49,50). Thus, symptoms cannot be attributed to cytotoxic effects of the virus. The fact that so many different strains of virus induce a common symptomatic profile led us to hypothesize that viral infection in some way triggers the release of inflammatory mediators that may, in turn, lead to the manifestation of nasal obstruction, rhinorrhea, and a sore throat. To begin to examine this hypothesis, we used the technique of experimental rhinovirus infection, in which an inoculum of live rhinovirus is introduced into the nasal cavities of volunteers whose sera do not already possess neutralizing antibodies directed towards the strain of virus to be used. This inoculation procedure leads to infection of virtually all subjects, as indicated by a rise in serum titer of neutralizing antibody or by the ability to culture virus from a nose or throat swab. Interestingly, only about 60% of infected subjects develop clinical symptoms (51). What differentiates subjects who become symptomatic (ill) from those who do not (nonill) is unknown.

To evaluate the involvement of inflammatory mediators in experimental colds, volunteers were inoculated with virus or placebo and then isolated in individual motel rooms. Subjects recorded symptom scores every 4 hours. Nasal lavages were performed prior to inoculation and every 4 hours for 5 days postinoculation and were analyzed for the presence of polymorphonuclear leukocytes and for various mediators and proteins (52). Of the 24 subjects from whom lavages were assayed for mediators, 5 were inoculated with placebo, and the remaining 19 could be shown to be infected using the definitions described above. Analysis of the symptoms recorded by these 19 subjects using the criteria of Jackson and coworkers (53) established that 11 of the infected individuals could be defined as ill, while the remaining 8 were nonill. Those individuals with symptomatic illnesses typically showed elevated symptom scores beginning 2 days after inoculation and persisting through the fourth day with a return towards baseline occurring by day 5.

Analysis of mediator measurements revealed that kinins were significantly elevated ($p < 0.03$) in lavages from subjects who were symptomatic, while kinin concentrations in lavages from the infected, nonill group were not different from controls. In the symptomatic group, kinins were first elevated at 4 a.m. on day 2, which was also the first time point at which symptom scores were increased. Prior to viral inoculation, kinin levels were usually in the range of 100-200 pg/ml, while during the days when subjects were symptomatic they peaked in the range of 2000-9000 pg/ml. An interesting diurnal variation in the pattern of kinin concentrations was observed with kinin levels peaking in the early morning and declining by afternoon. HPLC analysis of the kinins present in nasal lavages showed the presence of both Lys-bradykinin and bradykinin, with the latter peptide representing about 80% of the total. Increased kinin concentrations in the symptomatic group were associated with increases in polymorphonuclear leukocytes, albumin, and TAME-esterase activity. By contrast, no changes in the levels of histamine in nasal lavages were seen during symptomatic colds, suggesting that mast cell activation does not occur during rhinovirus infections. Further support for this was provided by measuring the concentrations of PGD_2, the major cyclooxygenase metabolite of human mast cells, in selected individuals. No changes in PGD_2 were observed in any subject. Thus, in experimental rhinovirus colds, kinin generation appears to occur independent of mast cell activation. Furthermore, we were able to demonstrate that total kinin levels correlated with symptom scores during experimental colds ($p < 0.01$).

In all the studies described above, we had examined the potential for kinin formation in experimental models. It was obviously important, however, to extend these observations to a natural disease state. To this end, we performed a prospective study of natural rhinovirus colds (54). One hundred individuals with no chronic diseases of the respiratory tract were recruited. No subject was taking chronic medications other than oral contraceptives. Prospective surveillance was conducted by having each subject maintain a log of the daily occurrence of respiratory and general symptoms. Nasal lavages were performed on each subject on each of 4 days when they were asymptomatic. Two-week periods were allowed between the collection of each of these specimens, which served as samples for baseline mediator measurements. Subjects were instructed to report to the study nurse for collection of nasal lavages for viral culture and mediator analysis at the first appearance of symptoms. A second lavage was usually performed on the following day. Mediator analysis was only performed on subjects who reported symptoms, were judged by the nurse to have an acute respiratory infection at that time, and whose symptoms could be attributed, by subsequent viral culture, to be due to a rhinovirus infection. Samples from 16 such subjects were analyzed. Kinin levels were significantly ($p < 0.01$) increased when subjects were infected and ill (mean = 724 pg/ml) compared to when they were asymptomatic (mean = 116 pg/ml). Increased kinin levels were associated with increased vascular permeability, as assessed by monitoring the levels of albumin in nasal lavages. No increases in histamine levels were observed during natural colds. Thus, data from our studies of natural rhinovirus colds confirmed the principal results observed in the experimental colds, namely that increased concentrations of kinins, but not histamine, in nasal secretions are associated with symptomatic rhinovirus infections.

V. BRADYKININ-INDUCED RHINITIS

A. Provocation Studies

Clearly, the demonstration that kinins are generated, and correlate with symptoms, during a variety of inflammatory conditions of the upper airways supports the hypothesis that these peptides may play a role in the pathogenesis of rhinitis. This data does not rule out the possibility, however, that kinin generation is an epiphenomenon unrelated to the manifestation of symptoms. The next step in testing the hypothesis that kinins may play a role in the development of symptoms was to determine if application of kinins to the nasal mucosa could induce a symptomatic response. It has been demonstrated that bradykinin is a potent bronchoconstrictor when administered to the lower airways of asthmatics but not normals (55-57) and that this peptide can induce retrosternal discomfort and cough in all subjects (57). There had been no evaluation, however, of the effects of kinins in the nasal cavity. We recruited 8 subjects, therefore, without regard to sex or atopic status and subjected them to a double-blind, crossover provocation study (58). Following a series of baseline lavages, subjects received a known diluent challenge followed after 10 minutes by a lavage. They were then challenged with four increasing doses of bradykinin or with repeated applications of placebo. Symptom scores were recorded at each stage of the protocol, and lavages were recovered for analysis of albumin and TAME-esterase activity (as monitors of increased vascular permeability). The 2 challenge days were separated by a minimum period of 1 week. A comparison of the symptoms induced (expressed as mean ± SEM) by provocation with bradykinin or placebo is depicted in Figure 2. As can be seen, bradykinin elicited a dose-dependent increase in symptom scores that was significant ($p < 0.05$) compared to placebo even at the lowest dose of bradykinin used. Although individual variation in the pattern of symptoms reported were seen, the principal symptoms noted were unilateral obstruction on the challenged side, rhinorrhea, and, in 7 of the 8 subjects, a sore throat persisting, in some cases, for up to 4 hours after challenge. Associated with the increase in symptoms, dose-dependent increases in the levels of albumin and TAME-esterase activity in lavages were also observed.

Since it has been reported that bradykinin is a secretagogue for histamine release from rodent mast cells (59,60), it was possible that bradykinin's ability to induce symptoms may be an indirect consequence of the release of histamine. No increase in the levels of histamine in nasal lavages were seen during kinin challenge, however, regardless of the atopic status of the subject. Thus, bradykinin does not induce histamine release from the human nasal mucosa. This is consistent with our own in vitro observations that bradykinin is not a secretagogue for any human histamine-containing cell tested (61).

In light of the subjective report that obstruction induced by bradykinin challenge was unilateral, subjects returned to the laboratory for a third visit and were subjected to an additional bradykinin challenge protocol in which nasal obstruction was measured objectively by anterior rhinomanometry. These experiments, in which lavages were not employed because they interfere with rhinomanometric measurements, confirmed that bradykinin-induced obstruction was, indeed, unilateral on the challenged side and that there was no observed reflex mechanism of contralateral obstruction.

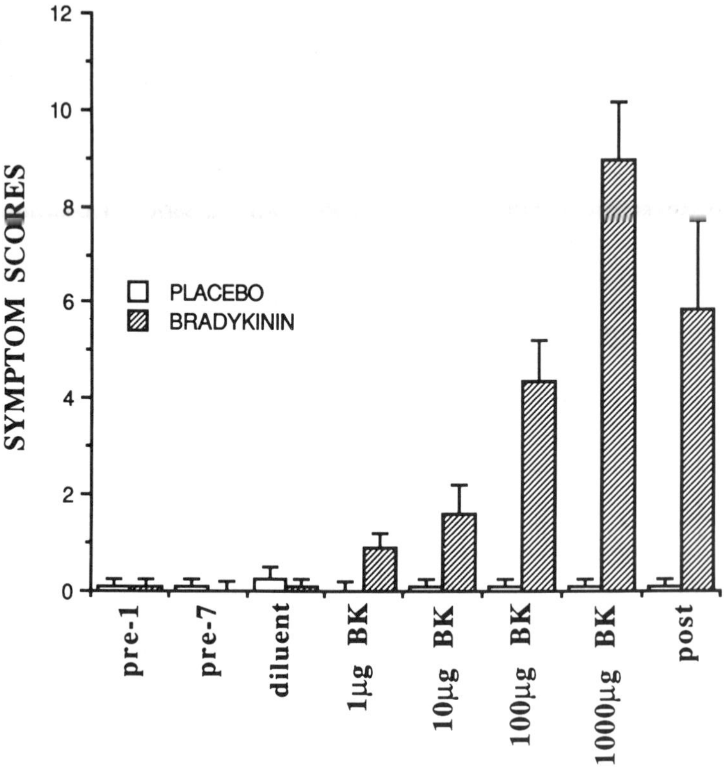

Figure 2 Comparison of symptoms induced upon provocation with bradykinin or placebo. Values are expressed as mean ± SEM. Symptom scores are significantly elevated compared to placebo at all doses of bradykinin.

Because our studies on kinin metabolism in nasal secretions had shown that the predominant pathway of kinin degradation was via the actions of a carboxypeptidase N-like enzyme that would remove the C-terminal arginine, it became necessary to consider the possibility that there may be significant accumulation of the product of this reaction, des-Arg^9-bradykinin, in the nasal cavity. This was of interest because of the work of Regoli and coworkers, who defined two kinin receptor subtypes (62,63). On the "classical" kinin receptor present on many types of smooth muscle, called a B2 receptor by Regoli, desArg^9-bradykinin is completely inactive. In terms of interaction with the other receptor subtype, called B1, however, desArg^9-bradykinin is more potent than the parent peptide. Thus, the possibility existed that if B1 receptors predominated in the nasal mucosa, the metabolism of bradykinin to desArg^9-bradykinin could result in the generation of an active moiety, rather than an inactive fragment. To evaluate the mechanism by which bradykinin caused nasal symptoms, therefore, we performed a double-blind study comparing the effects of provocation with bradykinin and desArg^9-bradykinin. The results confirmed our earlier observations that bradykinin induced a symptomatic response that was accompanied by a striking increase in vascular permeability. On the other hand desArg^9-bradykinin, even at an administered dose of 1 mg, failed to cause any symptoms or increased vascular permeability. Thus, the acute effects of bradykinin challenge are not mediated via B1 receptors. This does not rule out a possible role of this receptor subtype during chronic inflammatory states, however, since it has been shown that the B1 receptor can be induced by inflammatory stimuli (64).

B. Pharmacological Intervention Studies

Although the ability of kinins to induce rhinitis and sore throat, taken together with the descriptions of kinin generation in nasal secretions during allergic reactions and symptomatic rhinovirus infections, provides strong support for the hypothesis that kinins may be important mediators of inflammatory reactions of the upper airways, definitive verification of this hypothesis can only be achieved by demonstrating that blocking the actions of kinins during such reactions leads to symptomatic relief. In this regard, the model of nasal provocation with bradykinin provides a useful first step in the evaluation of pharmacological agents, since any agent that is expected to inhibit the actions of endogenously produced kinins should demonstrate efficacy in blocking the effects of exogenously administered bradykinin.

Because bradykinin is known to cause the release of prostaglandins from a variety of cell types (6-8), and because the actions of kinins in several tissues are reported to be mediated via prostanoids (65,66), we evaluated the possibility that the ability of bradykinin to induce symptoms of rhinitis may depend upon its ability to cause the release of cyclooxygenase metabolites of arachidonic acid. The effect of premedication with 650 mg of aspirin t.i.d. for 2½ days on the response to nasal provocation with bradykinin was examined. This dosage of aspirin was selected because previous studies in our laboratory had shown that it was adequate to completely inhibit the generation of PGD_2 during the immediate response to allergen challenge. Although, in our study of eight subjects, premedication with aspirin resulted in a trend toward lower symptom scores and a reduction in vascular leakage in response to kinin challenge, this trend was minimal and did not achieve statistical significance. Thus, prostaglandin generation is not a prerequisite for kinin-induced rhinitis, and cyclooxygenase inhibitors are unlikely to be useful agents in the evaluation of the role of kinins in the pathogenesis of rhinitis caused by allergen or viral exposure.

Clearly, the most direct way to interfere with the actions of kinins on target tissues is to prevent these peptides from occupying their specific receptors. Considerable excitement was generated, therefore, when the first generation of competitive antagonists for B2 kinin receptors were recently developed (67). One of these compounds, DArg[Hyp^3,$DPhe^7$]bradykinin (NPC 567), was selected for evaluation as a potentially useful agent for delineating the role of kinins in the pathogenesis of rhinitis. This compound had demonstrated the ability to antagonize the actions of bradykinin in several in vitro systems (68), while displaying less partial agonist tendencies than several other analogs. Nevertheless, before attempting to use this agent in our established models of human disease, it was important to document in vivo efficacy in blocking the response to nasal provocation with bradykinin.

We began by performing rising dose tolerance studies and established that, even at an administered dose of 2 mg per nostril, NPC 567 did not display partial agonist activity in the nasal cavity. Thus, not only did the antagonist fail to induce a symptomatic response, but it did not increase vascular permeability, as evidenced by the absence of elevated levels of albumin and TAME-esterase activity in nasal secretions. We then proceeded to examine the ability of the compound to block the effects of kinin challenge. Because NPC 567 has a relatively low affinity for kinin receptors (68), we selected our conditions to favor antagonism by administering 0.5 mg of drug or placebo into the nostril and, after a 5-minute period (to permit occupancy of receptors by the compound), we challenged with 20 μg of bradykinin. This low dose of bradykinin produces modest symptom scores but readily measurable increases in albumin and TAME-esterase activity. In a study of 12 subjects, NPC 567 had no significant effects on symptoms or the levels of albumin and TAME-esterase activity in nasal secretions following bradykinin challenge.

Since this antagonist is still readily susceptible to degradation by peptidases (see Chapter 6), it was possible that rapid degradation of the compound may have occurred during the 5 minute preadministration. To evaluate this possibility, we repeated the study but coadministered drug or placebo with the bradykinin. Again, the drug had no significant effect on bradykinin-induced symptoms or changes in vascular permeability. Finally, because of the compounds relatively weak potency, we performed a study in a limited number of individuals in which 2 mg of antagonist was used to try to inhibit the effects of nasal provocation with 20 μg of bradykinin, but the compound was still ineffective.

From these studies, we must conclude that NPC 567 is not a suitable compound with which to evaluate the role of kinins in allergen- or virus-induced rhinitis. The failure of the compound to antagonize a bradykinin challenge could be due to several reasons. Perhaps the two most likely explanations, however, involve the potency of the compound and the possibility of a novel kinin receptor subtype on which the compound is inactive. As mentioned above, NPC 567 has a relatively low affinity for the B2 kinin receptor, displaying a pA_2 value in the order of 6. Thus, it is almost three orders of magnitude weaker than bradykinin, and it may simply be impractical to achieve sufficient local concentrations of the compound in vivo in man to permit successful competition. On the other hand, our knowledge of kinin receptor subtypes is still developing along with new antagonists, and a recent report has demonstrated that guinea pig trachea contains a bradykinin binding site at which NPC 567 is ineffective in competing (69). It is feasible, therefore, that such a novel binding site may be important for kinin actions in the nasal cavity.

VI. SUMMARY

For compounds to be considered mediators of a disease condition, it is generally accepted that they must fulfill three criteria: (a) they should be present during symptomatic episodes and absent (or present in much reduced levels) when symptoms are absent, (b) administration of the compound to the appropriate site should induce relevant symptoms, and (c) interference in the actions of the compound should have a concomitant and appropriate effect on symptoms.

Our studies on the role of kinins in rhinitis have clearly documented that kinins are generated, and correlate with symptoms, during a variety of inflammatory conditions of the upper airways; and the symptom profile produced upon nasal provocation with bradykinin is clearly consistent with the symptoms noted during allergic rhinitis and colds. While these studies obviously provide strong support for a role of kinins in the pathogenesis of rhinitis, however, such a role cannot be established until the third, crucial criterion listed above is satisfied. In this regard, the failure of NPC 567 to block a kinin challenge was clearly a disappointment, not because it negates a role for kinins in the pathogenesis of rhinitis but because it means that this compound is not an appropriate tool with which to gain any additional insight into this issue.

It must be remembered, however, that the discovery of kinin antagonists is a fairly recent occurrence and, in analogy with the area of leukotriene antagonists, refinements in the structure, potency and stability of these compounds may be necessary before compounds with in vivo efficacy are available for study. The synthesis of more potent kinin antagonists is an area of active interest for several pharmaceutical companies and there are already promising developments in this regard. We remain convinced, therefore, that the availability of such compounds represents the most promising approach for delineating the involvement of kinins in airway inflammation. Moreover, if a role for kinins in the pathogenesis of allergic rhinitis and colds is established, potent and selective kinin antagonists may represent a novel therapeutic approach for symptomatic relief of these conditions.

ACKNOWLEDGMENTS

Dr. Proud acknowledges support from grant number HL 32272 from the National Institutes of Health. Dr. Churchill is a fellow of The American Lung Association.

REFERENCES

1. Elliott, D. F., E. W. Horton, and G. P. Lewis. Actions of pure bradykinin. *J. Physiol.* **153**:473-480 (1960).
2. Kellermeyer, R. W., and R. C. Graham. Kinins—possible physiologic and pathologic roles in man. *N. Engl. J. Med.* **279**:859-866 (1968).
3. Garcia-Leme, J. Bradykinin system, in: *Handbook of Experimental Pharmacology,* Vol. 50., *Inflammation* (J. R. Vane and S. H. Ferreira, eds.). Springer-Verlag, Berlin, pp. 464-522 (1978).
4. Marceau, F., A. Lussier, D. Regoli, and J. P. Giroud. Pharmacology of kinins: Their relevance to tissue injury and inflammation. *Gen. Pharmacol.* **14**:209-299 (1983).
5. Keele, C. A. Clinical and pathological aspects of kinins in man. *Proc. Roy. Soc. Biol.* **173**:361-369 (1969).
6. Hong, S. L., and L. Levine. Stimulation of prostaglandin biosynthesis by bradykinin and thrombin and their mechanisms of action on MC5-5 fibroblasts. *J. Biol. Chem.* **251**:5814-5816 (1976).
7. McIntyre, T. M., G. A. Zimmerman, K. Satoh, and S. M. Prescott. Cultured endothelial cells synthesize both platelet-activating factor and prostacyclin in response to histamine, bradykinin and adenosine-triphosphate. *J. Clin. Invest.* **76**:271-280 (1985).
8. Churchill, L., F. H. Chilton, J. H. Resau, R. Bascom, W. C. Hubbard, and D. Proud. Cyclooxygenase metabolism of endogenous arachidonic acid by

cultured human tracheal epithelial cells. *Am. Rev. Respir. Dis.* **140**:449-459 (1989).
9. Abe, K., N. Watanabe, N. Kumagai, T. Mouri, and K. Yoshinaga. Circulating plasma kinin in patients with bronchial asthma. *Experientia* **23**:626-627 (1967).
10. Scicli, A. G., T. Mindroiu, G. Scicli, and O. A. Carretero. Blood kinins, their concentration in normal subjects and in patients with congenital deficiency in plasma prekallikrein and kininogen. *J. Lab. Clin. Med.* **100**:81-93 (1982).
11. Ando, T., K. Shimamoto, Y. Nakahashi, T. Nishitani, S. Hosoda, H. Ishida, S. Tanaka, and O. Iimura. Blood kinin measurement by sensitive kinin radioimunnoassay and its clinical application. *Agents and Actions* **9**(Suppl.):222-226 (1982).
12. Smith, P. L., A. Kagey-Sobotka, E. R. Bleecker, R. Traystman, A. P. Kaplan, H. Gralnick, M. D. Valentine, S. Permutt, and L. M. Lichtenstein. Physiologic manifestations of human anaphylaxis. *J. Clin. Invest.* **66**:1072-1080 (1980).
13. Dolovich, J., N. Back, and C. E. Arbesman. Kinin-like activity in nasal secretions of allergic patients. *Int. Arch. Allergy* **38**:337-344 (1970).
14. Naclerio, R. M., H. L. Meier, A. Kagey-Sobotka, N. F. Adkinson, Jr., D. A. Meyers, P. S. Norman, and L. M. Lichtenstein. Mediator release after nasal airway challenge with allergen. *Am. Rev. Respir. Dis.* **128**:597-602 (1983).
15. Proud, D., A. Togias, R. M. Naclerio, S. A. Crush, P. S. Norman, and L. M. Lichtenstein. Kinins are generated in vivo following nasal airway challenge of allergic individuals with allergen. *J. Clin. Invest.* **72**:1678-1685 (1983).
16. Naclerio, R. M., D. Proud, A. G. Togias, A. Kagey-Sobotka, S. P. Peters, P. S. Creticos, N. F. Adkinson, Jr., P. S. Norman, and L. M. Lichtenstein. Mediators in nasal secretions of patients with allergic rhinitis. *Immunology and Allergy Practice* **VII**:212-219 (1985).
17. Naclerio, R. M., D. Proud, S. P. Peters, G. Silber, A. Kagey-Sobotka, N. F. Adkinson, Jr., and L. M. Lichtenstein. Inflammatory mediators in nasal secretions during induced rhinitis. *Clin. Allergy* **16**:101-110 (1986).
18. Schmaier, A. H., A. Zuckerberg, C. Silverman, J. Kuchibhotla, G. P. Tuszynski, and R. W. Colman. High molecular weight kininogen. A secreted platelet protein. *J. Clin. Invest.* **71**:1477-1489 (1983).
19. Schmaier, A. H., A. Kuo, D. Lundberg, S. Murray, and D. B. Cines. The expression of high molecular weight kininogen on human umbilical vein endothelial cells. *J. Biol. Chem.* **263**:16327-16333 (1988).
20. Gustafson, E. J., A. H. Schmaier, Y. T. Wachtfogel, N. Kaufman, U. Kuchich, and R. W. Colman. Human neutrophils contain and bind high molecular weight kininogen. *J. Clin. Invest.* **84**:28-35 (1989).
21. Proud, D., M. Perkins, J. V. Pierce, K. N. Yates, P. F. Highet, P. L. Herring, M. Mangkornkanok/Mark, R. Bahu, F. Carone, and J. J. Pisano. Characterization and localization of human renal kininogen. *J. Biol. Chem.* **256**: 16034-16039 (1981).

22. Proud, D., J. V. Pierce, and J. J. Pisano. Radioimmunoassay of human high molecular weight kininogen in normal and deficient plasmas. *J. Lab. Clin. Med.* **95**:563-574 (1980).
23. Baumgarten, C. R., A. G. Togias, R. M. Naclerio, L. M. Lichtenstein, P. S. Norman, and D. Proud. Plasma kallikrein during experimentally induced allergen challenge of allergic individuals. *J. Clin. Invest.* **76**:191-197 (1985).
24. Mandle, R., Jr., R. W. Colman, and A. P. Kaplan. Identification of prekallikrein and HMW-kininogen as a circulating complex in plasma. *Proc. Natl. Acad. Sci. USA* **73**:4179-4183 (1976).
25. Baumgarten, C. R., R. C. Nichols, R. M. Naclerio, L. M. Lichtenstein, P. S. Norman, and D. Proud. Plasma kallikrein during experimentally induced allergic rhinitis: Role in kinin formation and contribution to TAME-esterase activity in nasal secretions. *J. Immunol.* **137**:977-982 (1986).
26. Pierce, J. V., and J. A. Guimaraes. Further characterization of highly purified human plasma kininogens, in: *Chemistry and Biology of the Kallikrein-Kinin System in Health and Disease* (J. J. Pisano and K. F. Austen, eds.). DHEW Publ. No. (NIH)76-791, pp. 121-127 (1976).
27. Hojima, Y., C. G. Cochrane, R. C. Wiggins, K. F. Austen, and R. L. Stevens. In vitro activation of the contact (Hageman factor) system of plasma by heparin and chondroitin sulfate E. *Blood* **63**:1453-1459 (1984).
28. Webster, M. E., and J. V. Pierce. The nature of the kallidins released from human plasma by kallikreins and other enzymes. *Ann. N.Y. Acad. Sci.* **104**: 91-107 (1963).
29. Baumgarten, C. R., R. C. Nichols, R. M. Naclerio, and D. Proud. Concentrations of glandular kallikrein in human nasal secretions increase during experimentally-induced allergic rhinitis. *J. Immunol.* **137**:1323-1328 (1986).
30. Proud, D., C. R. Baumgarten, R. M. Naclerio, and L. M. Lichtenstein. The role of kinins in human allergic disease. *N. Engl. Reg. Allergy Proc.* **7**:213-213 (1986).
31. Proud, D., C. R. Baumgarten, R. M. Naclerio, and P. E. Ward. Kinin metabolism in nasal secretions during experimentally-induced allergic rhinitis. *J. Immunol.* **138**:428-434 (1987).
32. Blackley, C. H. Experimental researches on the causes and nature of *Catarrhus Aestivus* (hayfever or hayasthma). Balliere, Tindell and Cox, 1873. Reprinted by Dawson, London, pp. 77-81 (1959).
33. Austen, K. F., and R. P. Orange. Bronchial asthma: The possible role of the chemical mediators of immediate hypersensitivity in the pathogenesis of subacute chronic disease. *Am. Rev. Respir. Dis.* **112**:423-436 (1975).
34. Gleich, G. J. The late phase of the immunoglobulin E-mediated reaction: A link between anaphylaxis and common allergic disease? *J. Allergy Clin. Immunol.* **70**:160-169 (1982).
35. Kaliner, M. Hypotheses on the contribution of late phase allergic responses to the understanding of the treatment of allergic diseases. *J. Allergy Clin. Immunol.* **73**:311-314 (1984).

36. Naclerio, R. M., D. Proud, A. G. Togias, N. F. Adkinson, Jr., D. A. Meyers, A. Kagey-Sobotka, M. Plaut, P. S. Norman, and L. M. Lichtenstein. Inflammatory mediators in late antigen-induced rhinitis. *N. Engl. J. Med.* **313**:65-70 (1985).
37. MacGlashan, D. W., Jr., R. P. Schleimer, S. P. Peters, E. S. Schulman, G. K. Adams, A. Kagey-Sobotka, H. H. Newball, and L. M. Lichtenstein. Comparative studies of basophils and mast cells. *Fed. Proc.* **42**:2504-2509 (1983).
38. Bascom, R., M. Wachs, R. M. Naclerio, U. Pipkorn, S. J. Galli, and L. M. Lichtenstein. Basophil influx occurs after nasal antigen challenge: effects of topical corticosteroid pretreatment. *J. Allergy Clin. Immunol.* **81**:580-589 (1988).
39. Wasi, S., H. Z. Movat, E. Pass, and J. Y. C. Chan. Production, conversion and destruction of kinins by human neutrophil leukocyte proteases, in: *Neutral Proteases of Human Polymorphonuclear Leukocytes* (K. Havemann and A. Janoff, eds.). Urban & Schwarzenburg, Munich, pp. 245-260 (1978).
40. Painter, R. G., R. Dukes, J. Sullivan, R. Carter, E. G. Erdos, and A. R. Johnson. Function of neutral endopeptidase on the cell membrane of human neutrophils. *J. Biol. Chem.* **263**:9456-9461 (1988).
41. Pipkorn, U., D. Proud, L. M. Lichtenstein, R. P. Schleimer, S. P. Peters, N. F. Adkinson, Jr., A. Kagey-Sobotka, P. S. Norman, and R. M. Naclerio. Effect of short-term systemic glucocorticoid treatment on human nasal mediator release after antigen challenge. *J. Clin. Invest.* **80**:957-961 (1987).
42. Pipkorn, U., D. Proud, L. M. Lichtenstein, A. Kagey-Sobotka, P. S. Norman, and R. M. Naclerio. Inhibition of mediator release in allergic rhinitis by pretreatment with topical glucocorticosteroids. *N. Engl. J. Med.* **316**:1506-1510 (1987).
43. Togias, A. G., R. M. Naclerio, D. Proud, J. E. Fish, N. F. Adkinson, Jr., A. Kagey-Sobotka, P. S. Norman, and L. M. Lichtenstein. Nasal challenge with cold, dry air results in release of inflammatory mediators: Possible mast cell involvement. *J. Clin. Invest.* **76**:1375-1381 (1985).
44. Togias, A. G., D. Proud, L. M. Lichtenstein, A. Kagey-Sobotka, G. K. Adams, III, P. S. Norman, and R. M. Naclerio. The osmolality of nasal secretions increases in the inflammatory response to cold, dry air. *Am. Rev. Respir. Dis.* **137**:625-629 (1988).
45. Eggleston, P. A., A. Kagey-Sobotka, R. P. Schleimer, and L. M. Lichtenstein. Interaction between hyperosmolar and IgE-mediated histamine release from basophils and mast cells. *Am. Rev. Respir. Dis.* **130**:86-91 (1983).
46. Eggleston, P. A., A. Kagey-Sobotka, and L. M. Lichtenstein. A comparison of the osmotic activation of basophils and lung mast cells. *Am. Rev. Respir. Dis.* **135**:1043-1048 (1987).
47. Silber, G., D. Proud, J. Warner, R. Naclerio, A. Kagey-Sobotka, L. Lichtenstein, and P. Eggleston. In vivo release of inflammatory mediators by hyperosmolar solutions. *Am. Rev. Respir. Dis.* **137**:606-612 (1988).
48. Gwaltney, J. M., Jr., J. O. Hendley, G. Simon, and W. S. Jordan, Jr. Rhinovirus infections in an industrial population: I. The occurrence of illness. *N. Engl. J. Med.* **275**:1261-1268 (1966).

49. Douglas, R. J., Jr., B. R. Alford, and R. B. Couch. Atraumatic nasal biopsy for studies of respiratory virus infection in volunteers. *Antimicrob. Agents Chemother.* **8**:340-343 (1968).
50. Winther, B., B. Farr, R. B. Turner, J. O. Hendley, J. M. Gwaltney, Jr., and N. Mygind. Histopathologic examination and enumeration of polymorphonuclear leukocytes in the nasal mucosa during experimental rhinovirus colds. *Acta Otolaryngol. Suppl.* (Stockh) **413**:19-24.
51. Couch, R. B. Rhinoviruses, in: *Virology* (B. N. Lields, D. M. Knipes, R. M. Chanock, J. L. Melnick, B. Roizman, and R. E. Shope, eds.). Raven Press, New York, pp. 795-816 (1985).
52. Naclerio, R. M., D. Proud, L. M. Lichtenstein, A. Kagey-Sobotka, J. O. Hendley, J. Sorrentino, and J. M. Gwaltney, Jr. Kinins are generated during experimental rhinovirus colds. *J. Infect. Dis.* **157**:133-142 (1987).
53. Jackson, G. G., H. F. Dowling, I. G. Spiesman, and A. V. Boand. Transmission of the common cold to volunteers under controlled conditions. I. The common cold as a clinical entity. *Arch. Int. Med.* **101**:267-278 (1958).
54. Proud, D., R. M. Naclerio, J. M. Gwaltney and J. O. Hendley. Kinins are generated in nasal secretions during natural rhinovirus colds. *J. Infect. Dis.* **161**:120-123 (1990).
55. Herxheimer, H., and E. Stresemann. The effects of bradykinin aerosol in guinea pigs and man. *J. Physiol.* (Lond.) **158**:38-39 (1961).
56. Varonier, H. S., and R. Panzani. The effect of inhalation of bradykinin on healthy and atopic (asthmatic) children. *Int. Arch. Allergy Appl. Immunol.* **34**:293-296 (1968).
57. Fuller, R. W., C. M. S. Dixon, F. M. C. Cuss, and P. J. Barnes. Bradykinin-induced bronchoconstriction in humans. Mode of action. *Am. Rev. Respir. Dis.* **135**:176-180 (1987).
58. Proud, D., C. J. Reynolds, S. LaCapra, A. Kagey-Sobotka, L. M. Lichtenstein, and R. M. Naclerio. Nasal provocation with bradykinin induces symptoms of rhinitis and a sore throat, *Am. Rev. Respir. Dis.* **137**:613-616 (1988).
59. Johnson, A. R., and E. G. Erdos. Release of histamine from mast cells by vasoactive peptides. *Proc. Soc. Exp. Biol. Med.* **142**:1251-1256 (1973).
60. Ishizaka, T., M. Iwata, and K. Ishizaka. Release of histamine and arachidonate from mouse mast cells induced by glycosylation-enhancing factor and bradykinin. *J. Immunol.* **134**:1880-1887 (1985).
61. Lawrence, I. D., J. A. Warner, V. L. Cohan, L. M. Lichtenstein, A. Kagey-Sobotka, R. J. Vavrek, J. M. Stewart, and D. Proud. Induction of histamine release from human skin mast cells by bradykinin analogs. *Biochem. Pharmacol.* **38**:227-233 (1989).
62. Regoli, D., and J. Barabe. Pharmacologogy of bradykinin and related kinins. *Pharmacol. Rev.* **31**:1-46 (1980).
63. Regoli, D., F. Marceau, and J. Barabe. De novo formation of vascular receptors for bradykinin. *Can. J. Physiol. Pharmacol.* **56**:674-677 (1978).
64. Bouthillier, J., D. deBlois, and F. Marceau. Studies on the induction of pharmacological responses to des-Arg^9-bradykinin in vitro and in vivo. *Br. J. Pharmacol.* **92**:257-264 (1987).

65. McGiff, J. C. Interactions of prostaglandins with the kallikrein-kinin and renin-angiotensin systems. *Clin. Sci.* **59**:105s-116s (1980).
66. Musch, M. W., J. F. Kachur, R. J. Miller, M. Field, and J. S. Stoff. Bradykinin-stimulated electrolyte secretion in rabbit and guinea pig intestine. Involvement of arachidonic acid metabolites. *J. Clin. Invest.* **71**:1073-1083 (1983).
67. Vavrek, R. J., and J. M. Stewart. Competitive antagonists of bradykinin. *Peptides* **6**:161-164 (1985).
68. Steranka, L. R., S. G. Farmer, and R. M. Burch. Antagonists of B_2 bradykinin receptors. *FASEB J.* **3**:2019-2025 (1989).
69. Farmer, S. G., R. M. Burch, S. A. Meeker, and D. E. Wilkins. Evidence for a pulmonary B_3 bradykinin receptor. *Mol. Pharmacol.* **36**:1-8 (1989).

11

Bradykinin Antagonists in a Sheep Model of Allergic Asthma

William M. Abraham
Mount Sinai Medical Center
Miami Beach, Florida

I. INTRODUCTION

It has become increasingly apparent that asthma is an inflammatory disease of the airways, and, therefore, most recent experimental studies both in human subjects and in animal models have been directed at understanding the association between the airway inflammation and the airway dysfunction of asthma. This dysfunction is expressed as airway obstruction, airway hyperresponsiveness to a variety of stimuli, and a slowing of mucociliary clearance. One means of studying the interrelationships among these processes in the laboratory is to use controlled challenges with specific antigen. These studies can be designed such that the observed changes in pulmonary function can be correlated with the airway inflammatory response as assessed by bronchoalveolar lavage (both human subjects and animals) or by obtaining histologic sections (primarily animal studies). Using these techniques, it has become apparent that allergen challenge can elicit two types of airway responses: a single acute bronchial response or an acute bronchial response, which is followed 6-8 h later by a late response (1,2). Each pattern of airway response (i.e., the acute response only or both an acute and late response) is associated with a different inflammatory response, with the late response being characterized by the presence of eosinophils (3,4). Studies involving subjects or animals that develop both acute and late bronchial responses have been of special interest because the development of the late response has been associated with characteristics of chronic asthma (1,2) including refractoriness to β-adrenergic agents, a dependence on glucocorticosteroids, a heightened inflammatory response, and a prolonged and increased airway hyperresponsiveness (1,2,5-8). The increased airway responsiveness renders the airways more sensitive to subsequent exposures to allergens, viral infections, exercise, cold air, or other noxious airborne stimuli (e.g., pollutants), and so is thought to result in a worsening of symptoms (cough, bronchoconstriction, mucus accumulation).

To better understand these complex processes, we have studied a sheep model of allergic bronchoconstriction that shares certain pathophysiological similarities with those observed in asthmatic subjects (Table 1). Of particular interest is the identification of two subgroups of allergic sheep: those that develop only acute responses to inhaled *Ascaris suum* antigen (acute responders) and those that develop both acute and late responses after antigen challenge (dual responders) (9). The development of late responses in this animal model is associated with a more severe airway inflammatory response (7) and prolonged bronchial hyperresponsiveness (8). These similarities and the fact that antigen-induced airway responses in these animals are sensitive to pharmacological agents that are active in humans (10) suggest that this animal model may be useful both

Table 1 Similarities Between Allergic Sheep Model and Allergic Asthma

Natural allergy (positive skin sensitivity) (38)
Differential airway responsiveness between allergic and normal (nonallergic) groups (38,39)
Allergics bronchoconstrict to beta-blockers (40)
Allergics are hyperresponsive to bradykinin and sodium metabisulfite (25)
Allergics show acute bronchoconstriction (associated with hyperinflation) to inhaled antigen; readily reversible with β-adrenergic agents (38,41)
Allergic bronchoconstriction is associated with a prolonged slowing of mucociliary clearance (42)
Some allergic sheep, in addition to the acute response, develop a late bronchial response to antigen; the late response is not reversible with β-adrenergic agents (43)
Early and late responses are sensitive to antiallergic agents (9,44)
Late responses are sensitive to glucocorticoids (45)
Late responses are associated with airway inflammation (neutrophils and eosinophils) (7,46)
Late responses are associated with prolonged airway hyperresponsiveness (8)

as a preclinical predictor for active agents and as a model for elucidating the in vivo pathophysiological mechanisms of allergic airway disease.

Bradykinin has received increased attention as a putative mediator of asthma because asthmatic subjects are hyperresponsive to inhaled bradykinin (11-13) and recent studies have demonstrated the presence of immunoreactive kinins and kininogenase activity in bronchoalveolar (BAL) fluid from asthmatic subjects following allergen provocation (14). Increased immunoreactive kinins have also been found in nasal washings from patients with allergic rhinitis undergoing nasal allergen challenge (15). The exact role bradykinin plays in the pathophysiology of allergic airway disease is not well understood, but the recent availability of peptide analog antagonists of bradykinin (16) provide useful tools to begin to clarify these mechanisms.

In this chapter we will describe studies designed to assess the usefulness of one of these bradykinin antagonists, D-Arg[Hyp^3,D-Phe^7]bradykinin (NPC 567) (17), in modifying antigen-induced bronchial obstruction, bronchial hyperresponsiveness, and airway inflammation in the sheep model of allergic bronchoconstriction.

II. EFFECTS OF BRADYKININ IN SHEEP AIRWAYS

Before assessing the potential role of NPC 567 in allergen-induced responses, it was important to show that the actions of bradykinin in sheep airways were similar to those described in human airways. Bradykinin can induce cough in sheep (18), and inhaled bradykinin causes a short-lived (~20 min) bronchoconstriction that is dose dependent (19). Furthermore, sheep that are allergic to *Ascaris suum* antigen are ~6 times more sensitive to the constrictor effects of inhaled bradykinin than are nonallergic sheep (W. M. Abraham, unpublished observations). These observations are similar to those made in human subjects.

The mechanism of bradykinin-induced bronchoconstriction in human subjects is thought to be mediated, in part, through cholinergic reflex mechanisms, because the response can be blocked by the anticholinergic agents atropine and ipatropium bromide (11,13). Bradykinin-induced bronchoconstriction can be blocked by the antiallergic agents cromolyn sodium and nedocromil sodium (12) which, in addition to their well-known antiallergic properties, have been shown to inhibit bronchoconstriction caused by compounds (e.g., sulfur dioxide, sodium metabisulfite) that stimulate this cholinergic reflex (20-24). Bradykinin-induced bronchoconstriction has a similar pharmacologic profile in allergic sheep (25). Thus, blockade of bradykinin-induced bronchoconstriction was achieved by intravenously administered atropine or by nedocromil sodium aerosol. The protective effects of nedocromil sodium did not result from inhibition of histamine release because the histamine H-1 antagonist chlorpheniramine had no protective effect on the response to bradykinin (25). These findings suggest that bradykinin-induced bronchoconstriction in allergic sheep is mediated via a cholinergic reflex mechanism, similar to that proposed for humans.

Having established that bradykinin causes bronchoconstriction in sheep, it was important to show that the bradykinin antagonist NPC 567 could block this response. Pretreatment with inhaled NPC 567 blocked bradykinin-induced bronchoconstriction in a dose-dependent fashion (Fig. 1) (19). These observations indicate that there are functional bradykinin receptors in sheep airways, as has been suggested from ligand binding studies. These receptors appear to be located throughout the airways with the greatest distribution found in the distal airways (lung parenchyma) as compared to the proximal airways (tracheal smooth muscle) (26).

Because airway hyperresponsiveness is an important component of the pathophysiological response to antigen challenge, it was important to determine if doses of bradykinin that caused bronchoconstriction in allergic sheep also increased the animal's airway responsiveness to other bronchoconstricting agents. Bradykinin had inconsistent effects on airway respon-

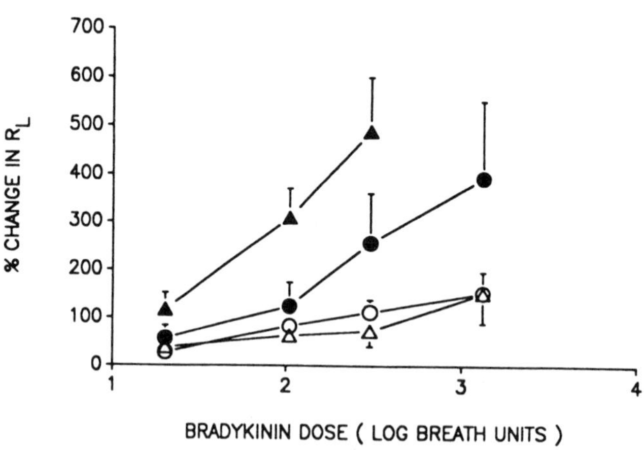

Figure 1 Dose-response curve to inhaled bradykinin in allergic sheep after placebo (▲), and after 20 breaths of 2 mg/ml (●), 5 mg/ml (Δ), and 10 mg/ml (○) NPC 567. Each point is the mean ± SE mean of six observations. Where not shown, SE mean lies within the symbol.

siveness assessed by carbachol dose-response curves. Similar results were obtained with inhaled substance P. These findings contrast with those obtained for the sensory neuropeptide, neurokinin A, which produced a significant leftward shift in the carbachol dose response curves of these allergic sheep (27). The lack of a direct effect of bradykinin and substance P on airway responsiveness was not surprising considering that neither of these peptides have been shown to produce hyperresponsiveness in man (28).

III. EFFECTS OF BRADYKININ ON ANTIGEN-INDUCED BRONCHOCONSTRICTION, INFLAMMATION, AND AIRWAY HYPERRESPONSIVENESS

After establishing that NPC 567 blocked bradykinin-induced bronchial responses in allergic sheep, the antagonist was used to determine if bradykinin contributed to allergen-induced responses in this model. The initial experiments tested the efficacy of the compound in acute responders (i.e., those sheep with only a single early response to inhaled antigen). Approximately 2 h after challenge when the antigen-induced bronchoconstriction has resolved, the sheep exhibit an increase in their airway responsiveness (Fig. 2). This hyperresponsive state has a duration of 2-6 h and is associated

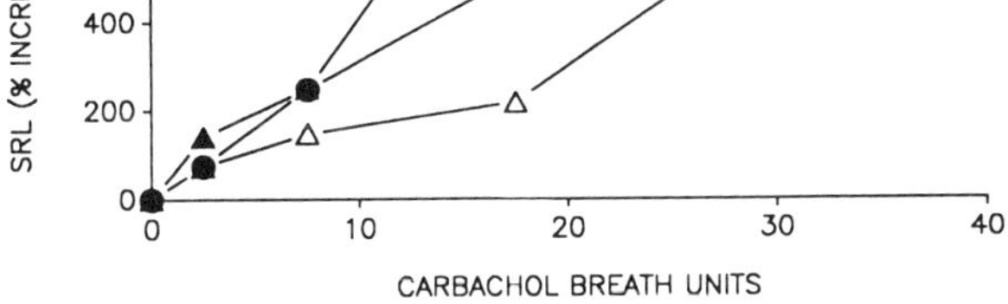

Figure 2 Change in airway responsiveness before and ~2 h after antigen challenge in allergic sheep. Airway responsiveness occurs after specific lung resistance (SR_L) has returned to normal. Baseline prechallenge curve (●--●); 2 h postchallenge curve (▲--▲); and 2 h postchallenge (Δ--Δ) when the sheep had been treated with NPC 567 (20 breaths 10 mg/ml 30 min before antigen challenge; 400 breaths of 2 mg/ml during antigen challenge). NPC 567 blocked the normal increase in airway responsiveness observed after antigen challenge.

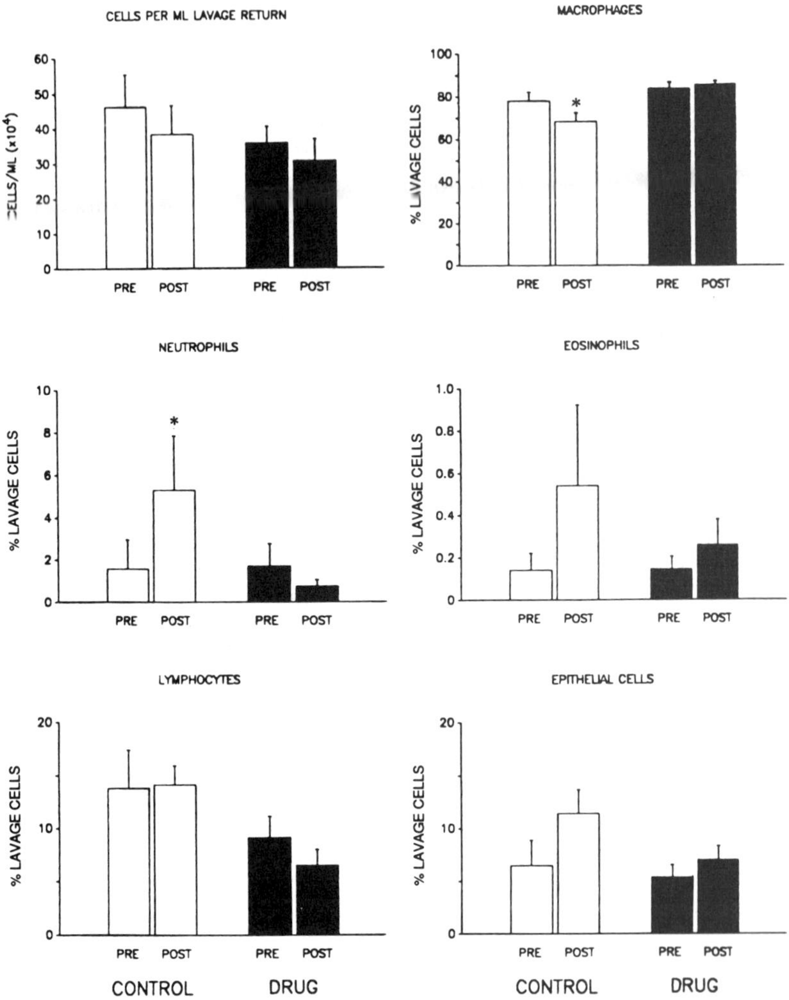

Figure 3 Results of BAL at baseline (Pre) and 2 h after antigen challenge (Post) in the control and drug-treated (NPC 567, 10 mg/ml) trials. NPC 567 reduced the influx of inflammatory cells (neutrophils and eosinophils) into the lung after antigen challenge. Values are mean ±SE, $n = 7$. *$p < 0.05$ vs. baseline (Pre).

with an influx of inflammatory cells into the airways as determined by BAL (19,29). NPC 567 given 30 min before antigen challenge and coadministered with the antigen had no effect on the acute bronchoconstrictor response to antigen. However, the drug did affect the subsequent development of the airway hyperresponsiveness (Fig. 2). The inhibition of the airway hyperresponsiveness was associated with a reduction in the post-antigen-induced inflammatory response in the airways (Fig. 3). Interestingly, if NPC 567 was given after the antigen challenge, but before the beginning of the postchallenge dose response curve, the drug had no effect on the subsequent development of airway hyperresponsiveness (19). Because the protective effect of the drug on airway responsiveness was seen only when the compound was used as a pretreatment and not when given after challenge, it was concluded that bradykinin is released during the early stages of airway anaphylaxis and that its role may be one of modulating the inflammatory response following antigen challenge. Furthermore, it is clear that although bradykinin is released early on it contributes little to the severity of the acute response to antigen.

The observations with NPC 567 are consistent with previous findings using this model (29) that indicate that the release of chemotactic mediators during the early stages of airway anaphylaxis is important for eliciting the development of this early onset of airway hyperresponsiveness. Because the direct chemotactic effects of bradykinin have not yet been described, one can only speculate on the mechanism by which NPC 567 affected the inflammatory cell influx and therefore the hyperresponsiveness. Possibilities include a modulatory effect of bradykinin on the release or the actions of other chemotactic mediators, such as platelet activating factor or leukotrine B_4 (LTB_4) known to be released following antigen challenge. Such interactions (i.e., between bradykinin and other potent chemotactic agents) could be important for maintaining vascular leakiness that is necessary for the full inflammatory response to occur (30).

IV. EFFECTS OF BRADYKININ ON ALLERGEN-INDUCED LATE RESPONSES AND INFLAMMATION

As discussed earlier, the late bronchial response which follows the acute response to allergen provocation is thought to be linked to factors that heighten the severity of asthma. The late response is associated with the recruitment of inflammatory cells to the airways and the release of chemical mediators (3,7,31-35). Furthermore, the airways of sheep that develop late responses are hyperresponsive at this time, such that the effects of spasmogenic mediators released during the late response are enhanced (36,37). Because the previous studies suggested that bradykinin may be important in promoting the secondary inflammatory events (i.e., cell influx and mediator release) that follow airway challenge with antigen, it was conceivable that bradykinin could contribute to the evolution of the late bronchial response by modulating these secondary inflammatory events. To study this problem, the effects of NPC 567 on antigen-induced bronchoconstriction, mediator release, and inflammation were determined.

In the control trial, antigen challenge resulted in an early bronchoconstrictor response that was associated with significant increases in the concentrations of immunoreactive (i)-kinins, TAME-esterase, prostaglandin (PG) D_2 and PGE_2 (Figs. 4,5). The late response was associated with significant increases in the concentrations of PGE_2, 6-keto PGF_1, thromboxane B_2, LTB_4, and LTC_4. i-Kinins were also significantly elevated during the late responses, but the concentration was less than that found during the early response. The late response was associated with a significant increase in the total percentage of granulocytes (neutrophils and eosinophils) in the BAL at 8 h postchallenge (Fig. 6). When the animals were

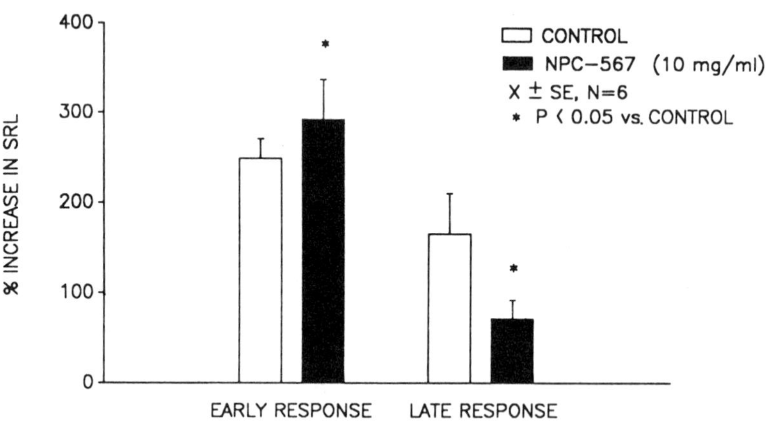

Figure 4 Effect of NPC 567 (20 breaths 10 mg/ml 30 min before antigen challenge, 400 breaths 2 mg/ml during challenge, and 20 breaths 10 mg/ml 4 h after challenge) on antigen-induced early and late responses in allergic sheep. NPC 567 had no effect on the acute bronchoconstrictor response represented as an increase in specific lung resistance (↑SR_L) but caused a significant inhibition of the late response. The lack of inhibition of the acute response and the blockade of the late response was correlated with mediator measurements obtained from BAL (see Fig. 5).

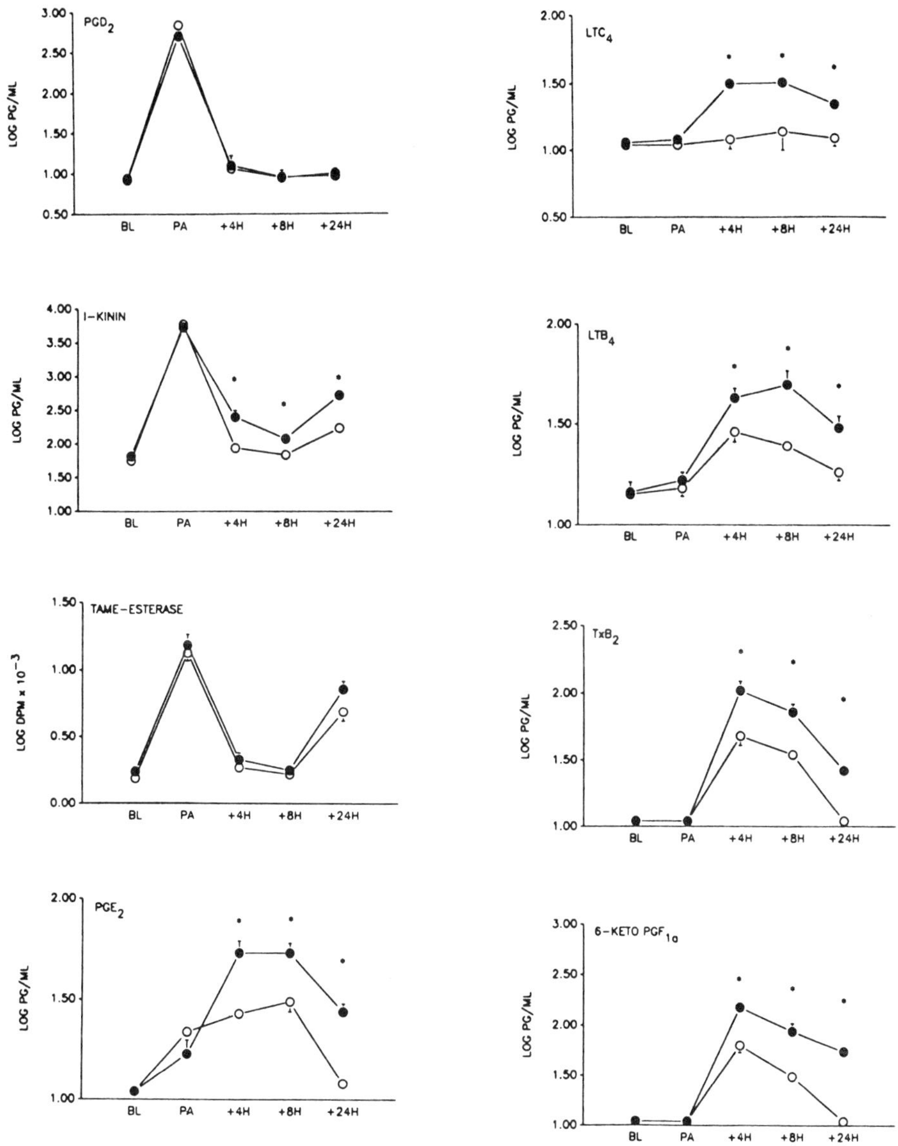

Figure 5 Mediator concentrations in BAL before and after antigen challenge in allergic sheep with and without NPC 567 (10 mg/ml) treatment. Concentrations are plotted as the log of the absolute value for the control trial (●) and for the NPC 567 trial (○). Values are mean ± SE for 6 sheep. Where not shown, SE lies within symbol. *$p < 0.05$ vs. NPC 567 trial. Baseline (BL), post ascaris (PA).

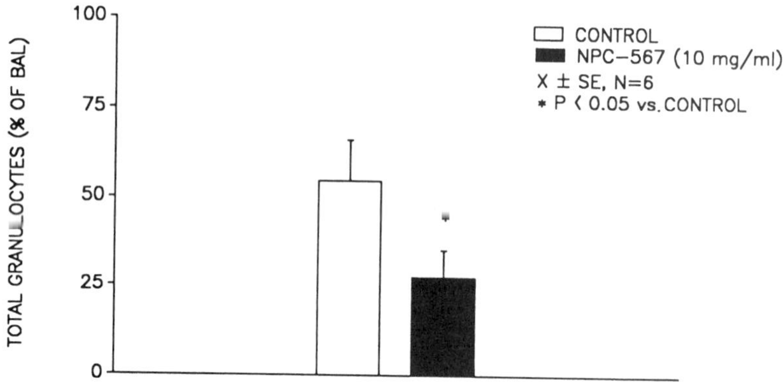

Figure 6 Effect of NPC 567 (10 mg/ml) on inflammatory cell influx in allergic sheep. NPC 567 significantly inhibited the granulocyte (expressed as percentage of neutrophils and eosinophils in BAL) infiltrate into sheep airways 4-8 h after challenge. This inhibition was associated with a reduction in the concentration of inflammatory mediators in the BAL (Fig. 5) and a reduction in the late responses (Fig. 4).

treated with NPC 567, there was no protection against the acute bronchial response to antigen (similar to the previous study). Consistent with this observation was the finding that concentrations of i-kinins, TAME-esterase, PGD_2, and PGE_2 were increased to levels similar to those seen in the control trial immediately after challenge (Fig. 5). During the late response, however, there was no secondary increase in the level of i-kinins, and the concentrations of all mediators associated with the late response were significantly reduced (Fig. 4,5). The blockade of the late response and the reduction in the mediator concentrations observed in the NPC 567-treated sheep were concomitant with a reduction in the total percentage of granulocytes in the BAL (Fig. 6).

These findings extend the previous observations using NPC 567 in acute responders and lend support to the argument that bradykinin plays a contributory role in post-antigen-induced inflammation and subsequent mediator release. The pathophysiological consequences of this inflammation appear to be the development of hyperresponsive airways and the late response.

It is important to note that NPC 567 reduced the release of all mediators and not just the spasmogenic leukotrienes (i.e., LTC_4, LTD_4) that have been proposed to mediate the late bronchial response in this model (31-33). Thus, while leukotriene antagonists and NPC 567 may provide similar protection against the late constrictor response in allergic sheep, the mechanisms of action appear quite different. The leukotriene antagonists prevent the action of a specific contractile mediator released from inflammatory cells, whereas the bradykinin antagonist attenuates overall mediator release by reducing the inflammatory cell influx.

The effects of NPC 567 were short-lived, however. Twenty-four hours after challenge, airway hyperresponsiveness was apparent, irrespective of whether the sheep received NPC 567 or not (Fig. 7). Interestingly, by 24 h the inflammatory response was similar in both groups, and both groups showed significant secondary elevations in i-kinins and TAME-esterase. Since the bradykinin antagonist is a peptide, it was not expected that a single pretreatment would provide protection over the entire 8 h time course of the study. Therefore, in these studies, the drug was administered not only before and during the antigen challenge, but at 4 h after challenge in an attempt to maximize its effects. It appears that even with this second treatment, drug levels were insufficient to provide protection for 24 h. It seemed likely, therefore, that additional treatments were necessary to combat the prolonged hyperresponsive state characteristically associated with the late response.

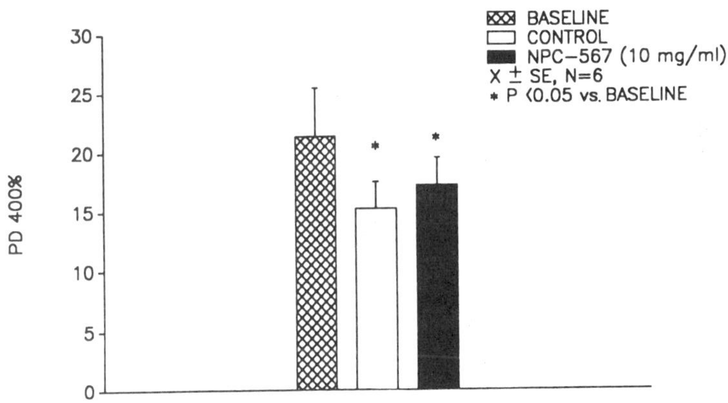

Figure 7 Effect of NPC 567 on airway responsiveness 24 h after antigen challenge in allergic sheep. Airway responsiveness was determined from carbachol dose-response curves (see Fig. 2) and is expressed as $PD_{400\%}$, i.e., the dose of carbachol in breath units that increases specific lung resistance by 400%. One breath unit of carbachol = 1 breath of 1% w/v carbachol. There was a significant decrease in $PD_{400\%}$ in both the control trial and the drug trial (NPC 567). Values are mean ± SE for 6 sheep. $^{*}p < 0.05$ vs. baseline dose-response curves.

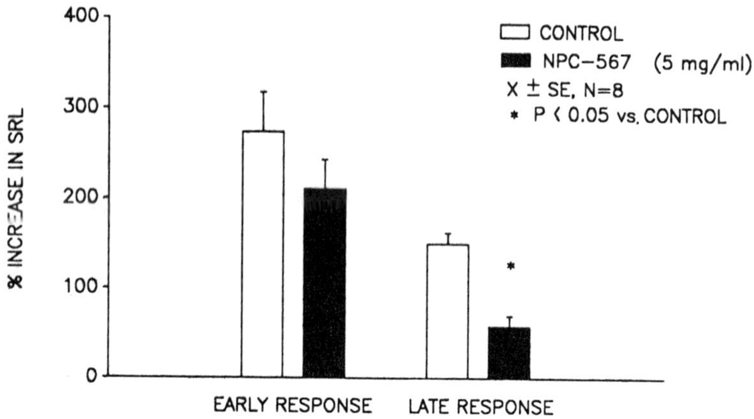

Figure 8 Effect of lower dose NPC 567 (20 breaths, 5 mg/ml 30 min before challenge; 400 breaths 1 mg/ml coadministered with antigen; and 20 breaths of 5 mg/ml given 4, 8 and 24 h after antigen challenge) on antigen-induced changes in specific lung resistance in allergic sheep. NPC 567 treatment did not prevent the early response as was seen previously, but blocked the late response. Values are mean ±SE for 8 sheep.

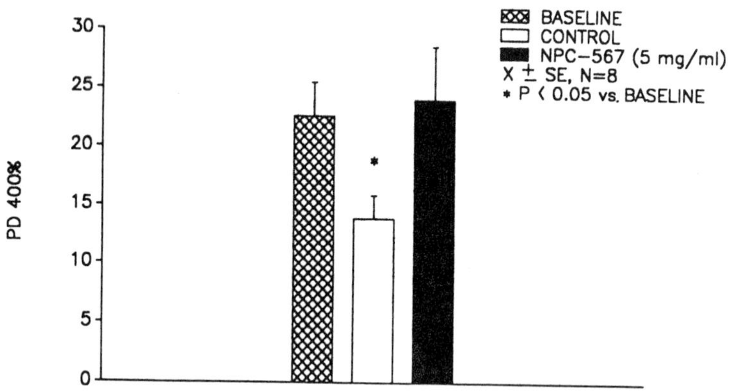

Figure 9 Effect of NPC 567 (5 mg/ml) on airway hyperresponsiveness 24 h after antigen challenge. Additional treatments of NPC 567 (as described in Fig. 8) blocked the hyperresponsiveness. Values are mean ±SE for 8 sheep.

To determine if subsequent doses of the antagonist could alleviate the airway hyperresponsiveness, as well as the late response, the study described above was repeated, except that the NPC 567 was given not only before, during, and 4 h after antigen challenge, but at 8 h and 24 h after challenge as well. Under these conditions, both the late response and the subsequent airway hyperresponsiveness were blocked (Fig. 8,9).

V. CONCLUSION

In summary, experiments using a well-characterized animal model of allergen-induced early and late responses that were designed to determine if the inflammatory mediator bradykinin plays a role in these pathophysiological responses have been described. Although it appears that bradykinin contributes little, if any, to the immediate bronchial response to inhaled antigen, the findings provides substantive evidence for the release of kinins and their modulatory role in allergen-induced inflammation and mediator release from these inflammatory cells that results in late responses and airway hyperresponsiveness. If similar findings are obtained in man, bradykinin antagonists may prove to be potentially useful in the therapy of inflammatory diseases of the airways, such as asthma.

REFERENCES

1. Pepys, J., and B. J. Hutchcroft. Bronchial provocation tests in the etiologic diagnosis and analysis of asthma. *Am. Rev. Respir. Dis.* **112**:829-859 (1975).
2. O'Byrne, P. M., J. Dolovich, and F. E. Hargreave. State of art: Late asthmatic responses. *Am. Rev. Respir. Dis.* **136**:740-751 (1987).
3. de Monchy, J. G. R., Kauffman, H. F., Venge, P., Koeter, G. H., Jansen, H. M., Sluiter, H. J. and de Vries, K. Bronchoalveolar eosinophilia during allergen-induced late asthmatic reactions. *Am. Rev. Respir. Dis.* **131**:373-376 (1985).
4. Fabbri, L. M., Boschetto, P., Zocca, E., Milani, G., Pivirotto, F., Plebani, M., Burlina, A., Licata, B. and Mapp, C. E. Bronchoalveolar neutrophilia during late asthmatic reactions induced by toluene diisocyanate. *Am. Rev. Respir. Dis.* **136**:36-42 (1987).
5. Cockcroft, D. W. and Murdock, K. Y. Comparative effects of inhaled salbutamol, sodium cromoglycate, and beclomethasone dipropionate on allergen-induced early asthmatic responses, late asthmatic responses, and increased bronchial responsiveness to histamine. *J. Allergy Clin. Immunol.* **79**:734-740 (1987).
6. Cartier, A., Thomson, N. C., Frith, P. A., Roberts, R. and Hargreave, F. E. Allergeninduced increase in bronchial responsiveness to histamine: Relationship to the late asthmatic response and change in airway caliber. *J. Allergy Clin. Immunol.* **70**:170-177 (1982).

7. Abraham, W. M., Sielczak, M. W., Wanner, A., Perruchoud, A. P., Blinder, L., Stevenson, J. S., Ahmed, A. and Yerger, L. D. Cellular markers of inflammation in the airways of allergic sheep with and without allergen-induced late responses. *Am. Rev. Respir. Dis.* **138**:1565-1571 (1988).
8. Lanes, S., Stevenson, J. S., Codias, E., Hernandez, A., Sielczak, M. W., Wanner, A. and Abraham, W. M. Indomethacin and FPL-57231 inhibit antigen-induced airway hyperresponsiveness in sheep. *J. Appl. Physiol.* **61**: 864-872 (1986).
9. Abraham, W. M., Delehunt, J. C., Yerger, L., and Marchette, B. Characterization of a late phase pulmonary response following antigen challenge in allergic sheep. *Am. Rev. Respir. Dis.* **128**:839-844 (1983).
10. Abraham, W. M. Pharmacology of allergen-induced early and late airway responses and antigen-induced airway hyperresponsiveness in allergic sheep. *Pul Pharmacol* **2**:33-40 (1989).
11. Simonsson, B. G., Skoogh, B.-E., Bergh, N. P., Andersson, R. and Svedmyr, N. In vivo and in vitro effect of bradykinin on bronchial motor tone in normal subjects and patients with airways obstruction. *Respiration* **30**:378-388 (1973).
12. Dixon, C. M. S. and Barnes, P. J. Bradykinin-induced bronchoconstriction: inhibition by nedocromil sodium and sodium cromoglycate. *Br. J. Clin. Pharmacol.* **27**:831-836 (1989).
13. Fuller, R. W., Dixon, C. S., Cuss, F. M. C. and Barnes, P. J. Bradykinin-induced bronchoconstriction in humans: Mode of action. *Am. Rev. Respir. Dis.* **135**:176-180 (1987).
14. Christiansen, S. C., Proud, D. and Cochrane, C. G. Detection of tissue kallikrein in the bronchoalveolar lavage fluid of asthmatic subjects. *J. Clin. Invest.* **79**:188-197 (1987).
15. Proud, D., Togias, A., Naclerio, R. M., Crush, S. A., Norman, P. S., and Lichtenstein, L. M. Kinins are generated in vivo following nasal airway challenge of allergic individuals with allergen. *J. Clin. Invest.* **72**:1678-1685 (1983).
16. Steranka, L. R., Farmer, S. G., and Burch, R. M. Antagonists of B_2 bradykinin receptors. *FASEB J* **3**:2019-2025 (1989).
17. Steranka, L. R., Manning, J. C., Dehaas, C. J., Ferkany, J. W., Borosky, S. A., Connor, J. R., Vavrek, R. J., Stewart, J. M., and Snyder, S. H. Bradykinin as a pain mediator: Receptors are localized in sensory neurons, and antagonists have analgesic actions. *Proc. Natl. Acad. Sci. USA* **850**:3245-3249 (1988).
18. Cortes, A., Ahmed, A., Ahmed, T. and Abraham, W. M. Citric acid and bradykinin produce cough in allergic sheep. *FASEB J.* **4**:A614 (1990).
19. Soler, M., Sielczak, M. W. and Abraham, W. M. A bradykinin-antagonist blocks antigen-induced airway hyperresponsiveness and inflammation in sheep. *Pul. Pharmacol.* **3**:9-15 (1990).
20. Dixon, M., Jackson, D. M. and Richards, I. M. The action of sodium cromoglycate on 'C' fibre endings in the dog lung. *Br. J. Pharmacol.* **70**:11-13 (1982).

21. Dixon, M., Jackson, D. M. and Richards, I. M. The effects of sodium cromoglycate on lung irritant receptors and left ventricular receptors in anaesthetised dog. *Br. J. Pharmacol.* **67**:569-574 (1979).
22. Jackson, D. M., Eady, R. P. and Farmer, J. B. The effect of nedocromil sodium on non-specific bronchial hyperreactivity in the dog. *Eur. J. Respir. Dis.* **69**(Suppl. 147):217-219 (1986).
23. Dixon, C. M. S., and P. W. Ind. Mechanism of metabisulphite induced bronchoconstriction, in: *Nedocromil Sodium (Tilade): Basic Research into Mechanisms of Action*. Proceedings from Societas Europaea Physiologicae Clinicae Respiratoriae, Lausanne (1989).
24. Dixon, C. M. S., and P. W. Ind. Sodium metabisulphite inhalation: Probe for non-mast cell activity of nedocromil sodium and sodium cromoglycate, in: *Nedocromil Sodium (Tilade): Basic Research into Mechanisms*. Proceedings from SEPCR, Lausanne (1989).
25. Abraham, W. M., Soler, M., Ahmed, A. and Cortes, A. Pharmacology of bradykinin-induced bronchoconstriction in allergic sheep. *FASEB J* **3**:275A. (1989). (Abstract)
26. Farmer, S. G., Burch, R. M., Meeker, S. M. and Wilkins, D. E. Evidence for a pulmonary B_3 bradykinin receptor. *Mol. Pharmacol.* **36**:1-8 (1989).
27. Abraham, W. M., Baugh, L. E., Harbeson, S. L., Cortes, A. and Ahmed, A. Airway effects of inhaled bradykinin, substance P and neurokinin A in allergic sheep. *Am. Rev. Respir. Dis.* **139**(4):A239 (1989). (Abstract)
28. Barnes, P. J., Chung, K. F., and Page, C. P. Inflammatory mediators and asthma. *Pharm. Rev.* **40**:49-84 (1988).
29. Soler, M., Sielczak, M. W. and Abraham, W. M. A PAF-antagonist blocks antigen-induced airway hyperresponsiveness and inflammation in sheep. *J. Appl. Physiol.* **67**:406-413 (1989).
30. Proud, D., and Kaplan, A. P. Kinin formation: Mechanisms and role in inflammatory disorders. *Ann. Rev. Immunol.* **6**:49-83 (1988).
31. Abraham, W. M. The importance of lipoxygenase products of arachidonic acid in allergen-induced late responses. *Am. Rev. Respir. Dis.* **135**:S49-S53 (1987).
32. Delehunt, J. C., Perruchoud, A. P., Yerger, L., Marchette, B., Stevenson, J. S. and Abraham, W. M. The role of SRS-A in the late bronchial response following antigen challenge in allergic sheep. *Am. Rev. Respri. Dis.* **130**:748-754 (1984).
33. Tagari, P., Abraham, W. M., McGolrick, J., Charleson, S., Soler, M., Ahmed, A., Cortes, A. and Ford-Hutchinson, A. W. Increased leukotriene E_4 excretion during antigen-induced bronchoconstriction in allergic sheep. *J. Appl. Physiol.* **68**:1321-1327 (1990).
34. Diaz, P., Gonzalez, M. C., Galleguillos, F. R., Ancic, P., Cromwell, O., Shepherd, D., Durham, S. R., Gleich, G. J. and Kay, A. B. Leukocytes and mediators in bronchoalveolar lavage during allergen-induced late phase asthmatic reactions. *Am. Rev. Respir. Dis.* **139**:1383-1389 (1989).
35. Okayama, H., Aikawa, T., Ohtsu, H., Sasaki, H. and Takishima, T. Leukotriene C_4 and B_4 in bronchoalveolar lavage fluid during biphasic allergic bronchoconstriction in sheep. *Am. Rev. Respir. Dis.* **139**:725-731 (1989).

36. Soler, M. and Abraham, W. M. Antigen-induced airway hyperresponsiveness develops independently from late responses in sheep. *Proceedings from the 8th Congress of the European Society of Pneumology* (1989). (Abstract).
37. Abraham, W. M., Ahmed, A. and Cortes, A. The effects of a leukotriene (LT)D_4 antagonist (MK-571) on LTD_4 and antigen-induced bronchoconstriction in allergic sheep. *Physiologist* **32**:161 (1989).
38. Wanner, A. and Reinhart, M. Respiratory mechanics in conscious sheep. *J. Appl. Physiol.* **44**:479-482 (1978).
39. Abraham, W. M., Oliver, W., Jr., Welker, M. J., King, M., Wanner, A., and Sackner, M. A. Differences in airway reactivity in normal and allergic sheep after exposure to sulfur dioxide. *J. Appl. Physiol.* **51**:1651-1656 (1981).
40. Wanner, A. and Abraham, W. M. Experimental models of asthma. *Lung* **160**:231-243 (1982).
41. Abraham, W. M., Oliver, W., Jr., King, M. M., Yerger, L. and Wanner, A. Effect of pharmacologic agents on antigen-induced decreases in specific lung conductance in sheep. *Am. Rev. Respir. Dis.* **124**:554-558 (1981).
42. Allegra, L., Abraham, W. M., Chapman, G. A. and Wanner, A. Duration of mucociliary dysfunction following antigen challenge. *J. Appl. Physiol.* **55**:726-730 (1983).
43. Wanner, A., T. Ahmed, and W. M. Abraham. Drug actions on mediators. Drug therapy for asthma, in: *Lung Biology and Health and Disease* (J. W. Jenne and S. Murphy, eds.). Marcel Dekker, New York, pp. 413-461 (1987).
44. Abraham, W. M., Stevenson, J. S., Eldridge, M., Garrido, R., and Nieves, L. Nedocromil sodium in allergen-induced bronchial responses and airway hyperresponsiveness in allergic sheep. *J. Appl. Physiol.* **65**(3):1062-1068 (1988).
45. Abraham, W. M., Lanes, S., Stevenson, J. S. and Yerger, L. D. Effect of an inhaled glucocorticosteroids (budesonide) on post-antigen induced increases in airway responsiveness. *Bull. Europ. Physiopath. Respir. Clin. Respir. Physiol.* **22**:387-392 (1986).
46. Abraham, W. M. The role of leukotrienes in allergen-induced late responses in allergic sheep. *Annals of the New York Academy of Sciences: Biology of the Leukotrienes* **524**:260-270 (1988).

Index

About the Editor

RONALD M. BURCH is Group Leader of the Pain, Inflammation and Bradykinin Antagonist Program at Nova Pharmaceutical Corporation, Baltimore, Maryland. He is the author or coauthor of nearly 80 journal articles or book chapters, serves as referee for 11 journals, and has three patents pending. A member of the American Federation for Clinical Research, American Medical Association, and American Society for Pharmacology and Experimental Therapeutics, he received the B.S. (1977) degrees in chemistry and marine biology from the College of Charleston, South Carolina, and Ph.D. (1981) in pharmacology and M.D. (1985) degrees from the Medical University of South Carolina, Charleston.